LETTERS
FROM THE
YOGA
MASTERS

Teachings Revealed through Correspondence
from Paramhansa Yogananda, Ramana Maharshi,
Swami Sivananda, and Others

MARION (MUGS) McCONNELL

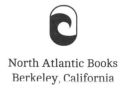

North Atlantic Books
Berkeley, California

Published by
North Atlantic Books
Berkeley, California

Cover art created from letters written by Swami Sivananda Saraswati of Rishikesh, Swami Satchidananda, Swami Vishnudevananda, Swami Shivananda Saraswati of Assam, Faye Wright (Sri Daya Mata) of Self-Realization Fellowship, and Dr. Hari Dickman (to author). Classic drawing of nadis circa nineteenth century Tibet is attributed to the prophet Ratnasara.

Cover design by Bill Zindel
Book design by Mary Ann Casler

Printed in the United States of America

Letters from the Yoga Masters: Teachings Revealed through Correspondence from Paramhansa Yogananda, Ramana Maharshi, Swami Sivananda, and Others is sponsored and published by the Society for the Study of Native Arts and Sciences (dba North Atlantic Books), an educational nonprofit based in Berkeley, California, that collaborates with partners to develop cross-cultural perspectives, nurture holistic views of art, science, the humanities, and healing, and seed personal and global transformation by publishing work on the relationship of body, spirit, and nature.

MEDICAL DISCLAIMER: The following information is intended for general information purposes only. Individuals should always see their health care provider before administering any suggestions made in this book. Any application of the material set forth in the following pages is at the reader's discretion and is his or her sole responsibility.

North Atlantic Books' publications are available through most bookstores. For further information, visit our website at www.northatlanticbooks.com or call 800-733-3000.

Library of Congress Cataloging-in-Publication Data
Names: McConnell, Marion, author.
Title: Letters from the yoga masters : teachings revealed through
  correspondence from Paramhansa Yogananda, Ramana Maharshi, Swami
  Sivananda, and others / Marion (Mugs) McConnell.
Description: Berkeley : North Atlantic Books, 2016.
Identifiers: LCCN 2015037866 | ISBN 9781623170356 (paperback) | ISBN
  9781623170363 (ebook)
Subjects: LCSH: Yoga. | Spiritual life. | Dickman, Hari,
  1895-1979—Correspondence. | Yogis—Correspondence. | BISAC: PHILOSOPHY /
  Eastern. | LITERARY COLLECTIONS / Essays. | HEALTH & FITNESS / Yoga.
Classification: LCC B132.Y6 M243 2016 | DDC 181/.45—dc23
LC record available at http://lccn.loc.gov/2015037866

1 2 3 4 5 6 7 8 United 20 19 18 17 16

For Hari, my beloved guide to the spirit.

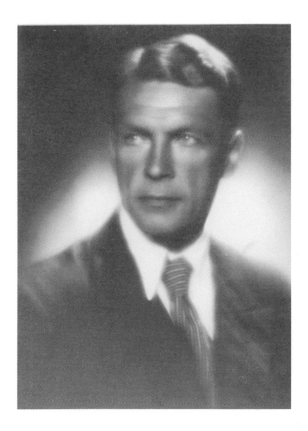

Dr. Hari Dickman, 1938. Photo credit: L. Alutis
Kreicberg.

ACKNOWLEDGMENTS

A BOOK DOESN'T WRITE ITSELF. It takes a lot of support from a lot of people. I had no idea this project would be so consuming, and without all the encouragement from my friends, students, and colleagues, this book would never have come to be.

From the very beginning of my years as a yoga teacher, I have tried to tell my students how blessed I am to have had Hari Dickman as my teacher. He was highly regarded by the greatest yoga masters of his time, and yet he remained humble and gentle. I am so fortunate to have been his student—I was his last student—with whom he willingly shared his knowledge and his M&M's. It has been my honor and my duty to pass on to others everything he taught me. His knowledge was hard won, gained during a time of censorship and war, refugee camps and homelessness. He worked obsessively at his yoga practice to earn the trust of many yoga masters so they would impart upon him the truths of this sacred path. This knowledge needs to be shared, not lost. This book is intended to let the world know about this lovely man, Hari Dickman. It is through the efforts of great yogis like him that we are able to enjoy the ancient truths of yoga today. And for this, we should all be grateful.

I thank Bob McConnell, my loving husband, for his endless support over the years it took to write this book, never complaining about papers and documents spread all over the house and office. He cooked numerous meals while I stared at the computer, and his only request was that every day we got out for a good walk together.

I am grateful to Mrs. Edie Thorslund, who for a brief time was my neighbor. She introduced me to yoga in 1973, when I was seventeen years old.

I would never have met Hari if Mrs. Velta Snikere-Wilson had not suggested that I study with him. In my search for a teacher, she shared his address with me. I have never met her—she is now in her nineties and continues to teach yoga in London, England.

Katherine DaSilva Jain opened her home to Hari in his last years, and then to me, so I could study with him. She also permitted me to copy Hari's letters after all my notes had been stolen. Without her generous spirit, this book could not have been written.

For many months, the late Doug Paterson helped me make photocopies of the letters as Katherine mailed them to me in small packages. I am grateful for the generous gift of his time—the hours we spent in front of the copier.

Gail Thompson tirelessly scanned in the photocopied letters so they will not be lost to fading. She spent more than a year scanning thousands of pages and labeling them by dates and author.

Doug Sutherland, my dear friend in New York City, whom I met on a bus right after I first met Hari, knows how much Hari has meant to my becoming who I am today. He has offered me constant encouragement to write this book.

Marsha Saldat and Helen and Steven Mikuska provided space in their homes for me to write in peace and quiet when life threw obstacles in my path. Helen's extensive yoga library became a huge asset while I was teaching in Calgary, away from my own library at home. We are so likeminded that our libraries are very similar!

When my computer crashed (as they inevitably do), Bill Gilbert of Villa Obregon rescued that day's most current copy of the manuscript. Jacque Morrow and Glen and Lois Worman of Kelowna promptly arranged the delivery of a new computer with an English keyboard to me in Mexico.

Jo C. Willems, my sister, spent hours creating line drawings and cleaning up images of the letters so they are readable. I cannot thank her enough for her creative spirit.

Swami Suryadevananda in Florida has been aware of Hari for some years through his work at the Divine Life Society in Rishikesh, India. His appreciation for Hari warms my heart. I am thankful to the Divine Life Society for giving me permission to use the photos of Hari doing asana in my book.

Dzintars Vilnis Korns found me through the internet during his passionate search to learn more about Hari and in his effort to preserve the history of yoga in Latvia. Dzintars's website documents much of Hari's past. It has been very helpful, and he freely shared his knowledge with me.

Thank you to Dr. Solveiga Krumina-Konkova, a leading researcher at the Institute of Philosophy and Sociology at the University of Latvia. She has devoted countless hours researching and documenting the history of the Yoga Society in Latvia and shared much of her information with me.

Dr. Vijay Pratap and Barbara Levitt of the SKY Foundation in Philadelphia helped me immensely with their review and feedback on portions of the manuscript, and their careful housing of the original letters in the Dr. Hari Dickman library.

Yogacharya Dr. Ananda Balayogi Bhavanani, chairman of the International Centre for Yoga Education and Research (ICYER) at Ananda Ashram, Pondicherry, India and chairman of Yoganjali Natyalayam, kindly assisted me with clarification on various mudras and techniques throughout the book. His expertise and his generosity with his time have been invaluable.

Brother Chidananda of Self-Realization Fellowship was very attentive and considerate in the painstaking process of permissions while ensuring the intended meaning behind certain statements was not lost. I am so grateful for his compassion through this process.

My first editor, Julie "Jools" Andrés, was passionate about making this book come to completion from the moment she heard about it. Her expertise and yogic knowledge made this possible. Her commitment to this book has kept me going even when I felt completely empty and defeated. I am so very grateful that she took this project on and has worked tirelessly with me to make it happen.

How can I ever thank the wonderful people at North Atlantic Books? Their encouragement and belief in this book propelled me forward through the challenging process of acquiring so many permissions. I am extremely grateful to Tim McKee and Louis Swaim and copy editor Jennifer Eastman for their clear, gentle, and honest feedback through the editing process. Thank you to Bill Zindel for the creation of the beautiful cover, which so perfectly reflects the content within. And thank you to Mary Ann Casler for the layout and design of the book, sharing the handwriting and typed content drawn from these fading letters that overflow with rich teachings. When I see these letters, I feel the energy of the swamis who wrote them, and I hope you experience a glimpse of that too.

Erich Schiffmann, thank you for your encouragement and your belief in me and this book, and for reminding me not to worry about how long it would take to write it.

Bernie Clark, Brenda Feuerstein, Mark Stephens, Neil Pearson, William Phillips, Nyaswami Gyandev McCord, Bill Francis Barry (Bharata), Mary-Louise Parkinson—thank you for your ideas, feedback, and corrections.

All my students and colleagues—you have kept me going on this project simply by your show of interest and words of encouragement. Thank you.

CONTENTS

Chapter 4 Pranayama 55

Chapter 5 Mudras and Bandhas 119

Chapter 6 Pratyahara and Dharana 139

Chapter 7 Dhyana 161

Chapter 8 Kundalini Awakening
and Samadhi   211

Chapter 9 Delicious Stories   227

LIST OF
ILLUSTRATIONS

Cover Photo: Letters from the Yoga Masters

Frontispiece: Dr. Hari Dickman, 1938

I.1. Letter to author from Hari, September 16, 1978.

I.2. Author and Hari studying in San Rafael, California, 1979. Photo: Mark Hovila.

1.1. *Skylight* heading, vol. 1, no. 2, spring/summer 1974.

1.2. Hari's letter to *Skylight*, vol. 1, no. 2, spring/summer 1974.

1.3. The Latvia Yoga Society: Hari is third from the left in the front row. Photo: http://tradition.lv/tradition/ljb.htm. Permission from Dzintars Vilnis Korns.

1.4. Article from the Divine Life Society acknowledging Hari for his translation services, 1939.

1.5. Photo of Paramhansa Yogananda. Photograph courtesy of Self-Realization Fellowship, Los Angeles, California.

1.6. Swami Yogananda's letter to Hari in Latvia, October 17, 1934.

1.7. First part of letter from Paramhansa Yogananda, January 31, 1946.

1.8. Later part of letter from Paramhansa Yogananda, January 31, 1946.

1.9. Handwritten note at bottom of letter from Paramhansa Yogananda, January 31, 1946.

E.1. Dr. Hari Dickman, January 1979, in San Rafael, California. Photo by author.
Author photo. Photo Credit, Keenan Geer, www.keenangeer.com
Note: each chapter ends with a small graphic, which comes from Swami Vishnu
    Tirth's letterhead.

FOREWORD

THIS IS AN EXTRAORDINARY BOOK. It is a shining jewel. Truly, it is priceless. You have found buried treasure.

Letters from the Yoga Masters: Teachings Revealed through Correspondence from Paramhansa Yogananda, Ramana Maharshi, Swami Sivananda, and Others is an intimate, endearing, and insightful look into the life of an amazing yogi-teacher, Dr. Hari Dickman.

Hari was the guru of another amazing yogi-teacher—the author of this book—Marion "Mugs" McConnell. I have known Mugs for quite a few years now. I am thrilled she is passing on the teachings she has garnered and cherished from her teacher. These are the teachings that Hari received via personal letters and correspondence with many of the yoga giants of his time.

Hari started the Latvian Yoga Society in the 1930s, before the Second World War. He was a devoted correspondent student of Ramana Maharshi, Yogananda, Swami Sivananda, and others. They instructed him through letters and books and even supplied him with teaching materials to use when he was in displaced-persons camps after the war. Eventually, Paramhansa Yogananda was able to bring Hari to the United States by sending him a minister's certificate to work at the Self-Realization Fellowship.

Mugs was just a teenager when the stars aligned for her first meeting with Hari. This book is written out of love and appreciation for both Hari and the teachings. Her love for him—and his for her—shines on every page. It has been her fortunate dharma to compile these teachings and shine additional light on how yoga came to the West. How fortunate for the rest of us!

Mugs was his last disciple. The relationship between Hari and Mugs was beautiful to witness. The love they had for one another, in their mutual interest in all things yoga, was inspiring.

This book includes techniques and stories that a vast array of yogis shared with Hari. Over one hundred yogis from several different lineages wrote him letters of instruction during his lifetime, and over fifty of them wrote regularly. These letters became their "textbooks." This is rare personal correspondence. Contained herein is a veritable treasure chest of spiritual wealth delivered personally via the written letter. And the teachings went beyond mere words. Paramhansa Yogananda drew a picture of a device made to assist in meditation. Swami Sivananda sent him gramophone recordings to aid his practice of *yoga nidra*. These are detailed teachings from many masters regarding pranayama, mudras, diet, philosophical discussion, inquiry, and theory, all interwoven with stories and personal anecdotes that support the techniques. It is an exciting read.

What a joy it is for me—and an honor—to be part of this love-filled historical gift of a book. It has enhanced my appreciation for how yoga flowered in the West. I have new insight into how it was lived by those who knew it. It has refreshed my faith in the yearning of the human heart for Truth and Love. The correspondence between Hari and his teachers is invaluable, no doubt. But equally inspiring is the intimate, innocent, loving relationship between Hari and Mugs.

I think many, many people will be fascinated by this insider's glimpse into this strand of the origins of yoga here in the West.

Read on! Enjoy the ride. Then share what you learn. You now are an integral part of the unfolding illumination!

Thank you, great masters. Thank you, Hari. Thank you, Mugs. Thank you, dear reader. Oh, and yes, thank you, life, source of it all.

OM!

With Love and Pranams,
Erich Schiffmann
Author of *Yoga: The Spirit and Practice of Moving into Stillness*
erichschiffmann.com
October 14, 2014

PREFACE

FOR MORE THAN THIRTY-FIVE YEARS, a large box of letters has moved with me through the phases of my life. This box holds old photocopies of more than 750 letters from over one hundred yoga masters, spanning the years from 1930 to 1979. The letters are grouped into different file folders, each one generally representing the teachings of a particular pathway of yoga, such as siddha yoga, natha yoga, or Sivananda yoga.

These letters were "textbooks" of my teacher, Dr. Hari Dickman, and they became my textbooks when he taught me. Over the years, as Hari advanced in his practice, he wrote to prominent yogis, asking about yogic techniques. The answers varied, depending on the pathway, as each pathway is a science of its own.

At some point in my own practice, two things occurred to me: first, why did so few people know of Dr. Dickman, who was a great yoga master, and second, as Hari's last disciple, perhaps it was my duty to share the information held in these letters. These thoughts became the impetus behind writing this book.

Had I known what a monstrous task I had embarked on, I never would have taken the first step. When Hari had a question, he asked several yoga masters at once. Their answers would often generate more questions, which would often result in several letters flowing between Hari and each master. More questions on the technique might arise months or years later, as Hari continued his practice. It is important to note here that Hari's "questions" are rarely seen, as I do not have copies of the letters he wrote. I followed the topics in the letters by looking at the month and year of the initial discussion, and then looked through the files of several other masters who wrote during that year to see if they also had addressed the same topic. It was an important but tedious process. Piecing the material together was like putting together the pieces of a jigsaw puzzle. I have only touched on the depths of wisdom held within the files. After all, it is one yogi's lifetime of study.

Few of the yoga masters who wrote these letters are alive today. Therefore, in order to acquire permission to include excerpts from these letters, I needed to contact the heirs of the authors of the letters or those in charge of their ashrams. This has been no small task, and in some cases, it was impossible. It took almost a year to track down and communicate with yogis through email, letters, late-night phone calls to India, and Facebook (yes, even Facebook!). Every effort has been made to honor each and every one of these generous and loving yoga masters, who dedicated so much time to teaching students outside of India.

Through this process, I learned how well Hari is remembered today by those yogis who are still alive, as well as by their students and the students of those yogis who have died, in India, Europe, Argentina, South Africa, and the United States. I am not the only one who loved him; many others have as well, who regarded him as a master of yoga and an equal.

I have met the most amazing people, who have taken such care and given so much time to ensure this book is a beautiful and just representation of Hari and the yoga masters who taught him. When I read this book, I feel my role in its production diminish. If feels as though I was merely the vehicle for the information to arrive on these pages.

I feel honored to have been Hari's last disciple. I feel honored to be the author of this book. I feel honored to have communicated with so many disciples of the yogis who taught Hari. It is my duty, my dharma, to share this with you.

Marion (Mugs) McConnell

INTRODUCTION

MOST OF THE WORDS IN THIS BOOK are from great yoga masters of the past. Some of my own thoughts and ideas are included, but the reason for this book is to share the wisdom of these masters as they shared it with my teacher, Dr. Hari Dickman,[1] who later shared it with me.

Dr. Dickman was known to many just as Hari. Hari devoted his life to the study of yoga. He once said to me that he was obsessed with yoga and could never get enough.

Most of Hari's yoga studies were completed through correspondence. World travel was uncommon when he began his studies, and Hari was never comfortable with it, so this correspondence was his primary mode of yoga instruction. He wrote letters to the prominent yoga masters of the time, requesting guidance for specific techniques, and they sent him books as well as letters with detailed instructions. Hari would then teach these techniques to his students in Latvia. In 1928 he became avidly involved with the Society of Parapsychology, which in 1934 was reregistered as the Center of Yoga Science in Latvia.[2]

During the Second World War, the Soviets invaded Latvia. Hari, his wife, Isabella, and her mother ended up living in camps for displaced persons.

They spent many years being moved from one camp to another until, in 1952, Hari and his wife and mother-in-law were brought to the United States through the blessings and help of Paramhansa Yogananda.

When Hari's wife, Isabella, passed away due to cancer in November 1974, they were living in Brooklyn, New York. Hari was eighty years old and lived a simple, yogic lifestyle. Due to their high regard for Hari and his devotion to the path of yoga, three yoga societies offered homes for him to live in: the Integral Yoga Institute of Sri Swami Satchidananda, the Swami Kuvalayananda Yoga Foundation (the SKY Foundation), and Yoga Organization for Research and Education (YORE). He chose to live with Katherine DaSilva, who was president of YORE at the time and a good friend of Hari's. She was soon to marry Jinendra Jain, and Jinendra welcomed Hari to their home, saying, "In India, it is considered a blessing to have the old people living with you. He is always welcome." Hari moved from Brooklyn to Rutherford, New Jersey, to join them. It wasn't long before Katherine and Jinendra were offered work in California, and in December 1975, Hari moved with them to San Rafael, where he lived out the remainder of his life.

My association with Dr. Hari Dickman began in July 1977, when, after four years of unguided personal yoga practice, I wrote to him from my home in Penticton, British Columbia, Canada. We began a regular correspondence, and most of my letters to him contained Suchard Milka chocolate, at his request. Hari loved chocolate, and he asked for only chocolate in return for his guidance. He soon determined I was predominantly a hatha yogi, and encouraged me to study with Swami Vishnudevananda, a fellow disciple and *gurubhai* (brother or sister under the same guru). In January 1978, enroute to the ashram in the Bahamas, I diverged to San Rafael, California to meet Hari in person. An immediate bond formed between us as he excitedly shared some tips on what to expect in ashram life, like daily pranayama and meditation.

Our regular correspondence continued until 1979, when he invited me to study with him in person. He was then eighty-four years old. He called me Bhanumati (the light that shines on everything), a spiritual name that Swami Vishnudevananda had given me.

During my stay with Hari in San Rafael, each day he would bring out specific letters from his files for us to discuss, and then we would work on the techniques described therein; I would take copious notes. Chocolate played a big role in our relationship, and it was not just for pleasure; it was also part of a spiritual ritual, as odd as that may seem. Each philosophy discussion was accompanied by a bowl of chocolate M&M's. His ultimate wisdom was balanced by a sweet innocence, displayed in his desire to not eat the brown M&M's—not one of the colors of the chakras, I suppose. So I would take care of getting rid of the brown ones.

I asked Hari one day, "Do you think that when you die, you will be enlightened and not have to come back again?" He replied, without hesitation, "Oh, no, I like chocolate too much."

Sometimes he justified his love of chocolate. The sweetest justification he ever gave, one that warmed my heart, was this:

A question may arise why, then, I still enjoy the Milka and do not always practice Pratyahara [withdrawal from the senses], which I have much practiced—and *with success*—in my life? I confess it is difficult to answer, and if answered, it will not be easy to understand by most people; maybe you, dear Bhanumati, might understand? It is the same [reason] as [why] some great Yogis used occasionally to smoke or to drink alcohol too. Sri Sri Ramakrishna said it is to keep to the earth. Otherwise, there is no desire, and the Jiva [soul], finding no joy in this life, flies away. Now I have two desires, viz., (1) a good, interesting book on Yoga, and (2) as you know, "Suchard Milka."

I have lost my house, garden, and my country (the Russian communist[s] robbed it); my brothers and my wife have passed away, so what remains, or to put it in other words, what is the use of my living on this earth anyway? [My life] would have a sense if I could share my knowledge and experiences in Yoga to people eager to know, but ... "such are few."[3]

When I write a letter, especially a spiritual one, and also when I get some books on Yoga, or some letter from a Yogi, I like to eat Milka, for these mentioned things make me feel happy, and I make something like a festival [of it], but as I don't drink, nor use drugs, so my substitute is Suchard Milka. Of course, you, dear Marion, need not follow in my footsteps.[4]

It all made sense, how the ritual of eating chocolate and reading spiritual knowledge was all that kept him here in his body, since nothing else was left.

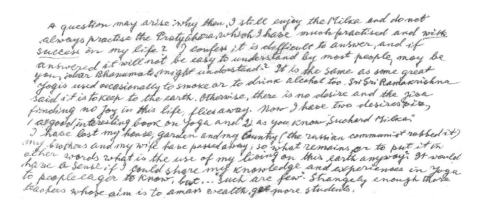

A question may arise: why then, I still enjoy the Milka and do not always practise the Pratyahora, which I have much practised and with success in my life? I confess it is difficult to answer, and if answered it will not be easy to understand by most people, may be you, dear Bhanumati, might understand? It is the same as some great yogis used occasionally to smoke or to drink alcohol too. Sri Sri Ramakrishna said it is to keep to the earth. Otherwise, there is no desire and the jiva finding no joy in this life, flies away. Now I have two desires viz., I a good interesting book on Yoga and 2) as you know "Suchard Milka." I have lost my house, garden and my country (the russian communist robbed it) my brothers and my wife have passed away; so what remains or to put it in other words what is the use of my living on this earth anyway? It would have a sense if I could share my knowledge and experiences in Yoga to people eager to know, but... such are few. Strangely enough those teachers whose aim is to amass wealth, get more students.

Figure I.1. Letter to author from Hari, September 16, 1978.

One day I had asked Hari to be my guru, completely expecting him to say yes, but instead, he flatly refused. "No," he said. "Being a guru is far too much responsibility." This was a great lesson in humility for me, and I have never forgotten it. A guru is one who guides you to the spirit, and that is a role not to be taken lightly. But I was disappointed at the time, since it was stated time and time again in the yogic texts that a serious student needed a guru. However, I have come to understand that Hari has been guiding me to the spirit all these years even though he wasn't my formal guru. In a letter to Hari, Paramhansa Yogananda, explained.

> Just as a dynamo [generator] spreads electricity in all the lights of the city, so the God-contacting devotee's spirit is spread to all those who are in tune with him. That is what I meant in the sentence, "I am always with you in Spirit." Those devotees who are in tune with their guru through unconditional devotion, obedience, and loyalty feel the constant flow of their teacher's blessings.[5]

When I returned to Canada, I moved into an apartment. I was robbed my first night there. All my notes were stolen. I thought they would end up in a garbage dumpster somewhere, because no one would even have a clue what they meant. I spent days searching dumpsters, clinging to a tiny hope that my notes would reappear, to no avail.

My only hope was to ask Katherine DaSilva Jain, Hari's dear friend and the keeper of the original letters, if she would let me photocopy them. She agreed. She sent me, one by one, the packets of letters from each author, just as Hari had organized them, and after the packets were copied, they were sent on to Dr. Vijayendra Pratap of the Swami Kuvalayananda Yoga (SKY) Foundation in Philadelphia, where the Hari Dickman Yoga Library has been named in Hari's honor. Some letters seem to have been lost en route, in the mail, but the remainder are held at SKY for safekeeping.[6]

Now I believe it is my dharma, my duty, to share with you a taste of the teachings passed on to me through these letters. I was Hari's last disciple, and these letters were our textbooks. He wanted me to share the teachings and encouraged me to write articles, especially about pranayama. These letters deserve to be shared, as they hold many techniques and wonderful stories from more than one hundred yogis covering over half a century. Many of these yogis have taught your teachers—or even you.

Hari knew me only near the end of his life, but for me, as a younger person, our correspondence and meeting was revelatory and altered my life path.

A Note on Transliteration

Regarding the Sanskrit transliteration in the letters: Please note that sometimes the *a* is dropped from the end of Sanskrit words, *v*'s are sometimes *w* or *b*. This is often related to how it is pronounced in a particular dialect rather than how it is actually spelled, since for many Indian yogis, English was a second language. For example, *rechaka* becomes *rechak*, *svar* becomes *swar*, and *vasana* can become *basan*.

In Sanskrit, the *a* is always pronounced at the end of the word, but in Hindi and some other Eastern languages, it is pronounced only if it is a long *a*.[7]

Likewise, the Sanskrit spiritual title Paramahansa (supreme swan) sometimes appears in its Bengali spelling, Paramhansa, with the middle *a* omitted. Although Paramahansa is the most common spelling today, I have used the Bengali spelling in the case of Paramhansa Yogananda, because his letterhead and all of his letters to Hari used Paramhansa.

Most of the correspondence is reproduced as it appears in the letters. However, in some instances, where copyright allowed, there has been some minor editing for clarity and flow.

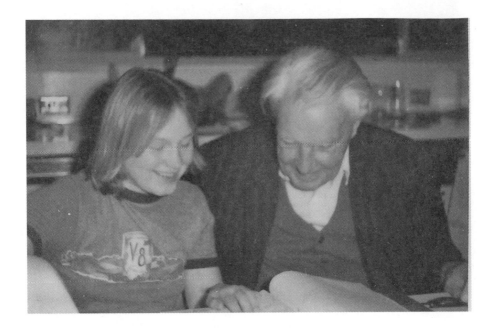

Figure I. 2. Author and Hari studying in San Rafael, California, 1979.
Photo: Mark Hovila.

While writing this book, I became aware that there is so much information in the 750-plus letters that I can barely scratch the surface in what I can
share with you. A lifetime of questions were asked, and the letters hold fifty
years of answers to those questions. I have had to make challenging choices
on what to include. I hope this book does Hari and his lineage of teachers
justice.

Chapter One

HARI AND THE
YOGA MASTERS

IT IS DIFFICULT FOR ME TO SHARE WITH YOU a full picture of who Sri Yogiraj Dr. Hari Dickman was, because the part that I know best is the portion of his life related to our yoga journey together. There was much about Hari that I never knew. What I can say is he was highly regarded and respected for his dedication to the practices of yoga by many of the yoga masters of the twentieth century. Many eventually considered him to be a yoga master.

While we studied together, Hari told me bits and pieces about his life. He was born in Latvia on July 4, 1895,[8] and his name was Harijs Dīkmanis. He said he started practicing yoga at the age of fourteen,[9] which would have been 1909. I cannot verify this, but the 1974 *Skylight Journal of Yoga* states of Dr. Dickman: "For more than 50 years he has studied both traditional, as well as modern, yoga under many of the great yogis who have travelled in the West."[10] Further, a letter dated February 5, 1965, from Shri S. S. Balshastri Phadke, a disciple of the Shri Shankaracharya lineage, states that Hari had been practicing yoga for a period of fifty years.[11] This would indicate that Hari's studies began at least as early as 1915.

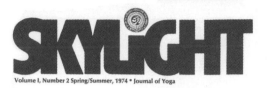

Volume I, Number 2 Spring/Summer, 1974 • Journal of Yoga

Figure 1.1. Skylight heading, vol. 1, no. 2, spring/summer 1974.

A LETTER FROM DR. HARI DICKMAN:

Dr. Dickman is a man who carries his 77 years lightly and with great dignity. For more than 50 years he has studied both traditional, as well as modern, yoga under many of the great yogis who have travelled in the West. He is a learned man, and a man who daily lives the yogic life. We are fortunate that his friendship pre-dates SKY Foundation founding. The Hari Dickman Yoga Library is named in his honor, We publish here a letter sent to commemorate our first anniversary. We will publish Dr. Dickman's observations from time to time in future issues.

Dear Members of the S.K.Y. Foundation,

Being unable to be present at the auspicious day of the Anniversary celebration of the founding of the SKY Foundation, I would like to substitute my physical presence with a few written words.

The SKY Foundation stands for teaching its members the scientific techniques of Yoga. It has already done a marvellous work in this field under the able guidance of Sri Dr. V. Pratap, a direct disciple of H. H. Sri Swami Kuvalayanandaji Maharaj, who in his turn was a direct disciple of the famous yogin of Malsar H. H. Sri Madhavadasji Maharaj.

Hatha Yoga has, in a rather short time, become very popular in the Western World, because its methods are very effective and yield tangible results even in a relatively short time. It imparts good health, cures otherwise, as incurable, pronounced diseases and makes the body look youthful even at an advanced age. And because of this Hatha Yoga has attracted the attention of the practical people of America and Europe.

But alas! these are really speaking only the by-products of practising this ancient System of Yoga. Though these by-products are very valuable indeed, they are not the ultimate aim of Yoga, be it Hatha Yoga or any other system of Yoga.

The distinguishing feature of Hatha Yoga lies in its stress on the mastery of the physical body, the nervous system and vital forces, and of course of the mind. As Yoga and Hatha Yoga in particular is a Science, or Vidya, it must have, and indeed has, a systematic empiric and graduated system by following which one can achieve its objective.

Now, what is the aim of Yoga including that of Hatha Yoga? The answer is given by various names i.e. Moksha, Mukti, Kaivalya, Samarasa etc. They point to the absolute freedom of the inner Self. Says Sri Gorakshanath in his Goraksha Shatakam:

"This is a ladder to Liberation, this is an escape from Death in as much as, the mind being turned away from illusion becomes attached to the Higher Self."

The path leading to that goal is summarized by Sri Gorakshanath as: Asana, Pranasamyama, Pratyahara, Dharana, Dhyana and Samadhi. It is incumbent for the earnest and sincere student of Hatha Yoga to know these steps of the ladder of Yoga, and after mastering one of them he must cautiously proceed to the following next one. To jump to the next step before mastering the preceeding one is a mistake to be avoided, and on the otherhand to stay permanently on only one before reaching the last one is also a grave mistake to be avoided if one wants to reach the final goal.

I wish all of you to proceed successfully and joyfully on the right path of Yoga under the expert guidance of the learned Sri Dr. Vijayendra Pratap.

OM SHANTI
Dr. Hari Dickman

Figure 1.2. Hari's letter to Skylight, vol. 1, no. 2, spring/summer 1974.

As an adult, he worked in Latvia as a customs officer, and at some point he married. Hari and his wife, Isabella—whom he called Tininch, which means *tiny*—did not have any children.

His surname, Dīkmanis, became westernized to Dickman and sometimes Dikman. His first name, Harijs, became Harry to most, and Hari (a name for Vishnu) to many of his yoga acquaintances. In his early letters to me, he signed them Harry, but as we became more familiar, he started using Hari. I don't know if "Hari" was a spiritual name given to him or if it was a natural process of change that occurred in the letters from some of the swamis. In 1976 Hari received from Baba Muktananda Swami the blessing of being called "Ek Acchha Purush" (One Pure Soul). As expressed to him by Arunachala Bhakta Bhagawal, from Sri Ramana Maharshi's ashram, "What more do you now need once you have received the highest blessing from him?"[12]

Hari received a doctorate of psychology and doctorate of metaphysics in 1962 from the College of Divine Metaphysics in Indianapolis, Indiana. From then on, he was referred to as Dr. Dickman. The president of the college, Dr. Henry Carns, wrote to Hari: "I would like to say that your examination papers were very unusual and excellent. We do not receive examination papers from every student that gives us the depth of perception and the personal Spiritual light that we found in certain parts of your examinations."[13]

Hari was a founding member, if not the founder, of the Scientific Center of Yoga in Riga, Latvia, which later became known as the Yoga Society. Sometimes it was referred to as the Yogoda Satsanga Society, a branch of Self-Realization Fellowship established by Paramhansa Yogananda, and sometimes as a branch of the Divine Life Society, which was founded by Swami Sivananda of Rishikesh. In 1935 the society was also considered to represent the Sri Yogendra Institute.[14] The Scientific Center of Yoga was in operation for about five years, until the start of the Second World War, when it was closed, and Hari believed the society's books had been destroyed: "When the Communists (Russian) invaded Latvia (after solemnly declaring that they will never occupy Latvia), the activities of the Yoga Society were suspended. The books on Yoga (we had them in Latvian, German, English, French, Sanskrit, Tamil, and Hindi languages) were confiscated and destroyed (sent to the paper mill)."[15]

I recently learned that not all these books were destroyed. A yogi from Latvia, Dzintars Vilnis Korns, informed me of this in the following email.

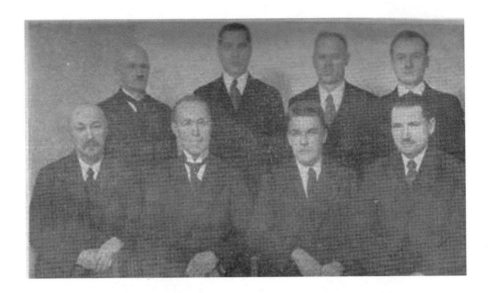

Figure 1.3. The Latvia Yoga Society: Hari third from the left in the front row. Photo: http://tradition.lv/tradition/ljb.htm. Permission from Dzintars Vilnis Korns.

Not all the books were burned. Important books do not burn so easily. I started at 1972 with Autogenic training, which was legal already at that time in Soviet Union, when I was fifteen years old. Step by step, I found contacts with people related to the Latvian Yoga Society. In beginning, these were discussions only, not real instructions or practice of Yoga. People were afraid to speak much with a guy so young, because it was an underground movement. But anyway, they tried to help me with my interests. When the former librarian of Latvian Yoga Society, Alfred Biezais, left this mortal world, somewhere about 1975 or 1976, ... his heirs tried to sell all of his library, because they did not have any interest in spiritual things or yoga. They tried to sell books illegally through Biezais's close friends, because it was impossible to do it legally, through secondhand bookshops or something like this. These books, of course, were forbidden. But the Soviet System had different grades of forbidden things. At this time, it was forbidden to distribute them, but not so firmly forbidden to have them. As a first-year student at a Latvian university, I couldn't buy many, so I bought only some. There were books translated by Dickman. So I met my first Yoga materials. A little later I found many other books translated by a team of former LYS members. Then I found people who could help me with books translated in the Soviet spiritual underground. But the first Yoga books I got were from former LYS heritage—so these books were my first Yoga teachers. All these were more or less underground activities, even till 1988. It was not as easy as in America that time.[16]

Hari translated many of the books in his Latvian Yoga Center. He told me he knew nine languages: Latvian, English, German, Russian, French, Bengali, Sanskrit, Hindi, and a little Polish. I suspect he knew Tamil as well. He taught himself many of these languages so he could read the yoga texts sent to him by various teachers. Many were in Sanskrit, Hindi, and Bengali. His skill with languages often led him to translate texts for Swami Sivananda, Sri Ramana Maharshi, and many others.

Although Hari communicated with and learned from nearly one hundred yogis, he considered three to be his main teachers: Paramhansa Yogananda, Swami Sivananda of Rishikesh, and Swami Vishnu Tirth.[17] He also studied in depth through letters with Swami Shivananda Saraswati of Assam and Sri Ramana Maharshi of Tiruvannamali, South India.[18]

A closer examination of Hari's relationship with the yogis he considered his main teachers will give you a clearer picture of how devoted he was to their teachings and how dedicated they were to teaching him. They considered him a very adept yogi.

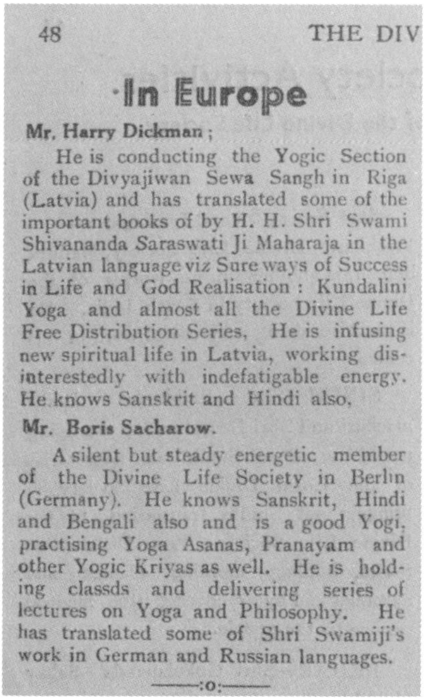

48   THE DIV

·In Europe

Mr. Harry Dickman ;

He is conducting the Yogic Section of the Divyajiwan Sewa Sangh in Riga (Latvia) and has translated some of the important books of by H. H. Shri Swami Shivananda Saraswati Ji Maharaja in the Latvian language viz Sure ways of Success in Life and God Realisation : Kundalini Yoga and almost all the Divine Life Free Distribution Series. He is infusing new spiritual life in Latvia, working disinterestedly with indefatigable energy. He knows Sanskrit and Hindi also.

Mr. Boris Sacharow.

A silent but steady energetic member of the Divine Life Society in Berlin (Germany). He knows Sanskrit, Hindi and Bengali also and is a good Yogi, practising Yoga Asanas, Pranayam and other Yogic Kriyas as well. He is holding classds and delivering series of lectures on Yoga and Philosophy. He has translated some of Shri Swamiji's work in German and Russian languages.

——:o:——

Figure 1.4. Article from the Divine Life Society acknowledging Hari for his translation services. 1939.

Paramhansa Yogananda

For some yoga masters, it was a contentious issue that Hari would study more than one yoga path. Many firmly believed that you must not mix the teachings, but rather stick to one path to avoid confusion, focus your attention, and attain perfection in that path. This was very true of Hari's relationship with Paramhansa Yogananda.

Paramhansa Yogananda was a disciple of Swami Sri Yukteswar Giri of Puri, India. In 1946 he wrote the spiritual classic *Autobiography of a Yogi*, introducing many westerners to the life of an enlightened yogi. He was devoted to teaching the ancient science of *kriya yoga* in its purest form. He founded the Self-Realization Fellowship (SRF) Headquarters at Mt. Washington, near Los Angeles, California. Today there are over five hundred SRF temples, retreats, and meditation centers worldwide.

Hari was devoted to Paramhansa Yogananda and felt his teachings were extremely valuable and effective. He honored and respected the fact that he was not permitted to teach kriya yoga to me or others without permission from SRF Headquarters in Los Angeles.[19] Hari made no exceptions, and his integrity made a huge impact on me; he set an infallible example of what I wanted to aspire to.

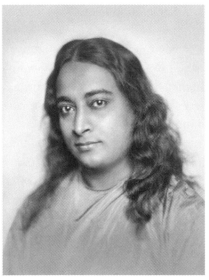

Paramhansa Yogananda taught Hari through letters, beginning some years prior to 1934 and continuing until his death in 1952. Thereafter, staff from SRF answered Hari's questions through letters until the fall of 1976.

The first preserved letter I have from Yogananda is dated October 1934, when he was still referred to as Swami Yogananda.

Dear Mr. Dickman: I was glad to receive your letter and crave your pardon for not replying it sooner,

Figure 1.5. Paramhansa Yogananda. Photo courtesy of Self-Realization Fellowship, Los Angeles, California.

due to the extreme number of letters waiting to be answered. I am so happy to know of your spiritual interest and of the intelligent questions that you have asked me.

Swami Yogananda then delves into clarifying Hari's questions on kriya yoga techniques. It is clear that they have already had a long-term relationship, as reference is made to Hari's "Yogoda Sat Sanga Center of Latvia."

Write whenever you can, and I shall make every effort to answer as soon as time permits. The new Yogoda Sat Sanga Center of Latvia will appear in the *Inner Culture Magazine* along with the rest of our centers.[20]

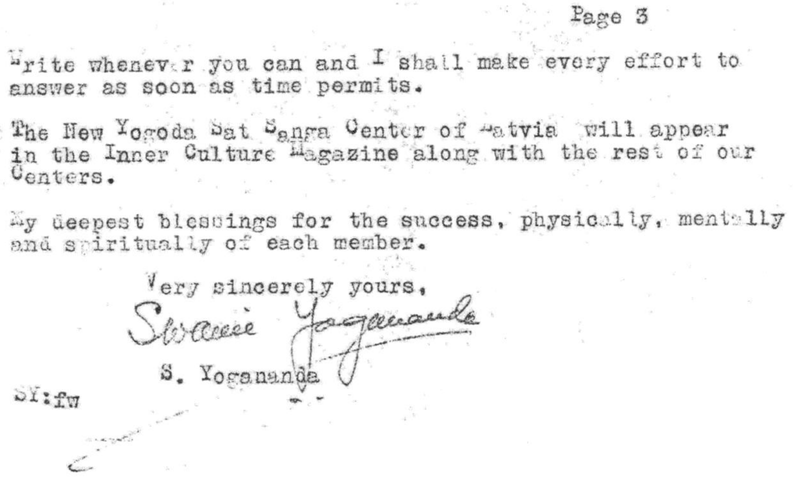

Page 3

Write whenever you can and I shall make every effort to answer as soon as time permits.

The New Yogoda Sat Sanga Center of Latvia will appear in the Inner Culture Magazine along with the rest of our Centers.

My deepest blessings for the success, physically, mentally and spiritually of each member.

Very sincerely yours,

S. Yogananda

SY:fw

Figure 1.6. Swami Yogananda's letter to Hari in Latvia, October 17, 1934.

A letter dated February 10, 1939, appears to be the last one from Paramhansa Yogananda to reach Hari in Latvia before the start of the Second World War. "In 1940 Latvia was occupied by the Bolshevik forces. The Yoga Society's work had to cease; their literature was confiscated. Postal communication too came to an end."[21]

Hari, who had been an officer in the czar's army, got a message that he and his wife were to be picked up by the Bolsheviks. If that were to happen, they could have been sent to Siberia. Along with Isabella's mother, they escaped out the back door while the Russians were coming in the front. It is unknown where they escaped to, nor how long it was until they made their way to a camp for displaced persons in Germany.

Displaced person (DP) camps were created after the war for the estimated eleven to twenty million refugees in Europe, many whom were survivors of Nazi concentration camps. Some were quickly returned to their homelands, but others had no countries or homes to return to and remained in the camps for many years. Most DP camps were closed by 1952, with the last camp closing in 1959. Conditions in camps varied and were sometimes harsh, simply because of the sheer number of people who lived in them. Many people were malnourished, living on fewer than 1,500 calories a day, and it was impossible to keep conditions sanitary, which resulted in the spread of disease.[22]

There is no evidence that letters were exchanged between Hari and any yogis during the war, but they resumed shortly after its end. Before and after the war, Paramhansa Yogananda corresponded tirelessly with Hari, answering his questions as Hari progressed through the SRF kriya yoga lessons. Paramhansa Yogananda's first letter to Hari after the war is dated January 1946 and was sent to 224/DP camp. This letter demonstrates his love for Hari and the students of yoga who had attended Hari's Latvian Yoga Center.

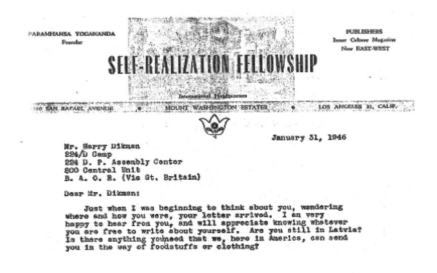

Figure 1.7. First part of letter from Paramhansa Yogananda, January 31, 1946.

Dear Mr. Dikman: Just when I was beginning to think about you, wondering where and how you were, your letter arrived. I am very happy to hear from you and will appreciate knowing whatever you are free to write about yourself. Are you still in Latvia? Is there anything you need that we, here in America, can send you in the way of foodstuffs or clothing?...

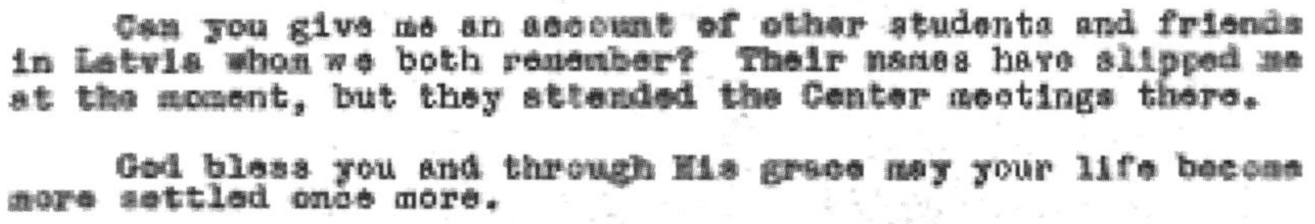

Can you give me an account of other students and friends in Latvia whom we both remember? Their names have slipped me at the moment, but they attended the Center meetings there.

God bless you and through His grace may your life become more settled once more.

Figure 1.8. Later part of letter from Paramhansa Yogananda, January 31, 1946.

Can you give me an account of other students and friends in Latvia whom we both remember? Their names have slipped me at the moment, but they attended the Center meetings there.

God bless you and through His grace may your life become more settled once more. With unceasing blessings, I am, Very sincerely yours, P. Yogananda

At the bottom of the letter, a note is added in Yogananda's handwriting.

It was most wonderful to hear from you & see you going strong in God. I prayed every week for your safety—I am glad beyond dreams you are safe. Let me know all about yourself and if you can start another centre of SRF in Latvia. With deepest love & blessings. P.Y.[23]

As mentioned earlier, Hari followed the teachings of more than one yoga master, and this created a little controversy.[24] In spite of this, Yogananda devoted himself to getting Hari and his wife, Isabella, out of the DP camps and into the United States, where Hari could work for the Self-Realization Fellowship. Until that move was arranged, Yogananda sent them care packages of powdered milk, canned goods, and yoga publications, though the maximum allowed weight of care packages was only five pounds.[25]

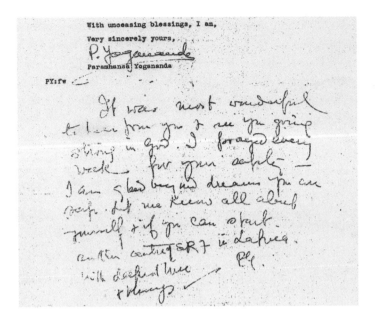

Figure 1.9. Handwritten note at bottom of letter from Paramhansa Yogananda, January 31, 1946.

Yogananda suggested that he mail Hari a certificate indicating that Hari was a minister for Self-Realization Fellowship, which would make Hari eligible to enter the United States as a minister.

> Dear Dr. Dikman: I have received your letter written February 27 and read its contents with great care. How many times during the war I thought of you and the other faithful students and prayed for your safety....
>
> If there is some difficulty in getting passage to America, you could tell the officials that you have been a minister of Self-Realization Fellowship, carrying on a Center in Latvia for a number of years, and as such, you should be eligible to enter the country as a minister....
>
> It has been my understanding that in the past you have followed Self-Realization Fellowship as well as other teachings. However, you must understand that if you have become active in the Fellowship there must be 100 percent loyalty to Self-Realization teachings

and its gurus. You must write me frankly about this. Otherwise, if you were to join the Fellowship, whether here or in India and teach something else, there would result great conflict and confusion. To mix teachings would only end in confusion for yourself and others. I write this because I have had similar experiences before, when some students have visited the Self-Realization Fellowship Centers and have taught something else—diluted the teachings—and thus, created great confusion and conflict among the members and Centers. Whatever you decide must come from your heart. I shall await your reply.

   With unceasing blessings and prayers that God will guide you, I remain, Very sincerely yours, Paramhansa Yogananda.

   P.S. If you so decide to wholly devote yourself as a minister of Self-Realization I will send you a minister's certificate as having carried on the centre in Latvia over two years (which will make you eligible to enter this country as a minister of SRF)—and then you could go back to India as a resident teacher in my Ranchi Yoga School or preach SRF in India. Please let me know your decision from your inner spirit immediately. Love & blessings, P.Y.[26]

The DP camp addresses on the letters changed as Hari, Isabella, and her mother were moved from one camp to another. Although Paramhansa Yogananda sent Hari a minister's certificate around July 1946,[27] there were many more requirements to be fulfilled before they could enter the United States.[28] In fact, the United States did not allow any displaced persons until after June 1948, followed by a second entry allowed after June 1950. It was considered to be a very bureaucratic process in which all refugees had to be sponsored.[29] A letter from 1948 indicates that there was a threat of Hari being sent to Russia, so Yogananda tried to arrange for Dr. Kennell, the leader of SRF's San Diego church, to arrange an affidavit for a priority emigration for Hari.

   It is too bad that we have been so long in working out something, but do not be discouraged. The Heavenly Father and the great gurus are watching over you, and as you are in tune so will you receive their guidance and help even throughout the worst difficulties....

   Delay was caused by complications but I am trying my utmost to get you here. With love, P.Y.[30]

Hari's knack for languages led him to work teaching English in the DP camps, and he also began lecturing and teaching yoga. Paramhansa Yogananda sent *East-West* magazines and materials to Hari,[31] along with a new set of the praecepta and instructions to be followed for conducting classes in the physical exercises and techniques.[32] It was probably one of the most important ways he spent his time, as it helped him and others to withstand the difficulties of life in the camps.

It was not until 1952 that Hari, Isabella, and her mother were finally able to leave the DP camps. They had endured at least six years moving from camp to camp. A February 1952 letter from Paramhansa Yogananda indicates that, at last, Hari had arrived in the United States. As far as Hari was concerned, Yogananda had saved his life.

Dear One, Years I prayed for your safe return to America when you wrote to know the art of Kriya—going out of the body—in case you were transferred to the wrong quarters of Germany. You always wanted to teach this work of SRF, a veteran in its teachings. Now, at this late hour, why do you want a job—it would be anyway a hand-to-mouth existence.

How many of you have crossed the sea—you, your wife, & who else—where is your mother-in-law? Is it your desire to be a national teacher of SRF & go from place to place or have a job—& do you think your wife & mother-in-law would not fit in the work. Or do you think that your wife & yourself & mother-in-law would not be satisfied at the headquarters, serving you with food, lodg[ing], & some pocket expenses. *I wish to know what is in your heart of hearts.* Please write at once everything after consulting your wife & mother-in-law, if she is with you.

It is all we can do these days with high cost of living … keeping body & soul together. [The] cost of living is more than what you get in jobs. We attained spiritual freedom through self-supporting ways—physical freedom. If I can help solve your problem through my humble efforts, I will be happy.

Do you lecture well—from spirit? Please let me know in enclosed envelope. With deepest love and blessings to you & all with you. Love, very sincerely yours, Paramhansa Yogananda.[33]

Hari told me about this journey crossing the sea when he revealed to me that he didn't like to travel. He said that he expressed his fears to Paramhansa Yogananda, who assured him that all would be fine. When Hari arrived at the dock, it was a very stormy day, and the sea was rough, but when the ship pulled out, the storm stopped, and the sea stayed calm all the way to New York. He accredited this calming of the sea to Paramhansa Yogananda.

The last letter to Hari from Paramhansa Yogananda was written a month later, on March 5, 1952. Hari still had not decided to come to SRF. It appears that Isabella was unsure about living in the communal environment at SRF, so Yogananda offered them a cottage at the Lake Shrine. He wanted Hari to come there and devote his life to one path, the path of SRF, and urged him to do so: "Now, after long deliberation, I feel in my faith in you, and your life's work remains—that you are preeminently fitted to spread SRF."[34]

Two days later, Paramhansa Yogananda passed away.

Hari and I talked about this. He loved Yogananda and regretted never getting to meet him in person, after being his disciple for eighteen years. I don't know what the reason was for Hari not going to work for Self-Realization Fellowship, though I am not sure it was a single thing. He certainly was considered by Yogananda to be adept enough to teach kriya yoga to others. Hari did say that it would be difficult for him to practice only one path of yoga, since all the paths he had studied offered him so much, and he was adept at the other paths as well. With the integrity that Hari demonstrated, perhaps this was his reason. He had to be true both to himself and to Paramhansa Yogananda.

Swami Sivananda Saraswati of Rishikesh

Hari was likewise devoted to Swami Sivananda of Rishikesh. Although I have no letters dated before 1946—which is likely due to the war—it seems they communicated with each other before the war broke out. Swami Sivananda clearly states in a letter of reference dated February 18, 1954, that he has known Hari for over fifteen years.[35]

Furthermore, a publisher's note on the back cover of *Yoga Chakravarty*, written by Hari for Swami Sivananda, states that Hari studied under Swami Sivananda since the inception of the Divine Life Society in 1936.

Sri H. Dickman belongs to Latvia. Those who have known him personally and who have studied his letters and other writings affirm that he should have been an Indian Yogi, re-incarnated now in the West to interpret Yoga to the West, and guide Westerners along the Path of Yoga. Very early in life he felt drawn to Yoga and Vedanta and with the characteristic thoroughness and sincerity of the Westerner, began practising Yoga.

As he progressed along the path, he obtained guidance from Indian Masters by correspondence. He is one of the earliest disciples and followers of Sri Swami Sivanandaji Maharaj, with whom he has been in regular correspondence ever since the inception of the Divine Life Society. Along with Srimatis Anna Plaudis and Anna Dolfij, he conducted the Divine Life Society Branch at Riga as the Latvian President.

He is himself an advanced Raja Yogi and has taught Yoga to several European Sadhakas [those who practice sadhana, "spiritual practices"]. He is a zealous Yoga-propagandist. He has translated Sri Swami Sivananda's Kundalini Yoga and Ten Upanishads into Latvian. He used to conduct Sadhana classes, on the beach in Europe and has rendered inestimable service to the cause of spread of Yoga-knowledge in the West. He is one of the few who have read all of Sri Swami Sivanandaji's works and thoroughly mastered them.

He is such an adept in meditation that he is able to practice Pratyahara, Dharana and Dhyana even in a bazar. He was able to stop the heartbeats, etc., through Pranayama. He is now in New York and continues his Sadhana for Self-realisation and also the glorious work of dissemination of spiritual knowledge.[36]

Yoga Chakravarty, written by Hari in the 1940s while he was in German DP camps, gives an account of Swami Sivananda's life and work for publication by the Divine Life Society. The above text is significant for many reasons. First, it points out how highly regarded Hari was—those who knew him said that he should have been an Indian yogi. It also expresses how advanced and adept he was in his practice. Second, there is the statement that Hari "obtained guidance from other Indian Masters." The fact that this is stated as a benefit rather than as a point of concern is notable. Unlike Paramhansa Yogananda, who diligently followed the teachings of his guru, Sri Yukteswar, and did everything he could to pass these teachings on in their purest form, Swami Sivananda never had that option. He was only with his guru for one day.

Prior to becoming a yogi, Swami Sivananda was known as Dr. Kuppuswami Iyer, a medical doctor in Malaya. Hari wrote in *Yoga Chakravarty* about the compassionate qualities of the doctor. "The Swami was a most sympathetic doctor. He tried to understand the feelings, troubles and anxieties of his patients. In serious cases he himself nursed his patients and administered medicines to them. If the patient happened to be poor, Dr. Kuppuswami did not take any fee from them for the treatment. He even provided them with clothing and money."[37]

We may wonder what would compel the doctor to leave his successful practice to live a life of renunciation. Hari went on to explain this.

> Once he treated a serious case of [a] sick Sannyasi. The Sannyasi had some rare manuscripts with whom he never wanted to part. But out of a sense of deep gratitude to Dr. Kuppuswami Iyer for his kind treatment he voluntarily offered those valuable manuscripts to the doctor. Those manuscripts contained the highest truths of Vedanta Philosophy. As the gunpowder easily catches fire, so the already spiritually inclined soul and by selfless-service [the] purified heart of the Swami caught the idea of renunciation."[38]

Hari continued to write about the doctor's pilgrimage that eventually led him to Rishikesh, which occurred after the Sannyasi saw *Brahma tejas*, the aura of Brahman or the Source itself, in the doctor's face.

> Dr. Kuppuswami had met several Sadhus during his wanderings but he did not ask till now any one of them to initiate him. But here was a Saint sent by Divine Providence. Brahma Tejas splashed from his austere but kind face. The Sannyasi said to the doctor: "Your face shows that you are born to fulfill a great mission. How I wish to initiate a person of your type, to be enrolled in the holy order of Paramahansa." The doctor at once felt that this is his divinely ordained Guru and gratefully accepted the Sannyasi's kind offer. The Sannyasi continued: "I am coming from Benares. My name is Viswananda. I have been a Sannyasi for a very long time. You are a proper Adhikari for initiation. I shall initiate you to-morrow morning." Early in the morning both the Guru and disciple took a bath in the holy river Ganges. The preceptor had already kept an ochre robe for his disciple. After proper rites and recitation of sacred Mantras Swami

Sivananda, for such was his spiritual name now, was initiated into the mysteries of "Tat Twam Asi" Mahavakya. The veil of Avidya was torn asunder and the Swami stood free and brilliant like the Sun.

This was the beginning of his glorious spiritual career for he was destined to be the Spiritual guide and Teacher not only of India but the world at large.

In the evening Sri Swami Viswananda (Swami Sivananda's Guruji) wanted to leave for Benares and addressed his disciple as follows: "I cannot remain here any longer. I have a big Ashram at Nadia. You may follow me if you like. I shall give you all conveniences for Sadhana." Swami Sivananda said: "Oh hallowed Teacher! My joy knows no bounds when I hear Thy honeyed words. I would like to remain here, if you would approve of it. My heart is captivated and charmed by the lofty Himalayas and Ganges." The Guru replied: "Yes, you can do so. May God bless you. May you become a dynamic Yogi."[39]

Imagine that! You become initiated as a swami, and the same day, your guru must leave and is not with you to guide and teach you. Swami Sivananda was awakened by his master, and from there he had to use his own inner strength and inspiration to study and practice. And he did. And this is what made him such a unique and special swami, especially for that time.

As we saw with Paramhansa Yogananda, most serious yogis study one path of yoga, one particular kind of sadhana, perfecting it without the distraction of exploring other paths. When you follow one course, it is a much more direct route to success. Swami Sivananda, however, sought out different yoga masters to teach him, undertaking extensive travel throughout India. "The Swami visited Badrinath and Kedarnath, travelled up to Rameshwar in extereme [sic] South India, as well as to Mount Kailas and Mansarowar lake in Tibet. The Swami has written an inspired book describing his experiences during his Yatra to Kailas and Mansarovar. The Swami paid also a visit to Sri Ramanashrama in Tiruvannamalai and Sri Aurobindo Ashrama in Pondichery where two famous Hindu Rishis and Yogins have their residences."[40]

By 1936, after twelve years of intense sadhana, Swami Sivananda established the Divine Life Society and built the Sivananda Nagar on the banks of the Ganges in Rishikesh. He continued to share his medical expertise, treating anyone who needed it. He became a guru for seekers of multiple interests, because he had achieved perfection in many paths of yoga. These multiple paths did not create confusion for him, for he understood deep in his soul how all paths lead to the same goal—the truth, the oneness, the union or yoga. Students of diverse aptitudes and temperaments flocked to him, as he was able to offer expert spiritual guidance in varied applications of yoga—jnana, hatha, raja, bhakti, and others.

Hari was one of those sadhakas who was drawn to Swami Sivananda. Their correspondence began around 1936 and continued until 1962. He was embraced as much as any disciple living in the swami's presence. There was no conflict with Hari corresponding or studying with other yoga masters, since Swami Sivananda understood this practice well.

It is interesting to note here that this open-mindedness of Swami Sivananda seems to have led him deep into his *sadguru* (true guru within), and he extended this attitude to his disciples. A letter to Hari from his gurubhai Swami Shivapremananda said, "Swami Sivanandaji never taught us anything specific and each of his monastic disciples picked up in his own way [knowledge] from where he could, some without substance and some [with] something of value and mainly from within themselves."[41]

He clarified this by saying that individuals react to practices differently, depending on their state of consciousness, and the teacher must suggest practices suited to each individual situation. At some point, one has enough experience to be his own guide, and he suggested Hari had achieved this.[42]

When we understand the word *guru* to mean "one who guides you to the spirit," this entirely makes sense. Swami Sivananda guided his disciples to their spirit, not in a rigid manner, but in a way that made sense to each of them. This is why the disciples of Sivananda all teach yoga in their own way. You can feel the threads of Sivananda Yoga wisdom in all of their teachings, but no two are exactly the same. Swami Sivananda was unique in that each one of his students could find his or her own path within, just as he had done through the guidance of his many mentors.

Swami Sivananda bestowed upon Hari the title of *Yogiraj* (King of Yoga), as is seen in a letter of reference he sent to Hari in 1954. This is an honorable title in the name of Siva and is given only to those who are considered yoga masters. At the same time, Swami Sivananda also awarded Hari with the sacred title *Star of the Divine Life Society.*[43]

Swami Sivananda encouraged all of his disciples to correspond with Hari and to visit him if they could, as they were gurubhais. One such visit is recounted in Swami Venkatesananda's booklet *The USA and Canada Revisited.*

"It was superwonderful to see Yogiraj Harry Dickman in the gathering. He is the seniormost European-disciple of Sri Gurudev and perhaps the greatest correspondent and most sincere student of Yoga. He is also the author of a biography of Gurudev. In his own simple, silent way he is spreading the teachings of Gurudev and the message of Yoga."[44]

Another visit is also referred to in this same booklet.

On the 6th of December, 1970, the Integral Yoga Institute (founded by Yogiraj Swami Satchidananda) gave a luncheon to which they invited Swami Vishnudevananda, Yogiraj Harry Dickman, [Swami Venkatesananda], Mr. Peter Max, and the Rabbi Gelberman.[45]

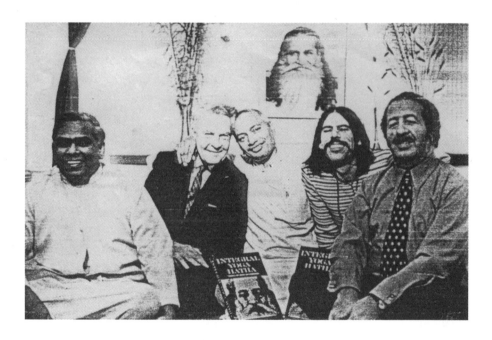

Figure 1.10. Photo of Hari with his gurubhais and friends (left to right): Swami Vishnudevananda, Dr. Hari Dickman, Swami Venkatesananda, Mr. Peter Max, Rabbi Gelberman, in front of a photo of Swami Satchidananda, December 6, 1970. Photographer unknown.

A reference letter written by Swami Sivananda in 1952, shortly after Hari arrived in the United States, introduced Hari to Dr. Robert Ernst Dickhoff.

It immensely delights me to introduce to your nobleself Sri Yogiraj Harry Dickman of Latvia who is at present staying in New York. Well known to me for over two decades, I have found in Sri Harry Dickman an ideal gentleman endowed with all noble and virtuous qualities. Further he was the President of the Latvian Branch of the Divine Life Society for many years and has taught Yoga to several European Sadhakas. An adept in Hatha Yoga, Sri Harry Dickman has made tremendous progress in Raja Yoga being gifted with a rare intuitional insight. He has translated my books "Kundalini Yoga" and "Ten Upanishads" into Latvian and his major work, a biography of mine, is awaiting publication.

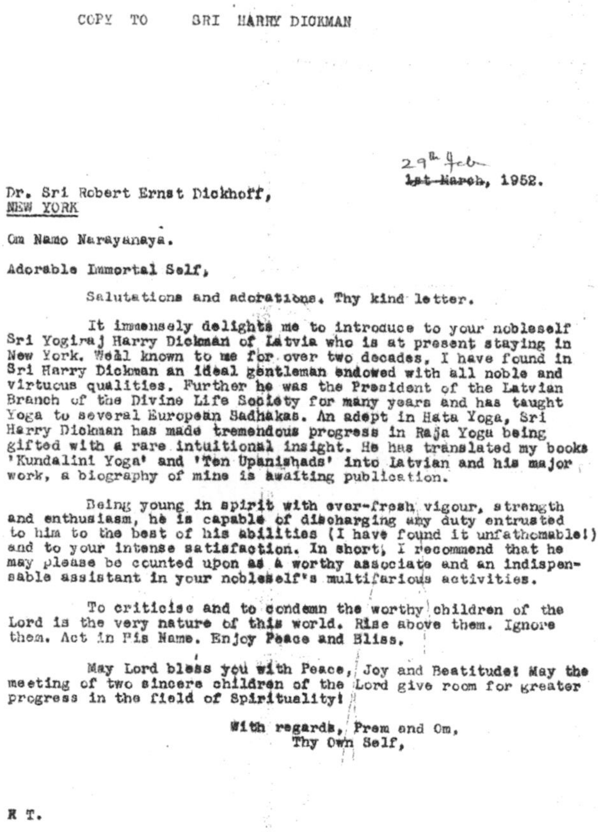

COPY TO   SRI HARRY DICKMAN

29th Feb
1st March, 1952.

Dr. Sri Robert Ernst Dickhoff,
NEW YORK

Om Namo Narayanaya.

Adorable Immortal Self,

Salutations and adorations. Thy kind letter.

It immensely delights me to introduce to your nobleself Sri Yogiraj Harry Dickman of Latvia who is at present staying in New York. Well known to me for over two decades, I have found in Sri Harry Dickman an ideal gentleman endowed with all noble and virtuous qualities. Further he was the President of the Latvian Branch of the Divine Life Society for many years and has taught Yoga to several European Sadhakas. An adept in Hata Yoga, Sri Harry Dickman has made tremendous progress in Raja Yoga being gifted with a rare intuitional insight. He has translated my books 'Kundalini Yoga' and 'Ten Upanishads' into Latvian and his major work, a biography of mine is awaiting publication.

Being young in spirit with ever-fresh vigour, strength and enthusiasm, he is capable of discharging any duty entrusted to him to the best of his abilities (I have found it unfathomable!) and to your intense satisfaction. In short, I recommend that he may please be counted upon as a worthy associate and an indispensable assistant in your nobleself's multifarious activities.

To criticise and to condemn the worthy children of the Lord is the very nature of this world. Rise above them. Ignore them. Act in His Name. Enjoy Peace and Bliss.

May Lord bless you with Peace, Joy and Beatitude! May the meeting of two sincere children of the Lord give room for greater progress in the field of Spirituality!

With regards, Prem and Om,
Thy Own Self,

R T.

Figure 1.11. Letter of reference for Hari written to Dr. Robert Ernst Dickhoff from Swami Sivananda, February 29, 1952.

Being young in spirit with ever-fresh vigour, strength and enthusiasm, he is capable of discharging any duty entrusted to him to the best of his abilities (I have found it unfathomable!) and to your intense satisfaction. In short, I recommend that he may please be counted upon as a worthy associate and an indispensable assistant in your nobleself's multifarious activities.[46]

Swami Sivananda wrote Hari another reference letter in 1954, which was apparently intended to help him start a school of yoga in New York.[47]

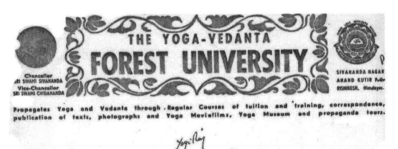

Figure 1.12. Another letter of reference for Hari from Swami Sivananda, February 18, 1954.

One can hardly believe that Hari and Swami Sivananda had never met in person! But that was the gift that Swami Sivananda gave to so many yogis through his intense desire to share his rich experience of inner spiritual life with other truth seekers. Hari was not alone, but rather part of a group of at least twenty other worldwide followers of Swami Sivananda studying through correspondence. You can read more about each of them in one of the Divine Life Society publications, *From Man to God-Man*, written by N. Ananthanarayanan.[48]

Sri Ramana Maharshi

One of Hari's earlier teachers was Bhagavan Sri Ramana Maharshi. I don't have any letters written to Hari from the Maharshi himself, but Hari told me he corresponded with him for years,[49] and there is evidence that he contributed instructions in yoga to Hari's yoga society in Latvia.[50] There are also very few letters remaining from the Sri Ramana Maharshi Ashram. I suspect most were destroyed or lost during the war. The earliest letter I have is from 1931, written by the Maharshi's disciple T. K. Sundaresa Iyer; the next is from 1933, from Niranjanananda Swamy, which included an interesting newspaper article. From then, the letters jump to 1947–1952, and finally there are three letters in 1976.

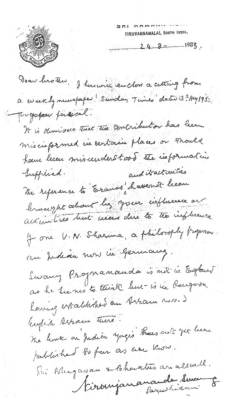

The newspaper article is from the *Sunday Times*, dated August 13, 1933 (city unknown), regarding the disciples who studied by correspondence with Sri Ramana Maharshi; Hari is included.

Figure 1.13. Letter from Niranjanananda Swamy, from Sri Ramana Ashram, August 8, 1933.

The foreign Bhaktas of Sri Ramana Maharshi are steadily on the increase, and some of them are striving not only for personal uplift, but to be of use to others, in their own circle.

Most of them have been visitors to the Ashram at Tiruvannamalai and lived there for a time. One, a London journalist, Mr. Raphael Hurst, was in residence there for full four months in 1931 and another, Swami Prajnananda, stayed a few weeks.... These constitute one group, persons who have a firsthand knowledge of the Maharshi; and there is another whose attachment to him was fostered only by books and letters.

The most prominent among them is Harry Dickman, a citizen of Latvia. Imbued with a spiritual trend, he had been a student of Indian Philosophy for some years before he heard of the Maharshi and got at his writings. From that time, he has been a close Bhakta, in regular correspondence, an inquirer and a Sadhak.

Mr. Dickman has built a circle around him of persons interested in Indian culture, and he never misses an opportunity to spread the light. Occasions like the birthday of the Maharshi are always utilized to hold classes and give lectures on his teachings or on kindred subjects. And such activities have brought him into contact with several kindred souls in Europe, one of them being the organiser of Eranos, a centre that was intended to be and has become a meeting ground for the East and West....

Of all of these, Mr. Dickman is perhaps the most enthusiastic, though it has not yet been his good fortune to see the Guru personally. Not only is he interesting a number of people in Maharshi's teachings, and popularizing his writings, but he has just brought out in the Latvian language, a rendering of Who Am I? and is now endeavouring to translate also the Upadesha Saram, another of Maharshi's works.[51]

The article mentions a few other notable students studying with Ramana Maharshi through his books and letters: Mrs. Olga Frobe-Kapteyn, who founded the Eranos Ashram in the Swiss Alps; Swami Prajnananda, a major in the British Army, who founded the English Ashram in Rangoon, India; and a London journalist, Mr. Raphael Hurst (misspelled as Hirst). Mr. Raphael Hurst is none other than Mr. Paul Brunton, renowned student of

SUNDAY TIMES, AUGUST 13, 1933

Maharshi's Foreign Bhaktas

An Expanding Circle

Ashram on Swiss Lake

The foreign Bhaktas of Sri Ramana Maharshi are steadily on the increase and some of them are striving not only for personal uplift, but to be of use to others, in their own circle.

Most of them have been visitors to the Ashram at Tiruvannamalai and lived there for a time. One, a London journalist, Mr. Raphael Hurst, was in residence there for full four months in 1931 and another, Swami Prajnananda stayed a few weeks, and before he came he had digested some Ashram literature and felt a great hankering to be there. These constitute one group, persons who have a firsthand knowledge of the Maharshi; and there is another whose attachment to him was fostered only by books and letters.

In Far Off Latvia

The most prominent among them is Harry Dikman, a citizen of Latvia. Imbued with a spiritual trend, he had been a student of Indian philosophy for some years before he heard of the Maharshi and got at his writings. From that time, he has been a close Bhakta, in regular correspondence, an inquirer and a Sadhak.

Mr. Dikman has built a circle around him, of persons interested in Indian culture and he never misses an opportunity to spread the light. Occasions like the birthday of the Maharshi are always utilised to hold classes and give lectures on his teachings or on kindred subjects. And such activities have brought him into contact with several kindred souls in Europe, one of them being the

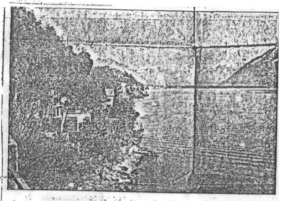

"Eranos", the *Ashram* situated amidst the picturesque scenes of the snow-clad Alps.

organiser of Eranos, a centre that was intended to be and has become a meeting ground for the East and West.

On The Alps

As the picture shows, this lodge is situated in ideal surroundings, on a lake at Ascona, Switzerland, with the snow-clad Alps at the back, a site that is said to resemble closely some Himalayan ashrams.

In a recent letter to the Ramanashram, Mrs. Olga Frobe-Kapteyn, its founder, writes of her plan "to establish there a kind of Ashram adapted to western needs and mentality" and expresses the hope that one or other of the Maharshi's disciples would go there.

All these Bhaktas are anxious to come to India and stay at the Ashram. Though they are getting the guidance they seek, they long to live by Maharshi's side.

Not in England

"I realise now," says Mr. Hirst in one of his recent letters, "that I made a mistake in not staying at the Ashram till the end of the year at least....I feel that I have made no spiritual progress all the time I have been back in England. The mental atmosphere of London is so materialistic and one must be so active that I find it very difficult to meditate now.........I realise that only at the Ashram could I meditate properly and make real progress. I realise that one must stay in the physical neighbourhood of the Guru for a long time before one is strong enough to resist the evil influences of the world.......My mind is made up to leave England for a long time one day perhaps for years —and stay with you."

As Interpreters

So is Prajnananda. He was an Major in the British Army, and after world-wide travels took up the life of a Buddhist monk. He was at the Ashram at the end of last winter and such were his experiences that he intends to return again this year.

Of all these, Mr. Dikman is perhaps the most enthusiastic, though it has not yet been his

Figure 1.14. Newspaper article about Ramana Maharshi's foreign students. *Sunday Times,* August 13, 1933, city unknown.

the Sri Ramana Maharshi and author of *In Search of Secret India,* published in 1934. It is interesting to note that Hari and Brunton were connected through at least one other guru as well. A 1977 issue of the *British Wheel of Yoga* points out that Hari "was a contemporary pupil with Paul Brunton under Sivananda at Rishikesh."

There are also other sources showing Hari as one of the Maharshi's disciples. One of Hari's Tamil texts acknowledges him and a few other Maharshi disciples.[52]

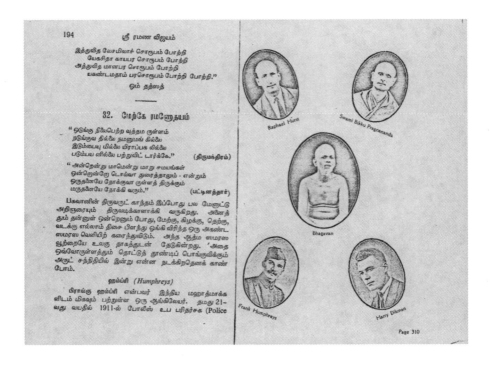

Figure 1.15. A Tamil text acknowledging students of Bhagavan Sri Ramana Maharshi. Title and publisher unknown.

About one year after Ramana Maharshi passed away, the president of Sri Ramana Ashram asked Hari to send them copies of the Maharshi's letters, since they contained valuable teachings that could otherwise be lost.

We are happy to have your letter of 3.5.51, along with the enclosures of copies of two letters, and thank you for the same. Our letter of the 16th Feb 1946 (the copy of which you sent) contains much interesting matter. It is such letters, if traced in your files, that will be useful for being published. One of the oldest devotees who was working in our office, says that most of the letters sent to you from our Asramam about the years 1929 to 1940 contain discussions and elucidations of remotest and [abstruse] points of philosophy and yoga as propounded by Sri Bhagawan. He considers these letters very valuable, as these were very closely scrutinized and sometimes dictated by Sri Bhagawan Himself.

Under such circumstances, we should be very happy if you will kindly endeavour to trace all the earlier letters and send us copies of the same. If we are fortunate to get these letters, these will be published for the benefit of the devotees of Sri Bhagawan.

We trust that by Sri Bhagawan's grace it would be possible for you to trace these letters for the benefit of prosperity.

—Niranjanananda Swamy[53]

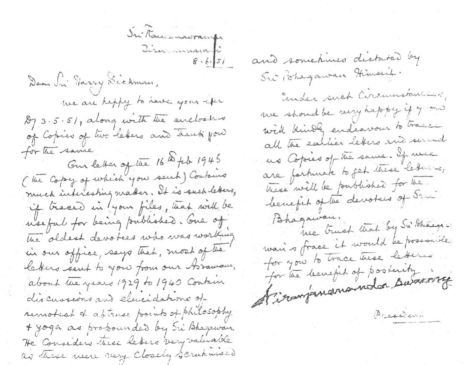

Figure 1.16. Letter from Niranjanananda Swamy from Sri Ramana Ashram, June 8, 1951.

It seems the disciples of this ashram were not the only ones seeking copies of the letters from their guru to Hari. In a letter dated May 16, 1975, a different Swami Niranjanananda, a disciple of Swami Satyananda Giri of the kriya yoga lineage, requested copies of letters the Maharshi sent to Hari between 1937 and 1971.

> Letters received by you from Beloved Guruji Maharaj are with you and, therefore, dates of these letters should be known to you because all communications were directly between you and Beloved Guruji Maharaj.[54]

So much knowledge was passed from the Maharshi and other gurus to their devoted disciple. Their letters were filled with details to ensure their practices were well understood. The gurus and masters and their disciples and servants all knew Hari. He was one of them, on the path, and they loved him.

Some of this knowledge is included in the pages that follow.

Chapter Two

THE EIGHT LIMBS
OF YOGA

HARI ORGANIZED THE LETTERS from his yoga teachers with love and precision. Each envelope was labeled with an overview of the contents. Letters were bundled together by author and ordered by date. He knew exactly where to go to find a letter covering a specific topic of interest.

We began our studies together by reviewing my notes taken during my time training in the ashram. There was much I did not understand yet, so I would formulate a list of questions from my notes, and then we would discuss them. He would pull information from letters that would support or correct my understanding. We would discuss contradictions in the methodology of different yoga paths, and he would explain how he would do the practice.

Often our discussions were purely philosophical. Many of the yoga teachings are deep and difficult to understand. It is as though hidden meanings become clear only as the layers of *maya*, "illusion," covering the true self within are slowly removed. Through study, meditation, contemplation, practice, and assimilation over time, the knowledge is revealed. I can attest to this, because even as I read the letters today, my understanding is very different than when Hari explained their meanings to me.

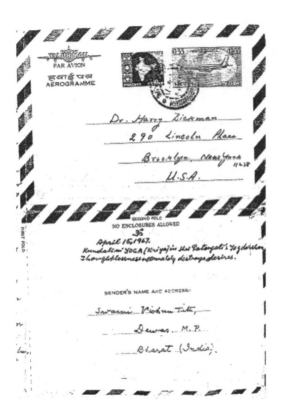

Figure 2.1. Letter demonstrating how Hari organized his letters by date and content for quick reference.

The eight limbs of yoga are a foundation for many paths of yoga, and the first two limbs are the foundation for success in the remaining limbs. These are the *yamas* and *niyamas,* the ethical restraints and observances, or inner and outer ethical practices. These encompass practices such as truthfulness, nonviolence, cleanliness, discipline, and steady study of the spirit; they underlie everything else we do in yoga, and those who don't master them are not really practicing yoga. Hari told me that Swami Sivananda said that it can take a lifetime to perfect one yama.

The letters I have chosen to include here illustrate many techniques that Hari and I discussed or practiced together. There are also letters covering techniques that Hari and I did not practice together but are ones that I have studied—through these letters—since his passing. This is how knowledge is delivered from one student to the next. It is my hope that readers will benefit from the wisdom Hari received from his teachers so it can be passed forward to the yogis of today and tomorrow.

Throughout the letters, you will hear reference to *ashtanga yoga,* the "eight limbs of yoga" as described in Patanjali's *Yoga Sutras.* The eight limbs are the

- *yamas*—ethical restraints, including *ahimsa* (nonviolence), *satya* (truthfulness), *asteya* (non-stealing), *brahmacharya* (non-excessiveness, generally related to sensual pleasures; celibacy), and *aparigraha* (non-possessiveness);
- *niyamas*—internal observances including *saucha* (purity), *santosha* (contentment), *tapas* (self-discipline), *svadhyaya* (self-study), and *ishvara pranidhana* (surrender to the Divine);
- *asanas*—postures;
- *pranayama*—control of the life force known as *prana;*
- *pratyahara*—withdrawal from the senses (to take us inward toward the true Self);
- *dharana*—concentration;
- *dhyana*—meditation; and
- *samadhi*—union with our God; enlightenment—the ultimate goal of yoga.

The majority of yoga pathways incorporate these eight limbs. Depending on the lineage, the asana limb is merely the proper seat for meditation and not a sequence of postures. It seems fitting that this letter from Mahant Dig Vijai Nath from the Gorakhnath Temple is the first to be presented, as it clearly explains these eight limbs of yoga.

I am highly pleased to learn from your ... letters that you are an earnest aspirant after *Moksha* [liberation] and that you feel a deep attraction for the *yoga* system, as taught by *Mahayogiswara* Adinath, Matsyendranath, and Gorakshanath. It is really gratifying to find that you have already studied a number of standard works on the system and that you are practicing *Ajapa-Yoga* [a meditation technique] and *Nada-anusandana* [a practice of concentrating on the inner tones of sound to raise the level of consciousness], which are two most important processes of *sadhana* [spiritual practices] of our school for a seeker of freedom from the bondages and sorrows of this world. You have not, of course, failed to note the warnings, given in the works on *Yoga,* that it is not safe to practice the esoteric *yogic* processes involving complicated forms of *Pranayama, Mudra, Bandha,* etc., except under the direct guidance of a competent *Guru.* Nor all such forms of discipline as are prescribed in the books of Yoga necessary or appropriate for every spiritual aspirant.

The yoga-system is a vast science and art of perfect self-mastery and self-refinement and self-elevation and self-illumination, based on a profound spiritual philosophy and a profound knowledge of human psychology and physiology and the cosmic order. It has discovered effective processes, by means of which a man can attain perfect control over his physical body, his nervous system, his vital forces, his sense-organs, his mental desires and passions and thoughts; he can immensely magnify his will-power, his intellectual capacity, his spiritual insight, the power of his sense-perception and mental vision; he can acquire powers which are normally regarded as miraculous and supernatural; he can exercise control over the forces of nature; he can travel with his physical body from one place to another without any conveyance; he can even create a number of physical bodies at the same time and perform different functions through them, and so on. We have seen and heard of several instances of such supernormal *yogic* powers even in our own time. But such siddhis [powers] are not essential for the attainment of *Moksha,* and hence the esoteric yogic processes leading to such *siddhis* are not generally practiced by *yogis* longing for Truth-realisation and *Moksha* by the shortest route. Hence the yogi-teachers of the present age try to prescribe comparatively simple non-technical formulas for the spiritual elevation of the aspirants under the present conditions of life.

Cultivation of will-power is very important not only for *yoga-sadhana,* but for every form of noble human endeavor. Here Will implies faith, urge, self-confidence, aspiration, determination, intensive effort. Will has to be strengthened, enlightened, and concentrated. Perfect self-mastery requires perfection of enlightened will-power. But this will-power can and has to be developed through its intensive application to some right purpose. For an aspirant for Yoga, will and effort has to be applied to the systematic discipline of the body, the senses, the vital forces, the mental propensities and excitements, [and] the intellectual thoughts, with the ultimate purpose of elevating the whole phenomenal being to the transcendent plane and realizing the unity of the self with the Supreme Spirit.

Yama and *Niyama* constitute the moral basis of yogic discipline, and these should be practiced by every spiritual aspirant with strong determination as far as practicable under the physical and social conditions under which an aspirant lives and moves.

A *yogi*, who has only *Moksha* as the ideal of his life and not the occult powers and experience, should choose one or two simple *asanas*—such as *Padmasana* [the lotus pose] and *Siddhasana* [the "adepts pose," the pose of those who have acquired siddhis]—for steadying his body and sit in one such posture as long as he conveniently can and practice calmness and tranquility of the body and the mind with thought concentrated on the Supreme Spirit.

A simple form of *Pranayama*, consisting in regular rhythmical slow and deep breathing, with mind concentrated on the *Ajapa-yoga* (which you are in the habit of practicing) is enough. Intricate forms of *Pranayama* and *Mudra* can be practiced only under expert guidance. *Pratyahara* and *Dharana* can be practiced in the form of withdrawing the senses and the mind from all sensuous objects and all worldly problems and inwardizing them and concentrating the attention either on the Indwelling Supreme Spirit or on the Image of some perfectly calm and tranquil *Mahayogi* [great yogi] absorbed in the deepest meditation. Gradually try to merge your ego in the all-pervading existence of the Supreme Spirit, Siva Who is the Absolute Reality and of Whom all the diverse orders of existences are phenomenal self-manifestations.

The prolonged practice of *Siddhasana* and rhythmical deep breathing and concentration together with the regulation of thought and word and deed in accordance with the principles of *Yama* and *Niyama* will certainly enable you to control your sexual excitements and all other excitements and worldly propensities. If, in spite of your best efforts, there are momentary lapses, don't mind them, don't brood over them; make a fresh determination to rise above such weaknesses and cheerfully and determinedly go on with your practices. Remember that the mind is the chief instrument of *yoga-sadhana* and that you have to pay special attention to the control and systematic discipline of the mind. The processes of control and discipline of *Prana*—the nervous system and vital organs—require special instruction and guidance. For the guidance of the initiated disciples in the right path according to their individual aptitudes, even the same *Guru* often gives [different] kinds of instructions with regard to subsidiary aspects of truths and practices. Hence you find apparent discrepancies in the authoritative texts. The inner significance is everywhere the same.[55]

All eight limbs are addressed through various techniques in the letters. And throughout, there is an understanding that the practice of the yamas and niyamas is an essential foundation for success in yoga. They may not be mentioned all the time, but without the ongoing practice of them, one's mind is not *sattvic*, "pure," and this is an essential ingredient for us to know God.

The yamas and niyamas help protect us from our egos. They help us to respect all of life and to be good and humble people. The ego is the strength upholding maya, the illusion that we are separate from God or any of God's creation, and it will fight to maintain its identity. The ego is manifested through our personalities, ever-changing with our moods and circumstances. If one becomes selfless or self-realized, the ego cannot survive, and it will not go down easily. The following letter from Brahmachari Animananda Dharmacharya explains the battle a yogi must fight in order to reach self-realization.

Generally, it is taken for granted that every devotee wants to see God. But, really speaking, it is not so. Most of the devotees hanker after miraculous power, and they get the same. There are 8 different kinds of Siddhis, which you have come across in the *Yoga Sutras* of Patanjali. They divert the mind of the devotee from God to the miracle. Hence, truly speaking, they are the real hindrances to [achieving] Self-Realization or full Self-Control. Self-Control means control over the Bigger Self, i.e., God, which means to become God Himself.

So, indirectly, you have asked me how to become God. Now in the path of Self-Realization stands the Ego or pseudo-soul. Really speaking, this Ego is doing sadhana.

At first stage of sadhana, the devotee gets success and proceeds leaps and bounds and attains a very high place in the spiritual world, due to the invisible help of the Guru. The devotee thinks that he himself has attained that place due to the force of sadhana. Then comes the supreme trial, i.e., a fatal combat between the Ego and the True Self. The Great Self puts the devotee in question to innumerable temptations, and the fight ensues between the devotee and the temptations. At the outset, the fight ends in favour of the devotee, i.e., the Ego wins the battle, but in the long run, the Ego of the devotee is sure to get defeated. One after another, a series of battles ensues, and you will be surprised to know that nearly in every occasion, the devotee finds himself helpless and condescends to surrender to all the temptations coming out of sex, anger, greed, delusion, pride, and jealousy. As long as the Ego thinks that he will win the next battle, he is sure to get defeated. Ultimately, the devotee feels himself so helpless that he finds no other alternative than to surrender [completely] to God. God now comes forward and renders help consciously—which is known as Guru-Kripa [the grace or blessing of the guru]. Then the devotee gets true mastery over Self, which is termed as Self-Control or Self-Realization. This is the true meaning of Self-Control. Now, dear Harry Dikman, do you understand why the rishis [saints or seers] had proclaimed this path is as sharp as the blade of [a] razor.[56]

The yamas and niyamas are covered in many other books and are touched on throughout the letters to Hari. Here I will focus only on ahimsa and brahmacharya, two topics discussed at length in the letters.

Ahimsa

All of the yamas and niyamas are approached through the eyes of ahimsa (nonviolence), for it is the foundation for all practices. Yogis must practice nonviolence toward others and themselves. No creature deserves anything less. The practice of nonviolence helps to tame the ego, reminding us that each of us has an equally important role in this manifested universe. Ahimsa is a difficult practice, because it permeates everything that we think, say, and do.

Watch your thoughts; they become words.
Watch your words; they become actions.
Watch your actions; they become habits.
Watch your habits; they become character.
Watch your character; it becomes your destiny.[57]

If we subscribe to the knowledge that we are made of molecules and that these molecules vibrate at varying speeds, then we acknowledge that we all exude a certain vibration. We transmit outwardly whatever values we embrace inwardly. As yogis, we are constantly trying to raise the level of our consciousness so we can transform our personalities to become more loving and accepting.

As you think, so you become. You are what you eat. These are yogic truths. Swami Shivananda Saraswati of Assam shared a long letter with Hari on ahimsa that reflects clearly his yogic view of how important it is—not just for each one of us personally, but also for the entire world we live in.

Mankind all over the world [has] to be initiated into this Yoga-religion of non-killing. Cruelty even to lower animals should be stopped. Every cruel action has its reaction. Political blood shed, conflagration of war, disease, premature death, tempest, earthquake and other natural calamities follow as a reaction to such cruelty to lower animals. Millions of butchered beasts, and birds, millions of fishes caught in water fail to take vengeance on human cruelty. So does nature take revenge on behalf of these victimized lower animals. [Nature's] destructive dance in the form of war, flood, earthquake, etc., will come to an end as soon as man would adopt this principle of non-killing as his creed; it is not an emotional talk or [idle] talk, it is the fundamental truth which all should know for the welfare of all human beings. Every sensible man should preach this non-killing truth throughout the world.

The Principles of non-violence [are inseparably] connected with food. The gross Parts in food constitute the body, while the finer Part constitutes the mind. That is why Sattwik [pure] food helps to develop Sattwik mind or divine mind, and Rajasik [stimulating] food tends to develop Rajasik mind, which is a mixture of higher and lower mentality. Tamasik [sedating] food tends to develop Tamasik mind, which is selfish, brutal, and ferocious. Thus, it is inevitable to take Sattwik food to become a Yogi or to attain divinity. The list of Sattwik food includes pulses, vegetables, roots such as potatoes, arum, etc., green leaves, milk curd, and little quantity of rice and bread. Rajasik food is a mixture of fleshfood, Sattwik food, and concentrated food, such as Ghee, butter, cheese, casein, powder-milk, and such other milk products, and sugar, etc. Tamasik food includes flesh food, concentrated food, decomposed food in major portion, and a little quantity of Sattwik food. Concentrated food or milk products, though [they] appear to be Sattwik food, in essence they are not; they are all Rajasik food, and like fleshfood, they are harmful for human system if their use is not kept in strict limitations.

All countries of the world should feel the need of taking Sattwik food in consideration of the fact that Sattwik food is good for health for Yoga and for the development of that mind, which should be free from violence, free from passion. It is desirable for all human beings to be initiated in the religion of non-killing. It is the crying need that ruthless cruelty of man to lower animals should be stopped one for all.

Cats and dogs do not touch pulse, bread, rice, etc., if they get meat and fish at their heart's content. Similarly human beings should abstain themselves from taking flesh-food if they get vegetarian food at their heart's content. Vegetarian food, like pulse, rice, and bread, etc., rich in [protein] but acidic in a nature, is not the natural food for cats and dogs. Thus, non-vegetarian food like meat, fish, and egg, rich in proteen [sic] but acidic in nature, are not natural food for human beings. In order to save man from the clutches of death at the time of scarcity of vegetarian food, nature has made provision for human stomach to digest certain quantity of flesh food. Now animals are free from the responsibility of mental elevation, but it is quite different with man. His object is to manifest divinity in life to become divine man, not beast man. This is the urge of Nature and in view of extending co-operation in hastening this urge, it is inevitable for human society to discard flesh food, and [the] killing of beasts, birds, and fish for human food should be prohibited. Flesh food makes human beings diseased in body and mind and makes human beings selfish brats.

Emperor Asoke strictly prohibited killing beasts, birds, and even fish for food in his whole [empire] since he realized, in his heart of hearts, the great utility of [Ahimsa] or non-killing of innocent animals for the welfare of all human races. Certainly in this age, man has no dearth of Vegetarian food. Hence, such demonic food saturated with blood is by no means his necessity. The human body is mainly constituted with alkaline blood in our body. Flesh food is not alkaline but acid in nature. Bodies of ferocious animals are made of acid blood, and this acid blood is the main factor in their body. Hence the natural food for tigers, jackels, dogs, and cats, etc., is flesh food. So this food cannot be beneficial for man. This is why men loving flesh food will inevitably have diseased body and their mind shall definitely be selfish and self centered—just like the ferocious animals.

[Two-thirds of the] people of India were Vegetarian, but now [the] number of vegetarians [is] decreasing day by day. In India at present age, Bengalees [*sic*] have been most addicted to flesh food. In consequence, we see health of Bengalis is very poor. Bengal suffers most from political strife, quarrelling, fighting, and killing, and all other anarchism are always prevalent in Bengal. On the other hand, there are natural calamities in Bengal more than other parts of India—famine, tempest, inundation, etc. Sometime ago 15 Laks (100,000) of people were washed away by furious sea in East-Bengal. We request Bengalees to change their habit of flesh food. If the killing of innocent beasts, birds, and fishes increases day by day in India, then the whole of India will be completely lost in the depth of sea by sudden earthquake. There is no place of ruthless cruel beastly men in the divine scheme of the creation.

The food[s] we take are changed into blood, and the blood constitutes our body. [The] Fine essence of blood constitute[s] our mind. From Sattwik food we get necessary alkaline blood. Supremacy of alkaline blood in [the] human body is not only good for health, it is very helpful, very essential to develop pure mind, holy mind and divine mind in men. Allopathic Doctors of our age are doing world of harm to human races prescribing flesh food and concentrated food such as butter, chhana, powdered milk for children even. These Doctors are completely ignorant of the science of food; they are completely ignorant what kind of food nourishes nerves and glands, what kind of food keeps our glandular activity normal and healthy. In non-vegetarian family of India, it was a custom not to allow children flesh food and concentrated food under twelve year of age. There is physiological reason behind this custom. Allopathic Doctors should know it and follow it for the welfare of all human society. To digest flesh food and concentrated food, extra secretion of the liver and other digestive glands is necessary. Immature liver and glands of the children cannot bear the strain of discharging extra secretion for long period, so their digestive glands gradually become weak and inactive. Their health breaks for life, their physical and mental growth hamper, [and] they become selfish and heartless brutes.

India adopted the replica of Asoke-Stambha as the national symbol, but the leaders of the State have neither the courage nor the capacity to enforce the non-violent policy of Asoke. They should boldly promulgate the non-violent policy of Asoke not to kill innocent animals for food in this holy country of holy men. Not only India but all the States of the world are drifting aimlessly like boats without the helmsman. Political leaders do not think, do not know what is the aim of human civilization.[58]

Understanding Brahmacharya

Brahmacharya is a topic that comes up for all serious yogis. As yoga has become so popular in our Western culture, brahmacharya has been defined as "moderation and balance in the pleasures of the senses" or "moderation in all things." This is a good discipline and beneficial to those with families who are on the yogic path. But what does *brahmacharya* actually mean? Historically, it has been translated as "celibacy." So what does *celibacy* mean, and why it is important to yogis?

The definition for *brahmacharya* in the Spoken Sanskrit dictionary is "chastity." In the *Merriam-Webster* dictionary, *chastity*, *celibacy*, and *continence* are considered synonyms. *Chastity* is defined as: (a) abstention from unlawful sexual intercourse; (b) abstention from all sexual intercourse; (c) purity in conduct and intention; and (d) restraint and simplicity in design or expression.

The *Merriam-Webster* definition for *celibacy* includes both (a) abstention from unlawful sexual intercourse, and (b) abstention from all sexual intercourse. And the definition for *continence* is the "abstention from all intercourse" as well as "the ability to retain a bodily discharge."

With these definitions in mind, I think we need to look into some of the research on brahmacharya that was understood back in the 1920s and 1930s. Let's take a look at the yogic journal *Yoga Mimamsa*, volume 3, published in April 1928 by the Kaivalyadhama Institute for Scientific Research, founded by Swami Kuvalayananda. This particular issue discusses, in detail, chastity, celibacy, and healthy sexual glands, and how they relate to the longevity of yogins.

In this journal, *chastity* and *continence* are synonymous, but *chastity* and *celibacy* are by no means considered the same. *Chastity* is considered the abstention from *unlawful* sexual intercourse, whereas *celibacy* is the abstention from *all* intercourse. For a yogin, all three—*chastity, celibacy,* and *continence*—would need to include definitions (c) and (d), above—purity of conduct and intention, and restraint and simplicity in design or expression.

Since brahmacharya is one of the five yamas from Patanjali's *Yoga Sutras,* the question is whether Patanjali is prescribing celibacy (total sexual abstinence) or chastity (abstention from unlawful sexual intercourse). *Yoga Mimamsa* states that "later Yogic tradition stands firmly for celibacy ... [but] ... there seems little doubt that Patanjali allows even chastity to be sufficient enough for Yogic development."[59] Their logic is found in *Yoga Sutras* 2.30–31. These two verses are translated by *Yoga Mimamsa:* "Inoffensiveness, truthfulness, non-stealing, continence, and non-receiving, are the Yamas.... These, when universal, that is, unbroken by time, place, purpose, and caste-rules, are great vows."[60]

The scholars behind *Yoga Mimamsa* explained why they felt these two verses allow for chastity as opposed to celibacy.

> The 30th Sutra simply lays down the five controls. The 31st prescribes the same, but in a stricter form, as it requires them to be practiced at all times and under all climes. Patanjali expressly calls this a stricter form, Mahavratam [a great vow or duty], suggesting thereby that the previous Sutra requires their practice only in a milder form. The stricter form of Brahmacharya is clearly celibacy, as is seen from the conditions of the 31st Sutra. But what is the milder form of Brahmacharya that the previous Sutra allows? It can be nothing else than chastity, as illegitimate intercourse, which is the only alternative, has absolutely no place in real Yoga.
>
> So, it is clear that Patanjali allows a married life to a Yogin, provided the marital bond is faithfully kept up, and provided within that bond strict moderation is observed according to the scriptural injunctions. But it seems that he looks upon such Brahmacharya as the minimum, because he also mentions celibacy (total

sexual abstinence) and calls it the maximum. So when the question, whether Brahmacharya in Yogins leads to longevity is to be scientifically examined, both chastity and celibacy will have to be taken into account.[61]

Scientists of the day (those not involved in yogic research) had found married life, guided by moderation, was the best way of keeping the sexual glands healthy, and healthy sexual glands benefited youthfulness and a long life. Excessive sex and venereal diseases were considered the most dangerous, and these were avoided through chastity and moderation.[62]

These same scientists considered celibacy an unhealthy option. Findings had shown that total abstinence led to premature old age and death and that the accumulation of internal sexual secretions could be toxic to the body. They argued the complete disuse of the sexual glands could lead to their atrophy and to possible nervous disorders, such as hysteria and neurasthenia.[63]

Given that these researchers found good support for the above arguments as to why celibacy was not healthy for the body and mind, how is it that Patanjali recommended celibacy for unmarried yogis? The answer lies in his advice to avoid the accumulation of internal sexual secretions through specific yogic practices that are healthy alternatives to sexual intercourse.

Researchers at Kaivalyadhama have found that effective practices for celibate yogis are *uddiyana, nauli, ashvini mudra, mula bandha,* and *sarvangasana.* The Kaivalyadhama researchers found that these practices promoted the activity of the lymphatic system, resulting in greater absorption of the internal sexual secretions and the building of tissues at large. When the absorbing activity of the lymphatic vessels and the secreting activity of the sexual glands are proportionate, there is no danger of accumulation. This, along with the other physiological benefits of yogic exercises, leads to a healthy and balanced body.[64] Hari told me the reabsorbed fluids transformed into *ojas,* a potent spiritual force that gives us vigor, vitality, and bodily strength.

One further note is made in *Yoga Mimamsa* on the topic of celibacy. The researchers at Kaivalyadhama point out that even without these yogic practices, celibacy would not produce any of the aforementioned negative effects, including the atrophy of these glands, if celibacy is chosen voluntarily and if one is truly celibate in the body, mind, and soul. In this case, there would be no desire. In their opinion, the damage is done by the suppression of the instinctive sexual desires. If there is no desire, every function in the body adjusts, attending to the balance between secretions and absorption. If the secretions are properly utilized, the glands continue their normal functions—it does not make any difference to the glands if the secretions are discharged through sexual relations or absorbed by the lymphatic system, as long as the balance is maintained. Whether celibate or chaste, when one is pure at heart, there is harmony and balance, and this will promote health and longevity.[65]

Hari and Brahmacharya

With the popularity of yoga in the world today, the expectation of restraining from all sexual intercourse hardly seems plausible. If you adopt Swami Kuvalayananda's interpretation of Patanjali's *Yoga Sutras* on brahmacharya, the allowance of chastity bridges yogic development from the ashrams of the East to the studios of the West, provided it is practiced alongside the required ethics and purity of heart.

It was no different for Hari. He completely dedicated his life to yoga and also to his wife, so the topic of brahmacharya came up fairly often in the letters, as he grappled with understanding the expectations of this yama.

Hari held Swami Kuvalayananda in very high esteem, due to the valuable results of his ongoing research published in *Yoga Mimamsa* from the Kaivalyadhama Institute. In a letter sent in September 1930, Swami Kuvalayananda addresses Hari's questions regarding brahmacharya. I do not know if Hari was married at that time.

> Regarding Brahmacharya, two or three ways may be suggested of controlling the awakened passion temporarily.
>
> The man may sit in cold water for about half an hour.
>
> He may immediately get himself in the company of a few friends and spend about an hour there.
>
> May take to some sublime literature that would exalt him to the ethereal region.[66]

In a letter dated November 2, 1933, he goes on to answer further questioning, recommending two techniques for controlling sexual urges, as well as offering the reminder that celibacy must also be practiced in the mind and the heart.

The exercises of Vajroli and Shakti-Chalana are the best for Brahmacharya....

Self-introspection is the best check applied to the mind that proposes wandering or entertaining any impious thoughts. The mind, if kept under observation, will always behave like an obedient pupil.[67]

The two techniques of *vajroli* and *shakti-chalana* are described in chapter 3 of the *Hatha Yoga Pradipika*. Swami Vishnudevananda says, in his commentary of this work, that it is not necessary to practice *vajroli mudra* if one is adept in *mula bandha*, because mula bandha will stop the sexual impulse from rising up in the first place.[68] But for the purpose of understanding vajroli, it is described as the physical contraction that draws water up through the urethra. It is accomplished in the same way that *basti* (a yogic enema) is performed, in which water is drawn up into the colon by the vacuum created from performing uddiyana or *nauli* (a deep exhalation held out while churning the rectus abdominis muscles). In the case of vajroli, one gradually increases the density of the liquid drawn up through the urethra, such as honey instead of water, until able to draw a sexual ejaculation backward.[69]

Shakti-chalana mudra is briefly described by Swami Vishnudevananda as sitting in *siddhasana*, performing *bhastrika pranayama*, and then bouncing the body up and down.[70] This is done to awaken the *kundalini*.

Swami Shivananda Saraswati of Assam described a process of vajroli mudra as used by some Tantrik yogis in a letter to Hari dated April 16, 1959.

How do we overcome passions? Our mind [is] encircled with six passions. These are sensuousness, anger, greed, attachment or ignorance, pride, and envy. These are the forms of our lower mind which are unfavourable to concentration. When we conquer these Shararipu ["six passions," also known as *shat-ripu*], our mind become[s] purified.

We can proceed to construct a building only when the foundation is firmly made; so also, there are some primary stages regarding this process of purifying our mind. The primary steps are the rules to be observed regarding taking diet and bath. The more hot the blood in the veins, the greater is the sex passion. There are the processes to keep this blood cool. All kinds of flesh food (egg, fish, meat, etc.) and concentrated food (butter, cake, cheese, ghee, sweet meats, etc.) make blood hot. Hence an a[s]cetic has to give up all these foods and will have to take plain diet.

Even in the cold countries, bath should be taken twice—once in the morning and once in the noon. Hot water is to be mixed with cold water in such a degree that [water that is] too cold is transformed into tolerably cold water. The temperature of this mixed water is to be [lower] than body temperature by one or two degrees. To take bath in this cold water will help you to keep your blood cool. The process of "pratyahar" should be accompanied with these processes of taking food and bath. Then only [the] mind can come under control and will be purified more and more. As the river flows to the ocean to be lost there, so also the self proceeds toward the self-realization, the self to be lost in itself.

The Hatha yogins have invented a wonderful physical process to rise up to the stage of samadhi for controlling sex-passions and to win over sex impulses. This process is still in vogue in some extinct form amongst a class of Tantriks and the "Sahajia Sampradayas" in this country.

The husband and wife [have] to practice this process at the very starting of the conjugal life. This is known as "[V]ajroli Mudra." This is a special process of sex-union without any discharge. One can easily win over sex-passions if one learns this process well. This passionless union transforms into divine union.

It is superfluous to state that the Jnanins and the Bhaktas of our country despise this process. This process becomes perverted rather for want of proper knowledge. So those who take recourse of this process are generally hated by the common people even. But those who are the real followers of this process, they care little for all these praises and blames, approval or disapproval, by others. As the process is risksome and is not liked by many, it is now going to be totally given up. The number of the followers of this process is now gradually decreasing.

Those who can control their sex-passions or impulses are very few in number. Most of the people are helpless, sufferers of the stings of sex-passions. He is really to be praised who could devise [a] physical process to win over the stings of sex-impulse. The fundamental point of all spiritualism is this—the control of passions and impulses, and control over mind. Unless you can do this much, no help is there. If this is the state, what harm is there if man can rise up to the purified state through this process of physical enjoyment, instead of going through the difficult process of self-strain and controlling mind. It seems that this "Bajroli Mudra" of Hatha Yoga is a challenge to all sorts of spiritualism.

We are the seekers of truth through Jnanapath [the path of knowledge], so we generally hate this physical process. Even the thought of this physical union seems to us to be vulgar. Still if we are to judge it unbiasedly, it can be said that as we have simplified the different difficult yogic processes and have made it easier for the common people, so also … [with] "Bajroli Mudra" … by simplifying and modifying it, I think it will be of great help to many pairs of the future.[71]

In September 1931, T. K. Sundaresa Iyer, a disciple of Ramana Maharshi based in Tiruvannamalai, wrote an extensive letter on brahmacharya to Hari. I remember well when Hari shared this letter with me as we discussed the yamas. I am led to believe that Hari was married at the time this letter was written to him, based on the letter's last bit of advice, which seems to include an allowance for chastity—the "minimum" amount of celibacy required for one to succeed both in yoga and in marriage.

Brahmacharya is, in its most perfect aspect, that state of one's being where enjoyment wells up from within and is not hankered after things around. In fact Absolute Consciousness is the real Brahmacharya, and what Brahmacharya is ordained as continence or celibacy is but a means toward the same. In its wider aspects, it is not merely abstinence from sexual intercourse, but [abstaining] from every activity of the senses that tend to draw us away from our living deep into the Self. Thus is seen the need for the selection of what words spoken, what tidings heard, what things felt by the physical body, what food or drink taken in, etc., may or may not tend to detract us from our effort to be our real selves. Viewed from this aspect, our own better halves, if they tend to create in us, a drawing out of our craving for sexual intercourse, are considered a drag on our progress. But knowing as we do, that women folk are but as much a manifestation of God as we are, if we but realize that it is not their fair skin or countenance that is their beauty, but the quality of their divine being, in essence, the same as the Self in us, then gradually the craving for the pleasures of the meeting of the flesh disappeared. In fact, this attitude of the mind ought to be developed in all its intensity.

But when in the initial stage, it is necessary to bear in mind that, in this respect, one must avoid the women folk when in an excited mood, in a heated or weak or exhausted condition of the body. For such are the moments when one is easily carried away.

Further, the moment the craving [creeps] up, if we but try to steady and go down a bit into our selves, the longing flies away quickly. Where this is impossible, an outward extension of ourselves, of course, by imagination, into a feeling of vast pleasure in divine nature would also have the same effect. Where even this fails, prayer intense and devout to God whom we adore, or to Guru, our divine Master, God's embodiment on earth, is sure to keep us on the path.

Above all, it is very necessary that the consciousness of our divinity should be so developed as to make us realize, every moment, that we are not the body, but the Supreme, one indivisible Being.

"I and my father are one" will help us much in this respect.

It is further important to bear in mind that all the qualities of a divine nature that go to make a perfect man are not obtained by trying to develop each quality one by one. It should then take ages for us to perfect ourselves. The God in us is the repository of all that is good and beautiful and only when we have lost or can [lose] our identity in Him do we begin to reflect outwardly the inner perfection. So the effort must be more [toward] the realisation of the All Beautiful in us, that we might lose the craving for the beauties and pleasure that are but transitory.

One thing more. A Sadhaka who is a householder, tho' himself beyond such cravings and temptations, has to break his rule occasionally out of concern for things beyond his control—perhaps his better half is not as well equipped as himself for the quest of the Higher. In such a case, occasional lapses, not more than one course a month, never harms the [Sadhaka] in his meditation. But even while in the act, he must not forget his real nature. It is hoped that these few lines will be of some help in solving your difficulties.[72]

In a letter sent to Hari in June 1946, it is clear that Paramhansa Yogananda views brahmacharya in the strictest sense of the word, regardless of marriage. "With regard to being married, marriage is no drawback so long as the husband and wife have one common goal—the pursuit of God and Self-realization."[73]

He added at the end of his letter a very personal postscript in his own handwriting.

> P.S. Many times, whenever I concentrated on you, I felt you had a mate. So it is not a surprise. If your wife is self-sacrificing and harmonious, it would be rather wonderful for both of you to go to India and settle at Ranchi after receiving the necessary adequate instructions here.
>
> Please let me know how soon you can come to America. If you and your wife both want to live like the ancient Rishis and their consorts—developing God's work of Self-Realization together [rather] than alone, you will find all things working nicely for you. It is better to live above the sex-pleasure even if you are married, like Gandhi has been after he took the vow of celibacy.[74]

On December 6, 1946, Yogananda continued:

> Most of the disciples are required to take the vow of celibacy, and while we have accepted married couples, it is emphasized that they live more on the plane of celibacy. If you and your wife are willing to abide by this rule, then I may seriously consider assuming the responsibility of bringing you both to this country.[75]

I have no doubt that Hari was fully celibate when I studied with him, and he was quite capable of a celibate life long before that. However, Hari would have needed to also consider the wishes of his wife, Isabella. Was this, along with the passing of Paramhansa Yogananda and Hari's desire to study many paths of yoga, the reason for his decision to not become a minister of the Self-Realization Fellowship?

Chapter Three

ASANA

DURING THE TIME I KNEW HARI, he wasn't much interested in teaching a lot of asana, so this is not the focus of this book. Once a week, a couple of students would join us, and he would lead us in an informative class, but his interests had long before shifted to other yoga pathways, such as laya yoga and kriya yoga. By this time, his focus was raja yoga. Hari said, "hatha yoga leads us to raja yoga." His guidance helped me not to feel guilty when I wasn't doing asana every day, but to appreciate the fact that I was drawn from the outer limbs toward the inner limbs of yoga.

Hari was very adept in asana and taught yoga on the beach in Latvia before the Second World War. He also taught yoga in Brooklyn, New York, once he settled there. Swami Sivananda's book *Practical Lessons in Yoga* was first published in 1938 and dedicated to students of yoga in the East and the West. The way he cites Hari as an example in this book shows that he already viewed him as an adept at yoga.

It is wrong to suppose that Yoga-Asanas are purely meant for the Indians and that they are ideally suited to Indian conditions. That it is not the case is proved by the following few instances.

Mr. Harry Dikman, the Director-Founder of the Yoga Centre in Riga, Latvia (Europe) is a good specialist in these Yoga-Asanas, Bandhas and Mudras and his opinion and advice to persons suffering from various kinds of diseases, curable and incurable, are increasingly becoming popular in Europe. I have not heard of another man either in Europe or in America, who takes such a keen and lively interest in this subject and is making researches in the same. You will be surprised to know that Mr. Harry Dikman is essentially a philosopher and a sage.[76]

Asana on the Beach in Latvia

In his book *Hatha Yoga (Illustrated)*, published in 1939, Swami Sivananda inserted many photos of Hari demonstrating various asanas and techniques on the beach in Latvia, including *sirsasana, urdvha padmasana, sarvangasana, vajrasaa, lolasana, padmasana,* and *uttida padmasana*. These photos show Hari's skill in these techniques.[77]

ILLUSTRATIONS

No.	Page No.	Exercises	Demonstrated by Yoga Experts
1	4	Sirshasan	
3	10	Oordhva Padmasan	
5	13	Sarvangasan	
23	46	Vajrasan	
29	63	Lolasan	Sri Harri Dikman, President,
32	79	Padmasan	The Divine Life Society,
33	81	Uttida Padmasan	Latvia, Riga, Europe.
42	137	Uddiyana Bandha	
46	158	Nauli Kriya	
47	160	,,	

Figure 3.1. List of asanas demonstrated by Hari, *Hatha Yoga (Illustrated)*, by Swami Sivananda, 1939, Divine Life Society, page xxxix.

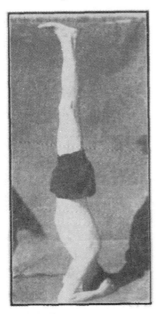

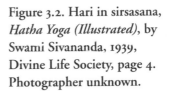

Figure 3.2. Hari in sirsasana, *Hatha Yoga (Illustrated)*, by Swami Sivananda, 1939, Divine Life Society, page 4. Photographer unknown.

ſ: SIRSHASAN (SIDE VIEW)

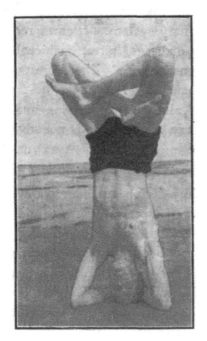

Figure 3.3. Hari in urdhva padmasana, *Hatha Yoga (Illustrated)*, by Swami Sivananda, 1939, Divine Life Society, page 10. Photographer unknown.

8. OORDHVA PADMASAN

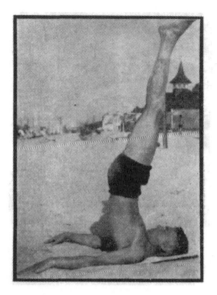

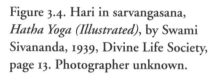

Figure 3.4. Hari in sarvangasana, *Hatha Yoga (Illustrated)*, by Swami Sivananda, 1939, Divine Life Society, page 13. Photographer unknown.

5.   SARVANGASAN

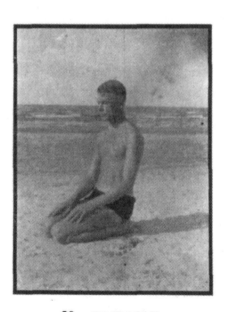

Figure 3.5. Hari in vajrasana, *Hatha Yoga (Illustrated)*, by Swami Sivananda, 1939, Divine Life Society, page 46. Photographer unknown.

23.   VAJRASAN

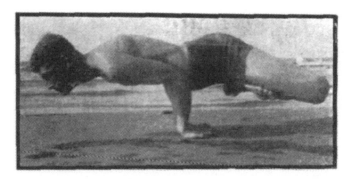

29. LOLASAN

Figure 3.6. Hari in lolasana, *Hatha Yoga (Illustrated)*, by Swami Sivananda, 1939, Divine Life Society, page 63. Photographer unknown.

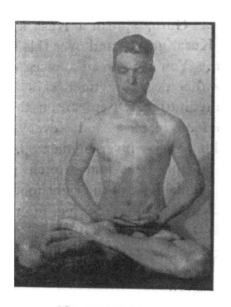

32. PADMASAN.

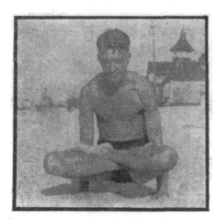

33. UTTIDA PADMASAN

Figure 3.7. Left: Hari in padmansana, *Hatha Yoga (Illustrated)*, by Swami Sivananda, 1939, Divine Life Society, page 79. Photographer unknown.

Figure 3.8. Right: Hari in uttida padmansana, *Hatha Yoga (Illustrated)*, by Swami Sivananda, 1939, Divine Life Society, page 81. Photographer unknown.

Chandra Namaskar

I would like to share a unique Chandra Namaskar that Hari taught me. I do not know where he learned it, so I call it Hari's moon salutation.

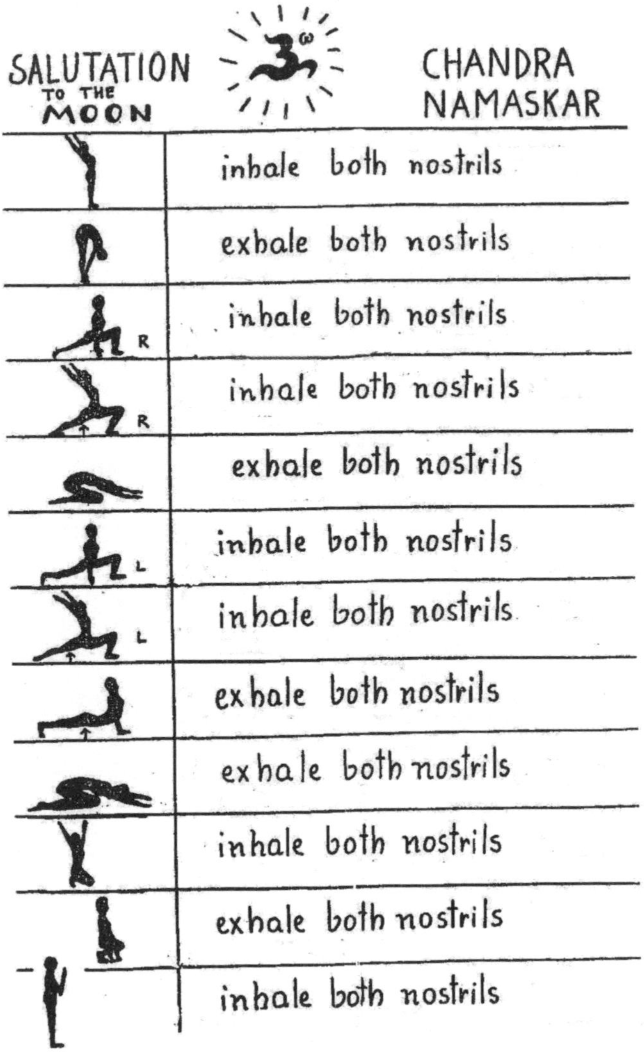

SALUTATION TO THE MOON	CHANDRA NAMASKAR
	inhale both nostrils
	exhale both nostrils
	inhale both nostrils
	inhale both nostrils
	exhale both nostrils
	inhale both nostrils
	inhale both nostrils
	exhale both nostrils
	exhale both nostrils
	inhale both nostrils
	exhale both nostrils
	inhale both nostrils

Figure 3.9. Chandra Namaskar handout Hari gave to the author. Source unknown.

His instructions for the process were:[78]

1. standing upright, inhale and arch back
2. exhale and bend forward
3. inhale and take the left leg back, exhale the left knee on floor
4. raise the left knee and point the left foot sideways to the West—inhale, raise the arms, and arch back
5. exhale and bring the right leg back, folding into child's pose with chin to the floor and arms stretched forward (I put my forehead on the floor to stimulate the third eye)
6. inhale and bring the left leg forward, exhale right knee to the floor
7. raise the right knee and point the right foot sideways to the East—inhale and raise the arms and arch back
8. exhale and take the left leg back, settling into a raised cobra, with only toes and hands on the floor—inhale and open the chest
9. exhale and return to child's pose with the toes tucked under
10. inhale upright onto knees, raise the arms and arch back
11. exhale and lift the knees into a squat on the toes, hands by your sides, and
12. inhale and raise up to standing with hands in prayer position.

Other than our weekly class in asana, our focus was on the other limbs of yoga, as described in the following chapters.

Chapter Four

PRANAYAMA

PRANAYAMA WAS HARI'S PASSION, and he was determined to teach me what he believed to be the correct way to breathe for yoga.[79] There are many ways to breathe, and even more opinions about which is the right way. The two basic practices that I regard as important in pranayama are exhaling from the lower lungs first and having a slight firmness below the navel during yogic breathing.

Exhale from the Lower Lungs

Dirga breath, or *mahat yoga pranayama* (great yogic breathing) is full yogic breathing, also known as the "three-part breath." A yogi utilizes as much of the lungs as possible, including the lower, middle, and upper areas of the lungs. These create the "three parts." For as long as I can remember, I was instructed to practice full yogic breathing by first inhaling into the lower lungs (upper abdominal region), then into the middle lungs (intercostal), and lastly into the upper lungs (clavicular). Exhalation began by drawing the abdomen inward to initiate the exhalation from the lower lungs, then the middle lungs, and lastly emptying the upper lungs. I learned this from Hari, as he was the first to instruct me in pranayama.

I was often asked by my students why I breathed in this fashion, when it seemed more logical to exhale from the upper lungs down to the lower lungs—much as a glass of water fills from the bottom to the top and then empties from the top to the bottom. I did not have an answer for a long time; I did it that way because I was taught that way, and it felt wonderful.

In 2010, Zena Ursuliak, a yoga teacher in Edmonton and a good friend of mine, came to Mexico to take a training I was leading. As a disciple of Swami Gitananda, she had a solid background in pranayama. When this question came up, she offered an excellent answer, which I paraphrase here: when we are talking about pranayama, we are talking about prana, the life force. During pranayama, we are directing this life force to specific areas. When we breathe in the manner described above, each area "holds" the prana for an equal length of time. The result is an even distribution of the prana.

Think of breathing in for a count of three: "one" for the *manipura chakra*, or solar plexus chakra, at the lower lungs; "two" for the *anahata chakra*, or heart chakra, at the middle lungs; and "three" for the *vishuddhi chakra*, or throat chakra, at the upper lungs. Then we exhale in the same fashion— "one" for the manipura chakra, "two" for the anahata chakra, and "three" for the vishuddhi chakra. With this approach, each of these energy centers receives the prana equally.

If you exhale from the top to the bottom, this is no longer true. The throat chakra holds the prana for the least amount of time, because it is the last to receive and the first to release the breath. This is our center of sweet, melodious voice, mantra, and expression of love, as directed by what lies in the heart.

The heart chakra holds the prana a little longer, as it is the second area to release the prana. Here is where the soul is said to reside, and our spiritual journey, as described in the Upanishads, is to get to know who dwells within this space.

Lastly, the manipura chakra, our power center, where our ego-personality resides, holds the prana the longest. Giving more prana to the ego-center may result in an imbalance of personal power. Our goal is to move into the spiritual world, where we know all material things are impermanent and are the cause of our pain and suffering.

So, when exhaling from the top to the bottom, the two higher, spiritual chakras absorb the life force for the least amount of time, and the center of ego and power gets the lion's share. There is already an imbalance of power in our world, and we do not need to feed that. More than anything, we need to align our personalities with our souls, so much so that our behavior reflects the spirit of love and compassion for all beings. Furthermore, psychic powers manifest as siddhis, and if they are not balanced by the compassion of the heart and the confidence to express that compassion, the siddhis are used for personal power. The siddhis are meant to be indicators of success in one's spiritual practice, nothing more, but the battle with the ego shows that it wants to claim them as its own.

Finally, according to Phil Liney from ICYER of Swami Gitananda lineage, it is not physically possible to exhale from the top of the lungs to the bottom—the diaphragm initiates both inhalation and exhalation, and therefore, even if we think we are exhaling from the top to the bottom, we are not. Mr. Liney suggests checking this out for yourself: take a breath in and then prepare to exhale from the top first. "Try contracting only your upper chest—you can't, the diaphragm will also be moving up. Now try contracting only your lower chest—you can, and for complete control, you should, then continue on to the middle chest then the upper chest."[80]

Controlled Lower Abdomen

Hari learned from Swami Kuvalayananda that in order to acquire the most oxygen value from your breathing, you must have a controlled abdomen. It may seem that a relaxed, protracted abdomen during inhalation would permit the diaphragm to descend lower and result in a greater expansion of the rib cage and intake of oxygen. However, after numerous experiments measuring pressure changes in pranayama, Swami Kuvalayananda and his fellow scientists at Kaivalyadhama Ashram found that "one is able to inhale larger quantities of oxygen when the abdomen is kept controlled than when the abdomen is kept protracted."[81] They found that although the diaphragm descends lower with the protracted abdomen, the ribs also become depressed, thus limiting the advantage gained by the lower descent of the diaphragm.

The scientists at Kaivalyadhama Ashram recommended this controlled abdomen in all pranayamas except ones like *kapalabhati* and *bhastrika,* in which the abdominal muscles are required for the quick, successive exhalations.[82] Therefore, I find it important to spend some time explaining how breathing with a controlled abdomen was taught to me.

First, let's explore the movement of the ribs with a relaxed, protracted abdomen. Sit comfortably with an erect spine, as in a seated *tadasana,* to allow for the most effective freedom of movement in the lungs, ribcage, and diaphragm. Relax the lower abdomen. Breathe in fully, filling first the lower lungs, middle lungs, then upper lungs. Exhale deeply by drawing in the abdomen to initiate the exhalation from the lower lungs, then the middle, and lastly the upper lungs. Repeat this several times, feeling the movement of the ribcage. Notice the movement of the perineum, or pelvic floor, during inhalation. There is a downward pressure or energy as the abdomen protracts during the inhalation.

Now try breathing with the lower abdomen slightly contracted. From your chosen seated position, lean forward and snuggle into your sitz bones (ischial tuberosity). Sit up and lean back onto them until you feel the lower abdominal muscles contact slightly to support you. This is a gentle mula bandha, and you can feel an upward pull on the pelvic floor. Observe your natural flow of breath for a moment as you become accustomed to this contraction. As you watch your breathing, notice that the expansion from the breath is above the navel now. Be sure to continue to lean back slightly onto your sitz bones—if you relax forward, you will lose the firmness below the navel.

Leaning back on the sitz bones is a technique I learned from Erich Schiffmann. It helps you to sit tall and straight, which is important for pranayama and meditation, but it also adds the slight support in the lower abdomen. Now, place one hand over the lower abdomen and gently contract the lower front abdominal muscles below the navel. Observe your natural flow of breath for a moment as you become accustomed to this contraction. As you watch your breathing, keep this area stable, with little or no movement, so the expansion from the breath is above the navel.

Once you are comfortable observing this breath, breathe in fully, without moving the lower abdomen, filling first the lower lungs above the navel, then the middle lungs, and lastly the upper lungs. Now exhale deeply by first drawing in the abdomen to initiate the exhalation from the lower lungs, then the middle and finally the upper lungs. Repeat this several times, being aware of the expansion above the navel. Feel the movement of the ribcage. See if you notice the greater expansion of the ribcage in this second technique. Notice that the movement of the perineum during inhalation is now an upward energy with this gentle mula bandha. I find that the body feels lighter with this mula bandha stabilizing the lower abdomen and the upward movement of the perineum, even during breath retention using the *bandhas* (locks).

Swami Kuvalayananda said that it was the "Western physical culturists" who recommend the abdominal muscles to be relaxed, allowing the abdomen to protract, whereas yogic technique requires these muscles to be controlled.[83] B. K. S. Iyengar, for example, in his book *Light on Yoga,* suggests that we "fill the lungs up to the brim." And Iyengar explains that "care should be taken not to bloat the abdomen in the process of inhalation. (Observe this in all the types of Pranayama.)"[84] I interpret this to support Swami Kuvalayananda's opinion.

Swami Sivananda of Rishikesh explained in a letter how this gentle firmness in the lower abdomen effects the kundalini.

> The technique of kumbhak [breath retention] in Sukh Purvak and Ujjayi is not difficult to understand if you bear [this] in mind: Special details of this process depends upon whether the Pranayam is done merely as a routine exercise for maintaining general health and vitality or whether it is done as a serious item of Kundalini Yoga to awaken the Kundalini. In the latter case it becomes a distinct Kriya of Hatha Yoga and it is in this aspect that the authorities you mention, have referred to it. Both Swami Suddhananda and Kuvalayananda and Yogendra are correct in their instruction. They have given the same instruction in different language.
>
> Kuvalayananda's "the abdominal muscles must be controlled or compressed during the process" automatically results in "the prana being pressed down so that it strikes the Muladhara" (as said by Swami Suddhananda).
>
> The same process is said by me, as "Send the current down to the Muladhara Chakra. Feel that the nerve-current is striking against the Muladhara Chakra and awakening the Kundalini." ... In actual practice, you will find that compression of the abdominal muscles itself forces the prana downward.[85]

As teachings are passed down to others over time, this finer detail may have been lost through many interpretations. Hari wished more yoga teachers were exposed to this practice of controlling the lower abdominal muscles in pranayama, particularly as students advance on their yogic path into the deeper practices of pranayama.

The word *pranayama* means "control the prana," the life force. There are many, many precautions given about practicing pranayama without the guidance of a guru or adept teacher. There is good reason for this.

To yogis, the physical body is known as the *sthula sharira.* Without the life force, it is merely molecules of matter put together, and it has no movement. It is a corpse. The astral body is called the *sukshma sharira*. This is the pranic body, the energetic body. This is an exact replica of the physical body and brings life to the physical body through the *pancha prana vayus*, or five forms of prana. All movement comes from prana. Prana moves through the seventy-two thousand astral nerves, or *nadis,* which are the nervous system in the physical body.

Breathing is generally an involuntary action under the control of the autonomic nervous system. The vagus nerve originates in the brain stem and, from there, sends fibers throughout the upper body, most significantly to the heart and lungs. The afferent nerves begin inhalation, and the efferent nerves begin exhalation, and the process of breathing continues automatically without us ever thinking about it.

It is a well-known fact to yogis that if we want to control the mind, we must control the breath. When we control the breath, we control the mind, and when the mind slows down to stillness, the prana can move into the central nadi, the *sushumna,* and the journey of Self-realization begins. Swami Sevananda of the Yogoda Sat-Sanga had a beautiful explanation why this is so.

> The Rishis have left the yoga practices purposely uncodified, for one not going through the first drills of continence, honesty, truthfulness, and other kindred virtues would ruin himself if he would practice the art himself. Further ... guidance at each step is necessary by a superior and master mind. So the knowledge of the yoga path is to be gained from one's own master and not through books. Still, I am going to give you some idea about the system.
>
> In the vedas, it is told that the first manifestation of Brahma, the unchangeable, is Prana (of which the Prana flowing through the nostrils is but a gross expression). Out of it originated Budhi [the discriminating aspect of the mind] and mind. So the different schools of Self realisation have taken hold of their stand on either the mind, Budhi, or Prana for reaching their goal to Brahma.
>
> The yogis concentrate all their attention to the control of the grossest Prana, or our breath, for it, they say, would reach us to its unpulsing side, the fixed Prana, which is no other than our real Self. Others try to control the mind or the Budhi, but the yogis think it is a very difficult course, if not unpracticable. Their reason is that samskaras [patterns of behavior] or seeds of our

Basana, or longing for pleasure, possession, etc., are embedded in the Prana. So as soon as we drive out one desire, another desire takes hold of the mind, and we are dragged to do an act that in our saner moments we would not dream of committing. So the best way, according to the yogis, is to control the breath, the master of mind, and as soon as it leaves the ordinary channel, the coming and going through the nostrils, and enters the sushumna passage and goes up and settles in Ajna Chakra, the mind evaporates, as it were, and the yogi enjoys the bliss of the first state of Self realization.[86]

A letter from Swami Vishnu Tirth supported this connection between the mind and prana.

The exercises of Pratyahar, Dharana, Dhyana, and Samadhi, including Pranayama, are all mental. Pranayam, as is generally understood, has nothing to do with breathing. Prana is not breath. Inhaled air cannot rise into the brain. Prana is that subtle force which controls breath and the whole system. And its currents can be directed simply mentally. When mind is concentrated on any plexus, say, Ajna Chakra, Prana will also follow. When the whole Prana from every part of the body becomes concentrated, i.e., [at the] Sahasrar, Nirbij Samadhi will ensue. The case of British Major Yeats Brown[87] cited by you is true, and serves as an illustration. Mind and Prana are closely interconnected mutually;... partial or complete control of either controls the other also to that extent.

Gita chapter 8 verses 11 and 12 require a yogi to concentrate his Prana and mind at the mid-brow (Ajna chakra) or in the Heart at the time of his death, [which alludes] to [a] similar practice.[88]

Hari would often say to me, "Where the mind goes, prana follows." This is the key to succeeding in our dharma, our life's purpose. When we focus our mind on any task, our energy, our life force, is directed to complete it. If our mind gets distracted, our energy dissipates into the distractions and is weakened. One yogi said this very well with regard to Hari's attempt to fit his yoga sadhana into his life of work and family—something many of us find a challenge.

As for what you write about your duties, etc., you take a common-sense view. We have nothing to say on that point. Where there is a will, there is a way. We can, if we are determined, make time for doing what we really love and wish to do. Our other pursuits are thereby automatically regulated.[89]

When we control our breathing, such as by extending the time it takes for our inhalations and exhalations or by holding the breath for any length of time, we affect the vagus nerve, and we are therefore affecting our nervous system and the heart, lungs, and brain. Physically, our pranayama will bring under control the impulses of the autonomic nervous system. Then the prana, the life force, is also controlled.

A small book Hari owned, *The Mysterious Kundalini*, was written by Vasant G. Rele to scientifically explain the kundalini energy as described in the tantra yoga text *The Serpent Power*, by Sir John Woodroofe. Hari studied both of these books extensively and encouraged me to as well. A passage from *The Mysterious Kundalini* supports the importance of pranayama and the regulation of breath in order for any serious yogi to achieve control over the body and to acquire siddhis, the yogic powers. Of course, these powers are not the goal of pranayama, but are a direct result of a successful practice.

We know that the respiratory act is under the control of the Vagus nerve, which has two sets of fibres, afferent and efferent; stimulation of the first stops expiration and produces inspiration; and stimulation of the second does the reverse. These fibres are excited to action by the alternate collapse and distension of the air vesicles of the lungs where the Vagus terminations are situated. Pranayama, then, is in effect a process of bringing under control the Vagus nerve, over which, normally, we have no control. One can understand the importance of this control when one knows that all the vital forces are more or less under the control of the Vagus nerve and its centre: and when this is achieved by Yoga, there is said to be nothing in nature that cannot be brought under the control of the performer and all the forces of nature will obey him as his slaves. When the ignorant see these powers of the Yogi, they call these miracles....

When a complete mastery over this rhythm and full expansion of the lungs is obtained, Prana, or energy, may be willed into any particular part of the body. The training of the will by Pranayama gives exercise to the mind, so that, in course of time, it acquires a capacity to respond to the higher vibrations and becomes what may be called super-conscious; such is the object of Pranayama in the science and philosophy of Yoga.[90]

Anyone who delves into the practice of pranayama without the proper prerequisites is asking for trouble. We absolutely must have a sincere effort to follow the yamas and niyamas, the yogic abstentions and observances that set the mind and thinking in a positive state. These ensure cleanliness of the body, through kriyas, for optimal health and a firm grounding in the spiritual studies of the Self. We must be stable in our asanas, so we are not disturbed by aches and pains during pranayama and meditation. We must be free from nervous disorders, heart disease, and lung disease. It is a package deal, and if you try to bypass the prerequisites, be prepared to experience negative effects.

It is no different than learning how to swim. First you must feel comfortable holding your breath under water, then opening your eyes under water. Then you must learn how to tread water in the shallows to prepare the muscles to support you. If you bypass any of the necessary steps, you can drown. So please, do not practice pranayama unwisely and without proper guidance.

This is not to say one should not practice proper breathing techniques from the beginning. Learning to use the full capacity of the lower, middle, and upper parts of our lungs is of great benefit to us all. Cleansing the nadis with *anuloma viloma,* alternate nostril breathing, is also an important practice that prepares one for advanced pranayama techniques. The *kapalabhati kriya* is important for cleaning the respiratory tract and helpful to do before asana and anuloma viloma. Keep in mind that all yoga practices should be comfortable to do with effort. Notice where your "edges of resistance" begin to appear, and then gradually increase your effort. Stay within a safe playing field and be content with steady but gradual progress.

It is through success in pranayama that a yogi may acquire the siddhis, supernatural powers. Although acquiring siddhis is clearly not the goal of yoga, they are important indicators that we are on the right path and doing things correctly toward success in yoga. Some of the following pranayama techniques will demonstrate this amazing control over prana.

Sri Swami Yogeshwaranand Saraswati from the Yoga Niketan Swargashram was a great resource on pranayama for Hari; he was a master of pranayama. He was considered a guru of the saints. Saints who spent many,

many years meditating in the Himalayas would go to the "Maharaj ji" to attain the ultimate experience of realisation of one's soul and God through his power.[91]

There are letters from this great yoga master to Hari from between 1963 and 1967, and there is good reason to believe that he wrote Hari even before then. One undated, handwritten letter is thirty pages long and covers fifty pranayama techniques.[92] It must have been written before February 1963, because on February 2, 1963, Swami Yogeshwaranand wrote to Hari with answers to questions inspired by those fifty pranayamas. He suggested Hari select a few of the pranayamas that were useful to him and persevere with those.[93]

I am so touched by the amount of time he took to share this information with Hari. He later compiled a book, titled *First Steps to Higher Yoga,* including these pranayamas, plus twenty more. It is very thorough and an excellent resource. The book extensively covers the first five limbs of yoga: yama, niyama, asana, pranayama, and mudra and pratyahara.[94]

I have drawn on many of the pranayamas in this thirty-page letter as a base for discussion. Certain pages throughout the letter have postscript notes on them, written in another language, almost like little secret instructions for Hari only, since he could read several languages.

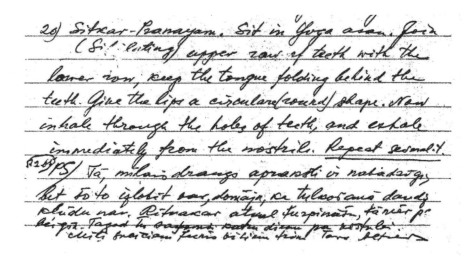

Figure 4.1. Letter from Swami Yogeshwaranand Saraswati showing comments in a language other than English. Date unknown.

Swami Yogeshwaranand begins with some important overall instructions, including his interpretation of Patanjali's *Yoga Sutras* 2.49–50 on regulating the control of prana, or breath: "Sutra: Regulating of breath in relation to desh (place), kāl (time) and saṅkhyā (number) into dirgh (long) and sukshm (subtle) by practicing bahya or rechak (outward), ābhyāntar or Purak (inward) and stambh or kumbhak (stopping) controls."[95]

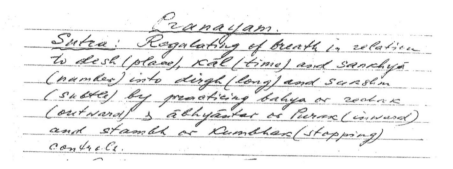

Figure 4.2. Letter from Swami Yogeshwaranand Saraswati describing over fifty pranayama techniques. Date unknown.

Desh, "place," refers to where you focus your attention during pranayama. Swami Yogeshwaranand calls this *desh paridrishti,* "considering the place of inner focus during pranayama." Examples would be exhaling up to the *nasika* (nose), inhaling down to the *muladhara* (root of the spine), and holding the breath at the *nabhi* (navel).

Kāl, "time," refers to counting the seconds or minutes during the process of inhalation and exhalation. Swami Yogeshwaranand calls this *kāl paridrishti,* "considering the ratio of time during pranayama." A common standard is a ratio of 1:4:2. For example, you inhale for 4 seconds, hold the breath for 16 seconds, and exhale for 8 seconds. Whatever number you choose for inhalation, the breath retention is held four times as long, and the exhalation is twice as long.

Saṅkhyā is the number of pranayama you practice, for example, you may practice twenty rounds of a particular technique at one sitting. Swami Yogeshwaranand calls this *saṅkhyā paridrishti,* "considering the number of rounds you practice pranayama." The purpose is to make your inhalations and exhalations longer and longer, gradually reducing several breaths into one.

Every man inhales about eight times and exhales about eight times every minute. One should reduce these 16 outward and inward breaths gradually into 4 then to 2, finally reducing into single breath. The release of breath should be such that the person close to him may not listen [to] the noise.[96]

To clarify, you regulate the flow of prana by gradually lengthening the inhalation *(puraka)* and exhalation *(rechaka)*. Each second equals one count. For example, inhale for a count of 15 (or 15 seconds), and then exhale for a count of 15. You gain control over the breath with the ability to stop it at any place during the length of time it takes for inhalation or exhalation. The breath is subtle when its movement is so gradual that no one near can hear the breath. Eventually your inhalation and exhalation are so long you may only take one inhalation per minute, or even less. Adept yogis are able to stop the breath completely for extended periods of time.

Swami Yogeshwaranand sent Hari five techniques for controlling the inward flow, outward flow, and stopping of the breath. It is important to note that visualization is key to understanding the "place" where the breath is. This *desh paridrishti* is to "look from the point of view" or the place where you focus your attention.[97] I have taken the liberty of adding a few words to clarify the instructions. Note: *vritti,* or *writti,* as he spells it, refers to the movement of the breath.

1. Bahya writti (outward movement of the breath): To reduce several natural exhaling breaths into one per minute.
2. Abhyāntar writti (inward movement of the breath): To reduce several inhaling breaths into one per minute.
3. Kumbhak writti (stopping the breath): To stop the breath wherever it is at any given moment, whether during inhalation or exhalation.
4. Bahyāntar (outward and inward): To regulate pranayama according to desh (place), kāl (time), and saṅkhyā (number) into outward and inward breath retention, or kumbhak.
5. Bahyāntarakshepi (outward, inward, stopping, and breathing): Take in a full breath. Begin to exhale the breath, and while it is in between the muladhar (root of spine) and the nabhi (navel), stop and hold the breath there until you begin feeling

restlessness. Then continue to exhale the air until it is between the nabhi (navel) and kanth (throat) and hold the breath outside, [as] long as you can. Now inhale in such a way that [it] first fills the place between muladhar and nabhi, and stop it here until you feel restlessness. Continue inhaling to fill the portion between the nabhi and hridaya (heart) and then stop it here. Finally fill the portion between hridaya and kanth (throat) and stop or hold the breath inside so long as you can.[98]

This process of visualization during pranayama is critical when we consider again that where the mind goes, the prana follows—the mind and the breath are interconnected, just as breath and prana are. If the mind wanders, the prana dissipates. Like a strong river splitting into several streams, the force or power behind the water is gone. If we focus the mind, we begin to directly focus and build the flow of prana.

During inhalation, visualize the prana flowing into the body via vishuddhi at the throat, down through the heart and the navel to the muladhara. The ajna and sahasrara chakras are above vishuddhi, so they are not part of the passageway for inhalation.[99] You can actually feel the passageway if you allow your mind to engage in the visualization. "The way in which rechak [and the] outward length of breath increases, is the same as in the process of purak—by inhaling, the [length of] breath will touch hridaya, nabhi, muladhar and finally pada tal (foot). This is dirgh-sukshm purak."[100]

Dirgh and *sukshm* (long and subtle) implies that you should extend your inhalations and exhalations as long as you comfortably can while keeping the breath barely perceptible. There is a tendency when we lengthen our inhalations, exhalations, and breath retentions to gasp and grab for the breath. There is no benefit in yoga to gasp desperately for air or to release the breath with a puff of force.

Swami Yogeshwaranand offers this instruction on how to practice making the flow of breath long and subtle.[101] Hang a piece of cotton gauze about a foot in front of your face. As you slowly exhale, try not to vibrate the gauze. If it does not move, then hang the gauze a little closer. Keep lengthening your exhalations as long as is comfortable, without moving the gauze. Do the same with your inhalations.

He calls this *sukshm shwas pranayama*. The *sukshma sharira* is the subtle or astral body. *Shwasa* is the breath. This pranayama helps us get our breath more and more subtle, so we do not disturb the external air as we breathe. Prana rides on the breath, so this technique is to help us get complete control of the breath and therefore control of the prana. I mentioned earlier that we aim to have control such that we need take only one complete breath per minute, or even just one inhalation per minute. With this control, *kevela kumbhaka* (an unintended breath retention) as well as deep meditation come more easily.

> Sukshm—Shwas—Pranayam (subtle inhaling-exhaling). Sit erect in Sukhasana. Sitting on the chair, put some cotton at about a foot away from nose. Now while inhaling, observe whether the cotton vibrates (this should be practiced in a place where is no fast air). While inhaling the length to which cotton vibrates, keep that length as a measure for inhaling 5 or 7 days. Do not inhale with more force than this. Now move the cotton 2 inches nearer and inhale in a way that the cotton may vibrate in the same manner, not more than that. Practice this as much that if the cotton placed just before the nose even then it may not vibrate.[102]

Hari taught me another method of controlling the breath and making it subtle. Place a lit candle at eye level. Use the ratio of 1:4:2 for your inhalation, retention, and exhalation. As you breathe in, do not cause the candle flame to flicker. Hold the breath, and do not disturb the flame as you transition into exhalation and throughout the entire flow of exhalation. Do not disturb the flame as you transition back into inhalation. The breath is silent and barely perceptible, measured by the stillness of the candle flame.

Kumbhak Pranayama with Bhavana

Bhavana means "concentrated thought," or a mental attitude related to love toward God. It is used to develop loving kindness, the connection between the mind and the heart. This technique, from Swami Shivananda Saraswati of Assam, known as *kumbhak pranayama with bhavana,* helps one to develop loving kindness by focusing the mind on the gods of the holy Hindu trinity. Pranayama can sometimes cause one to feel anxiousness. When I practice this technique with a concentrated mind, I feel loving peace extended toward myself and others. Practitioners can easily substitute Brahma, Vishnu, and Siva with another aspect of God to fit their personal spiritual path.

Indian Sadhaks generally think Brahma, Vishnu, and Shiva—the Gods of Trinity. When they practice these pranayam, with inhale they think Brahma, the Creator, whose colour is like Fire. Fire is the symbol of Creation.

When they retain the air (Kumbhak), they think Vishnu, the Preserving Deity, whose colour is Blue. Blue is symbol of Infinite.

When the air exhaled, they think Shiva, the Deity of Destruction, whose colour is white.

Bhavana of Brahma should be in navel region, Bhavana of Vishnu in heart region, Bhavana of Shiva in forehead region or Bhrumadhya.[103]

Here is my version of this technique. It can be practiced with alternate nostril breathing or breathing through both nostrils. The purpose is to connect the heart and mind through focused attention.

During inhalation, think of Brahma, the creator, whose color is red, like fire. Fire is the symbol of creation. Attention is held at the navel or manipura chakra. Sense all of creation around you. Consider lovingly your own personal creative energies and the life you have created for yourself.

While retaining the breath, think of Vishnu, the preserving deity, whose color is blue. Blue is the symbol of the Infinite. Attention is held at the heart region. Be aware of all that you preserve in your life. Consider lovingly what is worth preserving, and what it is time to let go of.

During exhalation, think of Siva, the deity of destruction, whose color is white. White is the symbol of purity. Attention is held at the bhrumadhya, the ajna chakra between the eyebrows. Lovingly, gently, let go of all that you no longer need to preserve, making way for new creation to enter into your life.

This technique engages the mind, so it does not wander or become distracted. Pure love is extended for each of these aspects in one's life—creation, preservation, and letting go of that which is no longer needed. It is very purifying, and it helps us to accept this natural flow of creation, preservation, and destruction as it occurs in all things manifested, including our personal lives.

Sahita Kumbhaka

Sahita kumbhaka is basically any pranayama practice in which we intentionally hold the breath. Here Swami Yogeshwaranand explained to Hari the practice using *japa* (repetition of a mantra) and the traditional counting to determine the proper ratio of inhalation, retention, and exhalation. He offered three options for these counts—short, medium, and long. The process described here is what I learned from Swami Vishnudevananda as anuloma viloma, alternate nostril breathing, which is described a little later;[104] others may know it as *nadi shodhana*. (Swami Yogeshwaranand offered other descriptions for anuloma viloma and nadi shodhana.)

> Sahit Kumbhak—this is of two kinds: 1) Sagarbh vritti 2) Nirgarbh (without).
>
> Sagarbh is that which is performed with the jap of OM or mantras with numbers. Nirgarbh (without) is that which is performed without jap.

Swami Yogeshwaranand goes on to explain that this pranayama can be short, medium, or long—referring to how long the count is for inhalation, retention, and exhalation. One must take time and gradually work toward the long count.

> (a) Kanishth (short). Sitting in abhyast asan [your accustomed seat], keep your neck and body upright, then, with the thumb of right hand, close the right nostril of the nose and repeat OM mentally 8 times (count on fingers or rosary) [while] performing purak (inhale) from left nostril. Then [close both nostrils and] do jap of OM 32 times. This is the time that should be taken for kumbhak. Then close the left nostril and do rechak [through the right nostril]—repeat OM x 16. Repeat the same exercise from the other nostril.
>
> (b) Madhyam (medium). Close the right nostril, perform Purak up to 16 jap of OM from the left nostril, then do kumbhak up to 64 jap, then perform rechak in a way that it may take time up to 32 jap. Rechak should be done by the right nostril. Repeat this from the right nostril.
>
> (c) Uttam (long). The whole method is like [the] previous one with the only difference in counting the numbers. Perform Purak

in 32, kumbhaka 128, and rechak 64 with the jap of OM. This could not be achieved in a day or two, develop it gradually.

The pranayama gives bodily activeness, one feels light, gives control over man (heart) and impulses.[105]

Please note that many of these pranayamas are advanced techniques, and it is not advisable to do them without the guidance of a qualified teacher or guru. Some may choose to practice these pranayamas without breath retention, which makes them much safer, and in which case you have no need to apply the bandhas, described below.

The Bandhas

At this time, I think it is important to explain the three *bandhas,* since serious practitioners use them during advanced pranayama practice.

Jalandhara bandha is applied during kumbhaka. Seated with an erect spine, the chin is lowered toward the jugular notch. Often referred to as the *throat lock,* it puts pressure on the nerve passing through the neck. This stimulation can create a trance-like state and slows down the heart. This bandha helps to press the *prana vayu* (inflowing breath) downward to meet with the *apana vayu* (outflowing breath). Swami Kuvalayananda strongly recommends that this bandha be applied during any long breath retention to protect the ears from any air rushing through the eustachian, or auditory, tubes to the internal ear once breath retention is released.[106]

I might add here *jihva bandha,* which is often used but rarely mentioned. It is a tongue lock applied during kumbhaka along with jalandhara bandha. It ensures a good seal where the nasal passages enter the throat, allowing no escape of air or prana. Touch the tip of the tongue behind the upper front teeth, then press the rest of the tongue against the upper palate all the way back into the throat to seal the air passage there. You can add this to your jalandhara bandha as you wish.

Mula bandha is the root lock and is aided when one sits in siddhasana, putting pressure on the perineum and anal sphincter. This helps to draw the apana vayu upward to meet with the prana vayu. It is applied during kumbhaka as well, although, as described earlier, it is also mildly applied during puraka in order to maintain a slight firmness below the navel.

Uddiyana bandha (diaphragmatic lock) is performed at the end of rechaka as an independent exercise to draw the joined prana and apana up the sushumna. However, it is also applied during the process of exhalation to slowly squeeze the breath out of the lungs, and then more strongly in the *bahya kumbhaka* (external retention of the breath—when breath is held out after an exhalation). *Uddiyana* means "flying or soaring up," which is the soaring up of prana through the spine to the sahasrara chakra. When practiced properly, the passage of the spine is opened for the currents of prana to rise, whereupon the union of prana and apana is accomplished. When the two combine, the mind becomes stilled, calmed, and thoughtless. One feels something like intoxication.[107]

Bandha traya is the term for engaging all three major bandhas together. During inhalation, there is a slight mula bandha. Jalandhara bandha is immediately applied and held during breath retention, along with a firm mula bandha. Uddiyana bandha is applied during exhalation, which helps prolong it. If bahya kumbhaka is performed, uddiyana is then applied then to draw the prana upward.

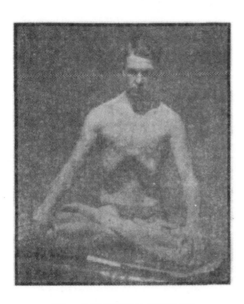

42.   UDDIYANA BANDHA

Figure 4.3. Hari performing uddiyana bandha, *Hatha Yoga (Illustrated)*, by Swami Sivananda, Divine Life Society, 1939, page 137.

Swami Vishnudevananda explained to Hari how to apply the bandhas.

Moola banda and jalandhara banda are done during retention, and udhayana alone is done during bahya kumbhaka or external retention. Bandhatraya consists of internal retention or anthara kumbak and bahya kumbak or external retention. As soon as you finish [inhalation], start jalandhara bandha. Pull the apana upward through moola bandha and prana downward through jalandhara bandha and unite prana and apana at the mooladhara chakra. When you do this, use your will power and take the united prana-apana along the central canal (sushumna) to Brahmarandhra [the place at the crown of the head where there is a soft spot in infants]. [Exhale]. While doing bahya kumbak, uddiyana is done. This makes one round.[108]

In Bandha Treya, during rechaka, naturally all Bandhas are un-locked and thus the united Prana Apana separates and goes to its original place. So the concentration will be only at Mooladhara dur-ing Rechaka. In Bhahya Kumbak, also there are all the three Band-has, even though the Uddiyana Bandha is prominent. As the Prana is not the physical breath, so even in Bhahyakumbaka the Prana can move in the Sushumna Nadi. More over, Uddiyana means Prana moves in the Sushumna.[109]

Swami Sivananda of Rishikesh added a beautiful visualization.

During the practice of Bandha Traya, for the first round, feel while inhaling that the Lord's Shakti is flowing into you; while retaining that, the Papa Purusha (Sinful Person) on the left side of the abdo-men is burnt; while you exhale, the ashes are thrown out of you. During the subsequent rounds feel that your entire body is filled by amrita (celestial nectar flowing into you) and that you are being transformed into God. Or, feel that the Prana and the Apana meet below the heart and their combined force is awakening the Kundal-ini. During the final Sunyaka [void, emptiness], be thoughtless.[110]

Swami Vishnu Tirth explained his technique.

Uddiyana is to be done with Rechak, i.e., while exhaling and with empty lungs. Mula bandha before Purak and Jalandhar after Purak, i.e., during inner kumbhak.[111]

Swami Sivananda explained how bandha traya should be applied for dif-ferent practitioners.

When Bandha Traya is done by a regular Pranayam practitioner as an accompaniment to his usual pranayama, there the breathing is done by alternating nostrils.

When a sadhak who is not having systematic pranayam as his routine sadhana taken up to the practice of Bandha Traya, he may breathe through both nostrils.

Whereas even if one is practicing pranayam, should he desire to do Bandha Traya as a separate exercise, then the breathing may be done through both nostrils. If done with pranayam, then the most suitable exercise is Sukh Purvak.

During actual sadhana time Bandha Traya may be done after asans and before Dhyana [meditation]. But at other ordinary times it may be done with advantage at any time that the stomach is light or empty.[112]

Pranayama Techniques

Pranayama was very important to Hari. He was a master at it and knew it was the best way to prepare oneself for the sacred mysteries of yoga. He believed traditional forms of pranayama were supported by the scientific research done by Swami Kuvalayananda at Kaivalyadhama and that modern adaptations were often erroneous.[113] He impressed me one day by showing me how to breathe into only one lung, explaining, "To inhale into one lung, one must relax the muscles on one side of the chest and tense the muscles on the other side of the chest. Concentrate on inhaling into the relaxed side." This kind of control and concentration was carried into all of the pranayama techniques he taught me, starting with *kapalabhati*.

Kapalabhati

In Sanskrit, *kapala* means "skull," and *bhati* means "luminous." Thus, kapalabhati is commonly known as "skull shining breath." Kapalabhati is a series of forceful exhalations with passive inhalations. It is one of the *shat karmas*, or six cleansing techniques, specifically for cleansing the respiratory system and removing phlegm. Using the diaphragm, each quick exhalation draws the abdominal muscles inward, and each passive exhalation releases the abdominal muscles back to normal. It is very important that with the exhalation, the abdomen draws inward, and on the inhalation, the abdomen relaxes. This technique strengthens the diaphragm and abdominal muscles while removing residual carbon dioxide, which can increase your energy levels.

In a letter to Hari, Swami Vishnudevananda explained the purpose of kapalabhati.

This is practised before starting pranayam so that the respiratory system is cleansed. It prepares for pranayam as it purifies the system thoroughly. It is mild and only [the] diaphragm works here. It is very useful before pranayam.[114]

Hari and I started with three rounds with 11 exhalations and increased gradually—by elevens—to 22, 33, 44, and up to 121 exhalations per round. Although only the diaphragm is at work, you will notice the pelvic floor rises with each exhalation, because our internal muscles are all connected. Hari and I would concentrate on visualizing each expulsion of breath against the muladhara chakra and then optionally hold mula bandha to activate the kundalini energy. Even during rests between each round we would hold our attention there.[115]

Even though Hari and I would practice pranayama after asana, we would do kapalabhati before doing asana. He said this exercise would produce a lot of oxygen in the body that would make our asana practice easier to do.

Swami Yogeshwaranand described it more like bhastrika, with equal force on the inhalation and exhalation. He did not indicate how many repetitions to do, but the process is clear—it can be done through both nostrils or alternating nostrils.

Kapal bhati Pranayam (Bellow type)

1. This is of two kinds. Sit in Siddhasan. Inhale and exhale forcefully and quickly like the bellows of a blacksmith.

2. Inhale gradually from the left nostril and exhale gradually from the right. Again inhale gradually from the right and exhale from the left.[116]

Sukha Purvak Pranayama

Swami Sivananda of Rishikesh refered often to *sukha purvak pranayama* in letters to Hari. He called it "easy, comfortable pranayama." Although the technique was not described in the letters, Swami Sivananda describes it in his book *The Science of Pranayama*. The text describes *Vishnu mudra*, a way of holding the hand to close the nostrils.

Sit on Padmasana or Siddhasana in your meditation room, before the picture of your Ishta Devata (presiding deity). Close the right nostril with the thumb. Draw in the air very, very slowly through the left nostril. Then close the left nostril also with little and ring fingers of the right hand. Retain the air as long as you can comfortably do. Then exhale very, very slowly through the [right] nostril after removing the thumb. Now half the process is over. Then draw air through the right nostril. Retain the air as before and exhale it very, very slowly through the left nostril. All these six processes constitute one Pranayama. Do 20 in the morning and 20 in the evening. Gradually increase the number. Have Bhava (mental attitude) that all the Daivi Sampat (divine qualities), e.g., mercy, love, forgiveness, Santi, joy, etc., are entering into your system along with the inspired air and all Asuri Sampat (devilish qualities) such as lust, anger, greed, etc., are being thrown out along with the expired air. Repeat Om or Gayatri mentally during Puraka, Kumbhaka and Rechaka.[117]

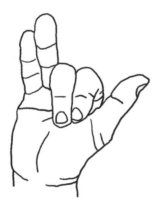

Figure 4.4. Vishnu mudra for performing sukha purvak pranayama. Drawing by Jo C. Willems.

Swami Suryadevananda explained to me that "easy, comfortable pranayama" did not mean that it was without effort, but rather that one should exert without struggle.

I feel the intention was to make it something friendlier and more comprehensive than a kriya or technique. Certain techniques are not suited to all, but all have the same goal: to purify oneself so that one's true nature could be seen. This in mind, it feels more approachable when you put it as "as long as comfortable" instead of a definite time to start. The key is not comfortable but "as long as" and then "comfortable." This is beautiful because in the same instruction there is "as long as" implying one should exert, and "comfortable" implying there should be no struggle. You have something specific with the druthers of ease at the same time—this masterstroke of dual instruction is all one really needs to know about the philosophy of practice of yoga in general. This keeps one from going to an extreme or getting complacent at the same time—in the same sentence. When the yogi does as long as, he will come to the anuloma viloma rhythm and if felt necessary, find his own rhythm beyond it. I feel that the anuloma viloma rhythm is just a guidance and not a rule, as each person is different in every way—a sort of good benchmark of sorts.

Further, I feel that one comes to all yoga practice with "yoga" first and not "practice." The goal is yoga—to discover the already underlying unity of all things. With this "as long as," the emphasis is on the yogi and not the technique, as otherwise, one can become a good specialist. In yoga, specialization is not the best thing, as specialization is the work of the ego. With "as long as"—the onus is on the yogi, and he can keep in mind why he is doing this in the first place—yoga.[118]

Nadi Shodhana

I didn't hear the term *nadi shodhana* until years after my training. Some claim it is a completely different technique than *anuloma viloma*, and others claim it is the same. As there are so many techniques in pranayama, and many variations on each of those techniques, not everyone will agree. Very often, names for pranayamas vary, just as they do in asana. For example, the standing forward bend pose is called *uttanasana* by some and *padahastasana* by others. The Sanskrit name usually describes what is going on in the pose— *uttanasana* translates as "intense stretch pose," which it is, and *padahastasana* means "hands to feet pose," which it also is.

Swami Yogeshwaranand offered a lovely variation of nadi shodhana, which could also be a variation of sukha purvak pranayama with a visualization added: block the right nostril and take a long, slow inhalation through the left nostril, visualizing the prana going right down to the muladhara chakra at the base of the spine. Close the left nostril and exhale slowly out the right nostril. Then inhale very slowly in the right nostril, visualizing the prana going right down to the muladhara chakra at the base of the spine. Then close the right nostril and exhale out the left nostril. This should be a comfortable process, without strain or stress. Concentrate on visualizing the flow of prana, and it will increase mental focus and calm the mind. This technique is extremely calming and beneficial for concentration and meditation. If you do this before *yoga nidra* (yoga sleep) you will have a very deep experience.

Swami Yogeshwaranand described nadi shodhana in a letter to Hari.

Nari Shodhan Pranayam (Nerve purification): Sit in Padmasan. Close/Press the right nostril, fill the air down to *muladhar*, without performing kumbhak, exhale from the right nostril gradually. Repeat the same way from the left nostril. Increase the number gradually.[119]

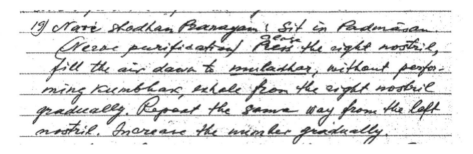

Figure 4.5. Letter from Swami Yogeshwaranand describing nadi shodhana, p. 14, undated.

Anuloma Viloma

Anuloma means "in order" or "with the grain," and *viloma* means "against the grain." In this pranayama, we are moving the breath contrary to the way we normally do. The timing for this uses a ratio of 1:4:2, for example, inhale through the left nostril for 8 seconds, retain the breath for 32 seconds, and exhale out the right nostril for 16 seconds. Then inhale through the right nostril for 8 seconds, retain the breath for 32 seconds, and exhale out the left nostril for 16 seconds. This is one round. Over time, increase to twenty rounds in a sitting. This ratio and count takes just under one minute per breath.

The main purpose of anuloma viloma is to purify the nadis, the energy channels in the nervous system of the subtle body.[120] It is said to balance the right and left brain hemispheres, calm the mind and thought waves, and eventually allow the prana to move into the sushumna, the central nadi.[121] One should exercise caution and start the practice without any breath retention at all, gradually building up according to comfort levels physically, mentally, and emotionally. This is an invaluable practice at any stage of your yoga journey. If it is done with a comfortable count, you will be more inclined to do a daily practice and may even look forward to it, as I do.

When I practiced anuloma viloma under the guidance of Swami Vishnudevananda, we were advised to practice on our own for twenty rounds during the first month in the ashram and gradually build up our count, using the 1:4:2 ratio.

After one month of individual practice, we gathered as a group for a daily practice using the above example of 8:32:16. Most of us found this too difficult, so the count was reduced to 7:28:14. I started to feel tingling in my body and some "jerking" during the practice. It felt similar to when I catch myself falling asleep, and I jerk awake, only I knew I was not falling asleep. I was absorbed and concentrated with the practice at hand. I wrote Hari and asked him what these jerking motions meant.

And now to your question regarding the prickly feelings in body and jerks when you practice Anuloma-Viloma pranayama. The jerks are due to *energy blocks*. They can be easily overcome by Shakti Yoga, but even without it, the systematic practice of Anuloma-Viloma pranayama will remove the energy blocks. It is rather good that you experience them. The jerk can remove the block. Otherwise a long continued (and not removed) [block] might cause some painful disease like arthritis, etc.

So please continue with Anuloma Viloma. One can do this pranayama even without kumbhaka, but the changing of the nostrils is, of course, necessary. It is called also Nadi Shoddhana or Nadi shuddhi—purification of the psycho-vital channels. These jerks also occur sometimes during meditation (when the Kundalini Shakti is roused and the Nadis (Naris) are not sufficiently purified.

Am glad that you, dear Bhanumati, have practically realized the need of Prana Shuddhi, i.e., the necessity of Anuloma-Viloma pranayama. So continue your Anuloma Viloma as you are doing it. Not too long a kumbhaka (retention of breath). Kumbhaka can be developed greatly, but it must be done *gradually*, systematically!

If one wants to develop kumbhaka, then proper vegetarian diet is highly advisable. But even vegetarian diet can be detrimental from yogic point. E.g., onion and garlic are more unfavorable (especially in regard to mental control) than meat.

But let us not forget the words of the Great Master (Jesus Christ) who said: It is not what comes in the body that makes you impure but that which comes out of it. Here evidently the Lord advises to put more attention to what kind of thoughts come out from our hearts than our mere dietetics (which of course have also some place in yogic curriculum, but we should not stress the lesser things in favour of the higher ones).[122]

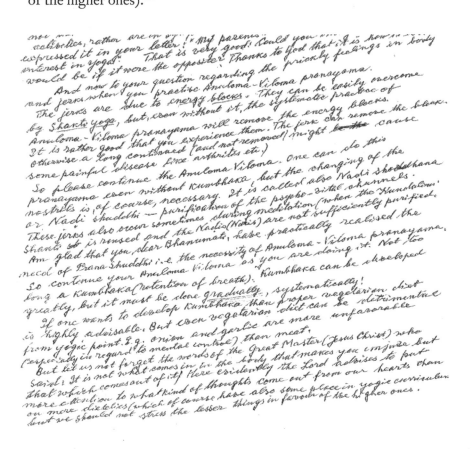

Figure 4.6. Letter to the author from Hari describing jerks felt during anuloma viloma, September 16, 1978.

Ujjayi

Ujjayi is one of the eight major kumbhakas discussed in the *Hatha Yoga Pradipika,* and I consider it an essential practice. Today ujjayi is most commonly understood to be practiced with exhalation through both nostrils. This makes it a very suitable pranayama for practicing during asana, while walking, or even lying down.[123] Practiced in this manner, it can be done in any position, anywhere.

However, there is a more traditional way to practice ujjayi, as described in the *Hatha Yoga Pradipika,* whereby one performs exhalation through only the left nostril.[124] The inhalation is done through both nostrils with a slightly closed glottis in order to create a low, smooth, and uniform sound. After kumbhaka, the right nostril is closed and the exhalation is done through the left nostril, the *ida nadi*—or the calming, feminine energy.

The name *ujjayi* implies "with sound." *Jaya* means "to conquer, succeed" and is a joyous sound for success—for example, *Jaya Ganesha!* Greetings in ancient India consisted of the word *jaya* and were pronounced loudly.[125] (Even now, when we greet someone we are pleased to see, the greeting is said with some enthusiasm and usually a little loudly.) Most importantly, *ujjayi* means "to lead one to success."[126]

We should not underestimate the effects of slightly closing the glottis in this pranayama. Ujjayi stimulates the throat area and the parasympathetic nervous system. This is the area of the vishuddhi chakra, where our silent thoughts and intentions become vocalized. Ujjayi cultivates sweetness of voice and calmness of mind. We are more likely to say the right thing when we are calm, and we are more likely to succeed when we say the right thing.

In a letter, Swami Yogeshwaranand said that the inhalation should fill the area with prana only from the heart chakra to the throat chakra, and then be retained there. The prana is held between the throat and the heart—no lower. He then conveyed an interesting way of exhalation to Hari: move the air from the throat into the mouth and then exhale out the left nostril. When we perform kumbhaka with jalandhara bandha, we feel the air locked at the throat. Using your mind's eye, you can indeed move the breath into the mouth before exhaling out the left nostril. It has quite an interesting effect.

Ujjayi Pranayam: Sit in abhyast asan [accustomed seat], inhale from the both nostrils gradually. Fill the air only from hridaya (heart) to kanth (throat), do Jalandhar bandha. Perform kumbhaka up to your capacity. And than [*sic*] exhale from the left nostril gradually. While performing kumbhaka air should not go down beyond hridaya. From throat, bringing the air into mouth, exhale gradually from the left nose.[127]

Hari wrote back, asking if he should contract the abdomen in order to prevent the air from moving below the heart. Swami Yogeswaranand responded, "No, abdomen in no case be contracted or drawn in while doing Ujjayi Pranayama."[128]

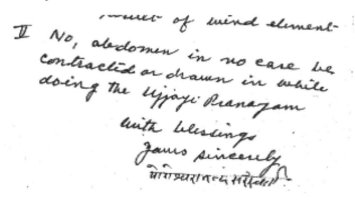

Figure 4.7. Comment in letter from Swami Yogeshwaranand, 1965.

Hari told me to hold the slight contraction below the navel along with mula bandha and concentrate on the muladhara chakra to awaken the kundalini. Once kundalini is awakened, the concentration should change to the ajna chakra.[129]

Surya Bheda

Surya is the sun, and in this pranayama, the inhalation is always done through the right nostril and exhalation is always done through the left. It is therefore a warming pranayama and should not be done when one is already too warm. It aids in digestion and removes impurities through perspiration.

Here is how I do this technique, following Swami Yogeshwaranand's description. Sitting in your accustomed seat, inhale through the right nostril, producing a little noise, which just means there is a soft sound created as the breath moves. Take the breath all the way down from the throat to the stomach, feeling as though the body is filled with air from the head right to the feet. Retain the breath as long as is comfortable, or until you feel restless. Then close the right nostril and exhale slowly out the left nostril, producing a soft sound. Gradually work up to thirty-one rounds of this pranayama.

Energetically, I imagine the prana flowing from the vishuddhi chakra at the throat to the manipura chakra at the solar plexus during each inhalation. During kumbhaka, I feel the prana permeate every region, from head to toes. As I exhale, I imagine the prana moving upward from the manipura chakra at the solar plexus all the up to the vishuddhi chakra at the throat and then out the left nostril.

Regarding bandhas with this pranayama, Hari taught me to curl the tongue back into the throat (a variation of khechari mudra) to help raise the kundalini.[130] Swami Sivananda of Rishikesh told Hari, "There is no Uddiyana bandha in Soorya Bedha Pranayam. Moola bandha starts at the beginning of the inhalation and continues till the end of Kumbhak. Jalandhara Bandha starts at the beginning of kumbhak. So during retention both the Bandhas should be practiced."[131]

> Surya Bhedi: Sitting in abhyast asan, perform purak from surya nadi (right) producing a little noise. Having filled the air in kanth [throat], hridaya [heart] and udar (stomach), perform kumbhaka up to your capacity. While performing this, one should have a feeling that the air is filled in the body from head to the feet. When you begin to feel restlessness, then close the right nostril and perform rechak from Chandra nadi with speed (left nostril) producing noise. In this Pranayam, purak is from the Surya nari (right nostril) and rechak from the Chandra nari (left nostril) is performed repeatedly.
>
> First day perform one pranayama [then] with the gap of every one or two days, increase one by one up to 31.
>
> This pranayama helps awakening of Kundalini, increases life, checks the old ages.[132]

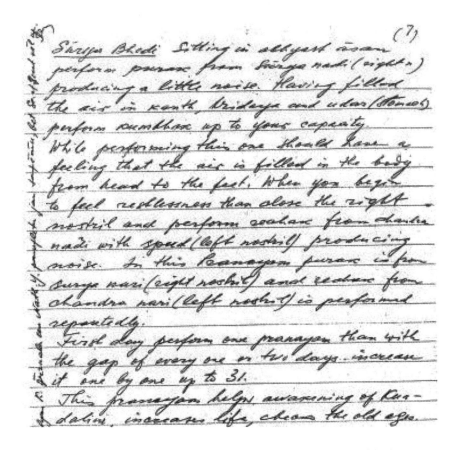

Figure 4.8. Letter from Swami Yogeshwaranand describing surya bhedi,
p. 7, undated.

Bhastrika

Bhastrika is also one of the eight major kumbhakas of the *Hatha Yoga Pradipika*. It is similar to kapalabhati except there is equal force on the inhalations and exhalations, whereas kapalabhati has a passive inhalation followed
by a quick and forceful exhalation. Bhastrika is said to arouse the kundalini
quickly due to its purifying affects and enables the prana to break through
the three *granthis,* or psychic knots, in the sushumna.[133]

Hari said it was important to have movement in the throat during this
pranayama, meaning that the skin over the jugular notch should move
slightly as a result of the breath passing through the throat. Concentrate on
the muladhara chakra and imagine that every exhalation hits there.[134]

Swami Vishnudevananda gave a specific order in which to practice bhastrika in relation to other techniques in order to pierce the granthis.

> Bhastrika should be done after anuloma and viloma pranayam (or sukha poorvak), ujjayi, suryabheda. Bhastrika is very essential after the above purificatory pranayamas to open the granthis or knots. This is the only way to break the granthis easily.[135]

Sometimes bhastrika is taught by breathing through both nostrils, sometimes only through the left nostril, sometimes only through the right nostril, and sometimes by alternating between the left and right nostrils. Swami Brahmananda, who published *Jyotsna*, the first commentary of the *Hatha Yoga Pradipika*, in 1893, describes three of the above practices in his commentary. In his "alternating nostrils" practice, he suggests several repetitions of rapidly inhaling through the right nostril and exhaling through the left nostril until one is tired, then take one last deep inhale through the right nostril, perform kumbhaka, and exhale out the left nostril. Then do the reverse, always inhaling through the left nostril and exhaling through the right nostril.[136] All are variations of bhastrika.

Swami Yogeshwaranand also described bhastrika, and what I like about his technique is that he brings awareness to feeling the breath on your fingers. Note that he makes reference to a photo in a book of his (which he does not name by title), though there is a good photo in his *First Steps to Higher Yoga*.[137]

> Sit in posture of abhyast asan. Close the right nostril with the fingers [i.e., thumb] of right hand. Lift the right elbow up to the shoulder level. Keep the left hand on the left knee.... Now perform purak and rechak forcefully producing noise from the nostrils. The force of inhaling [and] exhaling of breath should be felt on the fingers. In this way, perform purak and rechak at least 8 to 10 times. After this, perform abhyantar kumbhak [breath retention held after inhalation] and be in the state of kumbhak as long as you can. Then *exhale from the left nostril*. While exhaling, close the right nostril by the thumb. Perform the above three times from each nostril and increase the number daily. Some teachers advise that while in kumbhak, Jalandhara bandha should be also performed.

It is advised that weak persons should not perform it for longer period. One should do it by judging his own capacity, otherwise it may cause headache, cough, etc. One who practices the above pranayama must consume milk and butter according to his needs. Otherwise blood could appear in his cough.

Perform it carefully and never do it beyond your capacity. It awakens Kundalini, opens the gate of sushumna, reduces weight of the body.[138]

The *Hatha Yoga Pradipika* gives these same warnings for pranayama in general. In 2:14–17, it states that in the early stages of practice, we must eat the right food, use the bandhas properly, and take time to slowly control the prana. Just as we must take time to tame lions, elephants, and tigers—since without careful approach and keen awareness, they can kill the practitioner—we must also take time to control the prana. With the right practice and diet, pranayama can free us from many diseases, but with the wrong practice, the result can be headaches, ear and eye aches, as well as cough, asthma, and other diseases.[139]

Swami Shivapremananda offered Hari some good alternative advice for this intense practice.

Daily practice of kapalabhati will give [resistance] to cold weather. Bhastrika is, of course, the best but should be done only when the lungs are strong. I think you could practice something in between, i.e., a stronger version of Kapalabhati and a milder form of Bhastrika.

Breathe deeply three or four times, then begin sharp exhalation, giving a lift not only to the diaphragm (as in Kapalabhati) but the force of exhalation should involve a mild form of ashwini mudra [contraction of anal sphincter] and mula bandha, as it were, in the process of squeezing the whole abdomen up. There will also be a mild vibration in the chest by contraction of the trachea and bronchii, with the feeling of current moving up to the inside of the throat, while exhaling. While inhaling, there is no sound of trachea, of course (because no contraction of it is involved), but it is slightly more forceful than in Kapalabhati, in which inhalation is automatic. The sound of exhalation in the beginning of Bhastrika is different than that of later for the simple reason that the building up of the pressure as one continues produces a different kind of vibration. Do this only 20 times, then deep breathe three or four times and, inhaling three quarters of lung capacity, do kumbhaka for one minute. Do as many rounds as you wish without feeling tired or spasm in the chest. As I said, it is better not to do full Bhastrika, but vary in between Kapalabhati and Bhastrika until you feel that your lungs are strong enough.

God bless you, Hari Maharaj. Keep in good health. You are wise enough to know that pranayama should not be overdone.[140]

Sitali and Sitkari

Sitali is a cooling breath and extremely beneficial during the warm seasons, because it quickly cools down the body. Normally, when we inhale through the nose, the breath is slightly warmed as it passes through the nasal passages and into the body. In this pranayama, we inhale through the mouth to avoid warming the air as it is drawn in. The tongue is rolled like a tube, and the breath is drawn in through this tube. You can feel the cool air at the back of the throat. Close the mouth and retain the breath as long as is comfortable, and then exhale out through both nostrils.

The external air must be cooler than the body temperature in order for this pranayama to have the desired effect of reducing the body temperature. It doesn't take long to work.

In 1983 I backpacked with my sister from Mexico to Canada on the Continental Divide. There was one stretch near Rawlins, Wyoming, where we walked for seven days without seeing a tree. In these very hot desert conditions, I would set up a tarp with a reflective Mylar side toward the sun to create some shade to do this pranayama. I found it very effective for cooling.

Swami Vishnudevananda added some interesting points for the practice of this cooling breath, including kumbhaka and a ratio for counting.

The ratio of Puraka, Kumbhaka, and Rechaka can be 1:2:2. The abdominal muscles should be held firm, and though not actually pressed behind as in Uddiyana, [they] should not be in a relaxed position. But when you start the exhalation, you will have to exert pressure in the abdomen and contract it as in other Pranayamas. During exhalation, of course, the abdomen will go in first and then only the chest. This applies to all Pranayamas. Sitali is a cooler. There-fore, the aspirant is advised to concentrate at tip of the nose, on the Moon.[141]

The *Hatha Yoga Pradipika* claims this pranayama will destroy diseases of the abdomen and spleen, as well as other diseases, including fever, bilious-ness, hunger, thirst, and the effects of bad poisons.[142] I do not recommend it for persons with asthma, as the incoming air is neither filtered nor warmed, and this could result in an asthma attack.

Sitkari pranayama is often used as an alternative to sitali for those who cannot roll their tongue into a tube. Open the mouth and place the tip of the tongue behind the top front teeth. This creates a bit of a smile, and there should be space on either side of the tongue. When inhaling through these spaces, there will be a hissing sound.

Although there is no mention in the *Hatha Yoga Pradipika* of a breath retention in this technique,[143] Swami Kuvalayananda said there should be kumbhaka simply because of the fact that sitkari is included with the eight kumbhakas, which implies there is breath retention.[144] Swami Yogeshwa-ranand, however, clearly dropped the kumbhaka.

> Sit in Siddhasan posture. Inhale just like in Sitali from the hole of the stretched tongue, producing a whistling noise. Now without per-forming kumbhak, exhale from the both nostrils immediately. This pranayam develops physical beauty, among other things.[145]

Bhramari

Bhramari pranayama is commonly known as "bee humming breath." It gets its name because the breathing is accompanied with a humming sound pro-duced in the palate during the exhalation. This is the easiest and most com-fortable practice for most people. Occasionally it is taught with the humming sound produced on the inhalation as well, as described in the *Hatha Yoga Pradipika*,[146] but Hari suggested not teaching that in the beginning. He prac-ticed humming only during exhalation. He made the exhalation as long as possible, which has the same benefits of a kumbhaka.[147]

Bhramari is performed with both inhalation and exhalation through both nostrils. Swami Kuvalayananda described the inhalation as a high humming

sound, resembling the sound of a male bee, and the exhalation as a low humming sound, resembling a female bee.[148]

Swami Sivananda of Rishikesh also taught Hari bhramari pranayama
with sound produced during both inhalation and exhalation. He added a natural kumbhaka, that is, a natural state of suspending the breath, not a long,
controlled kumbhaka.[149]

Swami Gitananda suggested that the sound produced on inhalation
should be palatal, resembling the sound of a male bee, thus called *bhramara*
(the *A* being the masculine word ending). The sound produced on exhalation should be a nasal sound, resembling that of a female bee, and therefore
called *bhramari* (the *I* being the the feminine ending).[150]

Swami Satchidananda said that producing the sound during inhalation is
optional. He suggested practitioners produce the sound only during exhalation until they have perfect mastery of this, and only then trying it during
inhalation as well, though it may be discontinued if too difficult. He also
clearly stated that the sound in bhramari pranayama is produced in the palate, not in the nose.

> You are correct in saying that the bee sound in Bhramari Pranayam
> is produced in the palate and never in the nose. The exact place for
> the sound is in the junction where the nasal opening branches out
> from the throat.
>
> The inhalation should be done in a normal way, neither too
> slow nor too quick, and the exhalation as slowly as possible. Both
> the process[es] are performed through the nostrils (both) and not
> through the mouth. There is no kumbhaka and matras [the count
> measuring how long each breath should be] for Bhramari except the
> one long kumbhaka at the end.[151]

Swami Satchidananda added that concentration of the mind during
bhramari should be on the sound produced. The practice can be carried on
as long as one is comfortably able to. To end the practice, there is one long,
deep inhalation followed by a breath retention, held without difficulty, then a
slow exhalation. The reason for no other kumbhaka or counting with breath
is so the technique can be very relaxing.[152]

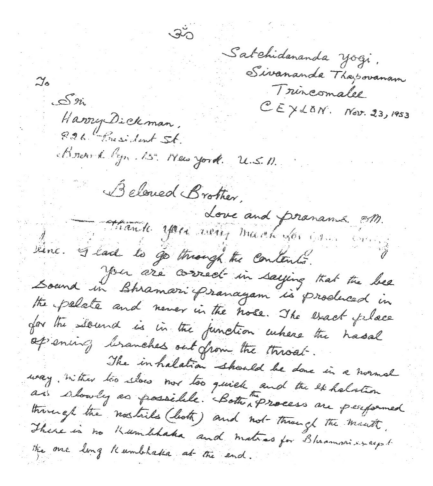

Figure 4.9. Letter from Swami Satchidananda regarding bhramari pranayama, 1953.

Swami Yogeshwaranand added a different twist to this sacred prana-yama—inhalation through the left nostril alone, which I love. I believe that when he referred to hearing "other sounds" in this letter, he meant the inter-nal sounds of the anahata chakra. (Discussed below.)

Bhramari Pranayam (bee humming). Sitting in posture of virasan [hero pose], close the right nostril and perform purak (through the left nostril). When the air is filled, do kumbhaka for a few moments. Then, producing a humming noise like that of a [bumblebee], do re-chak gradually and slowly. Prolong rechak as long as you can, while concentrating to the produced humming sound. By practice, gradually you shall begin to hear other sounds also with that one. Increase it gradually. The above pranayama gives richness and sweetness to the voice. The breath becomes long and noiseless. It gives peace to the mind and heart, and power of concentration.[153]

I was taught a form of bhramari breath by a family in New Delhi while my husband and I were in India. They included the *yoni mudra* (blocking out the senses): block the ears with the thumbs, the eyes with the index fingers, the nose with the middle fingers, the upper lip with the ring fingers and the lower lip with the baby fingers. (Though the nose is only symbolically closed, so one can still breathe.) I was taught to inhale through both nostrils without humming, and then block my senses with yoni mudra and exhale, producing the humming sound (which is the *M* sound of Om). Repeat it again, exactly the same way, and then on the third repetition, instead of humming, say "Om" out loud for the entire length of the exhalation. Adding yoni mudra to the practice of bhramari makes me full of beautiful internal vibrations.

Repetition of the mantra Om is a powerful practice in and of itself. Swami Sivananda of Rishikesh said, "Om is the greatest mantra. When repeated with absolute full faith and sincerity, it will give what all other mantras can bestow."[154]

In the *Gheranda Samhita,* one of the three classic texts on hatha yoga (along with the *Hatha Yoga Pradipika* and the *Siva Samhita*), bhramari is done while closing the ears with the hands during inhalation and kumbhaka. With external sounds blocked, we begin to hear internal sounds in the right ear, such as crickets, a lute, thunder, drums, and so on. According to the *Gheranda Samhita,* the last sound to be heard is that of the anahata or heart chakra, the "unstruck sound," referred to as a "resonance." From this resonance comes a light, and by immersing the mind in that light, one attains samadhi.[155]

There is no mention in the *Gheranda Samhita* of making a humming sound, as there is in the *Hatha Yoga Pradipika.* It only refers to listening for these internal sounds. I believe that these are two sides of the same coin, just as a mantra can be repeated both verbally *(vachika japa)* or mentally *(manasika japa)*. Whether one is making the humming sound or listening for the internal sounds by closing off the external sounds, the result is the same. Hari could hear these internal sounds back in 1953, if not before.[156]

To practice pratyahara and withdraw from the senses takes us deep into our heart chakra, where the soul resides. This knowledge always takes me back to the teachings of Thomas Ashley-Farrand, my teacher of mantra (who also goes by the name Namadeva Acharya). He taught that sound is the initial manifestation of God, even before light. This manifestation is the word Om, the primordial sound.

> In the Gospel of John it says, "In the beginning was the Word. And the Word was with God and the Word was God." Talk about a powerful statement summarizing the power of sound!
>   In Genesis we find, "And God said, let there be light."[157]

Swami Sivananda called this *nada* (sound).

> The primal sound or the first vibration from which all creation has emanated is Nada. It is the first emanative stage in the projection of the universe (creation). Nada is the first manifestation of the unmanifested Absolute. It is Omkara or Sabda-Brahman. It is also the mystic inner sound on which the Yogi concentrates.[158]

This is a simple but powerful pranayama. It is considered a corrective pranayama to tone up certain parts of the body or the nervous system.[159] The energetic effect of this pranayama is that the anahata and vishuddhi chakras are stimulated so that the sounds that emanate from the throat are positive and kind, coming from a peaceful heart. The humming sound has a calming effect on the mind. It is the Om sound vibrating within. As when we hum to a baby, calming it so it can sleep, so we hum ourselves into the inner quiet, immersing our minds with those inner sounds and the resonance of our hearts until a light appears, and we immerse our minds in that, too, until there is nothing but bliss!

Murccha

Murccha means "loss of awareness." Swami Kuvalayananda said that with a steady daily practice, this pranayama would lead to a "stupor" or "a mental condition of mind that is not only pleasant but also helpful in concentration, as it excludes all sensory disturbances and leaves the mind free from associating ideas."[160] There are two distinct aspects to this pranayama—jalandhara bandha is held firmly, and it is held during the exhalation. The successful practice of these two features in murccha pranayama should result in a blissful state of consciousness.

He went on to explain why this works. When we lower the chin toward the jugular notch in jalandhara bandha, pressure is applied to the carotid arteries and sinuses on the sides of the neck. This stimulation slows down the heart. The classical yogis of India call the carotid sinus *vijnana nadi,* or the nerve of higher consciousness.[161] Normally, when we hold our breath for any length of time, our natural response is to panic and want to breathe. When jalandhara bandha is perfected, it counters this effect, creating an inner calm.

The *Siva Samhita* 5:36–38 says, "Sitting in the padmasana posture, renouncing the society of men, let the Yogi press the two vijnana nadis (the vessels of consciousness, perhaps coronal arteries) with his two fingers. By obtaining success in this, he becomes all happiness and unstained; therefore, let him endeavor with all his might, in order to ensure success. He who practices this always, obtains success within a short time; he gets also vayu-siddhi [mastery over the vayus or vital airs] in course of time."[162]

To practice murccha in the method described by Swami Kuvalayananda, one takes a deep inhalation followed by a "tightly fixed" jalandhara bandha during kumbhaka. When ready to exhale, jalandhara bandha is loosened only enough to allow for a very slow passage of outgoing air, extending the exhalation as long as possible. Over time, practicing a large number of rounds every day will bring about the desired results.

There is no matra, count or ratio, for inhalation and exhalation in murccha, according to Swami Sivananda. He advised Hari not to practice murccha or bhramari and not to prescribe them to his students. He said that Hari had done enough hatha yoga, and it was more important to meditate on the Supreme only, as this is what ultimately gives knowledge and breaks the bonds of karma.[163]

Interestingly, Swami Yogeshwaranand provided Hari with a very different description of this pranayama, although this is partly because he omitted some details. The inhalation is not actually mentioned in his letter, and more surprisingly, he says nothing at all about holding jalandhara bandha during breath retention or exhalation. A much clearer description of this pranayama, including inhalation and jalandhara banda, is in his book *First Steps to Higher Yoga,* which I highly recommend for serious practitioners of yoga.[164] I like that he adds a *drishti* (place where you focus your attention). He said the eyes should be focused on the ajna chakra.

> Murchha Pranayam. Sitting in posture of Padmasan, close the right nostril [inhale through the left] and perform kumbhaka. Try to eradicate [all thoughts from] your mind ... and feel as if you are becoming unconsciousness. Keep your glance in the centre of eye brows. Retain kumbhaka as long as you can, then exhale from both nostrils slowly and gradually. While performing kumbhak, avoid thinking and feel as if your heart and mind are becoming unconscious. Practice the same from the left nostril also [close the left nostril and inhale through the right]. The name Murcha (unconscious) has been given to this pranayama according to its benefits. By practicing above, one achieves peace and rest, and mind becomes un-turmoiled [without turmoil].[165]

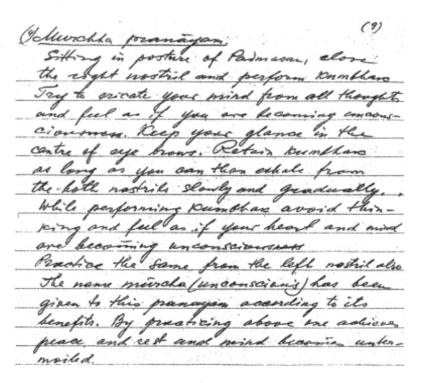

Figure 4.10. Letter from Swami Yogeshwaranand describing murccha pranayama, p. 9, undated.

I know Hari asked S. S. Goswami about murccha, because it is mentioned in a letter from 1962.

> Murccha is an advanced process which cannot be [taught] from a book. Personal instruction will be necessary and only very advanced pupils can learn it. This is why the technique has not been included in the book.[166]

He clearly avoided giving detail of this pranayama, perhaps intentionally, since he could not teach Hari in person.

One final note on murccha: in Swami Vishnudevananda's commentary to the *Hatha Yoga Pradipika*, he indicates that it is a minor pranayama, a light variety of yogic breathing used to acquire a trance state—one of the five *avasthas*, or states of consciousness.[167]

Plavini Pranayama

Plavini is a pranayama that enables one to "float." This particular pranayama lowers the effect of gravity on the body significantly below normal, so one can almost float on the surface of water like a lotus leaf. This is accomplished by taking air into the stomach by swallowing it. Dr. Swami Gitananda Giri called this practice of floating on water *plavini mudra*, although the end goal is not to float on water but rather to break the gravitational attraction of the earth and achieve the siddhi (power) of levitation.[168] Through practice, one can swallow enough air that the stomach and abdomen inflate so tightly that tapping them will create a sonorous sound. After filling the stomach with air, the yogi then fills the lungs as well with a deep inhalation, followed by kumbhaka for as long as comfortable, then exhales. Several rounds of pranayama are repeated before emptying the air from the stomach.[169]

Hari queried Swami Vishnudevananda about this pranayama and received a detailed description of the process.

> Though simple, the technique is a highly complicated one, for the simple fact that it relates to an involuntary physical process and bringing it within one's own volition. Sit on Padma or Siddha Asan. Sip a little water; keep it in the mouth for a few seconds. Now gently and consciously swallow this water. Concentrate all your attention on the throat now and mentally take note of the process of

swallowing. Do this without water the next time. Make sure to get the same "swallowing-noise" when you "swallow" without water. If you get it, you know that you are swallowing air, though the throat is not made to do this job [ordinarily]. What normally closes during the process of breathing has to be consciously and voluntarily kept open during Plavini; in other words, instead of the air reaching the lungs as it normally and involuntarily does, you should make it reach the stomach. THIS MUST BE DONE ON COMPLETELY EMPTY STOMACH, and the intestines also should be free from any clogging matter. Therefore, kindly practice this in the early morning, after answering calls of nature; and take no solid food after 3 p.m. the previous day. Otherwise the air swallowed may not easily pass out through the anus; and it is essential that the air is not unduly detained in the stomach. Drink half a glass of water before you commence the practice; it will prepare the passage for the air.

With the air inside the abdomen, you will be able to float on water (as you see in the enclosed illustration, a picture taken while I was afloat with Plavini Pranayama). In fact, you can never be drowned!

Now to remove the air from the stomach. Practise Mayurasan [peacock pose, in which the upper arms and elbows press into the stomach area while balancing on them]. After a few minutes, do [Sirsasan], preferably with Uddiyana Bandha.... The air will come out little by little through the anus. Again do Mayurasan, and then again [Sirsasan]. Repeat the process (with Agnisara in between) till all the air is expelled.

The air should not be expelled immediately after swallowing. Wait for at least fifteen to twenty minutes so that the air will pass through the stomach into the intestines and the colons and will not be accumulated in the stomach. When the air is only in the stomach and has not passed into the intestines, your effort to expel it might injure the valve between the stomach and the intestines.

In the beginning stages, the air will after a few seconds of the swallowing, escape through the throat itself in the form of eructations [burping]. As a matter of fact, this itself is a sign that you have caught the right technique. As you progress, however, you should try not to allow the air to escape this way and by the combined exercise of the will and practice of Jalandhara Bandha, try to retain the air within.

Re: Plavini. If the glottis is fully closed when you swallow the air, the air will not go into the lungs at all. Practice will enable you to reach perfection in this.[170]

I will just note here that Swami Kuvalayananda[171] and Dr. Swami Gitananda[172] both permited the air to be removed from the stomach through burping.

Madhya Rechaka Pranayama

Sometimes one of the shat karmas (six cleansing techniques) like nauli, *madhya rechaka* falls into the category of a pranayama because it involves tremendous breath control, a strong exhalation followed by a bahya kumbhaka (external breath retention). *Madhya* means "middle" or "medium." In this case, the breath is retained after a deep exhalation along with the protrusion of the rectus abdominis, as in nauli.

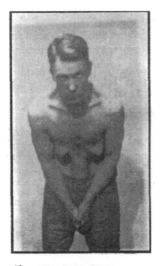

46.   MADHYAMA NAULI

Figure 4.11. Hari performing madhyama nauli, *Hatha Yoga (Illustrated),* by Swami Sivananda, Divine Life Society, 1939, page 158. Photographer unknown.

Because of this deep exhalation and external breath retention, Swami Yogeshwaranand classified madhya rechaka as a pranayama—a technique for the control of prana. He described the protrusion of the rectus abdominis using the word *sole.* It is unclear what he meant by this; perhaps he was referring to the fish or perhaps there was a language barrier.

Madhya rechaka benefits digestion and the removal of wastes in the intestines. Efficient removal of wastes is important for overall health of the body and mind. The strong upward pull of the necessary uddiyana bandha draws the prana upward.

Hari said that when performing any of the following rechak pranayamas (madhya as well as dakshina and vamana, discussed below), it is important to tense the shoulder and clavical muscles so they protrude and are isolated. This is clearly shown in the photos.[173]

(Middle exhaling) Sit in swastikasan or abhyastasan, exhale all the air of the stomach, then raise the portion between navel and 1st ribs so that it may stand out like a sole [?]. Perform bahya kumbhak up to your capacity and stamina.

It is good for all diseases of the intestines.[174]

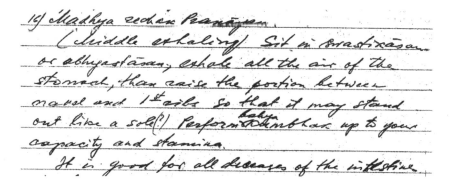

Figure 4.12. Letter from Swami Yogeshwaranand describing madhya rechak pranayama, undated.

Dakshina and Vamana Rechaka Pranayamas

These two pranayamas are done the same way madhya rechaka pranayama is, except the protrusion of the rectus abdominis is drawn over to the right *(dakshina nauli)* and then to the left *(vamana nauli)*. They can be done sitting or standing.

Deeply exhale and hold the breath out while drawing the stomach back toward the spine and up under the rib cage as far as possible (uddiyana bandha). Then, relax the rectus abdominis muscles forward and pull them to the right. This gives us dakshina nauli. Hold as long as is comfortably possible, release uddiyana bandha and breathe in slowly. Relax a moment and then repeat the process, pulling the rectus abdominis over to the left side for vamana nauli.

According to Swami Sivananda, in his book *Hatha Yoga (Illustrated)*, you should bend or lean a little to the right side to draw the rectus abdominis in that direction, and visa versa. The book included a photo of Hari performing dakshina and vamana nauli while standing with hands firmly clasped together. Hari taught me to press my hands down on my thighs, just above my knees, instead of clasping my hands together, and I find this makes it easier to achieve a strong uddiyana with nauli. To take the rectus abdominis from one side to the other, simply press more firmly on the thigh of the desired side.

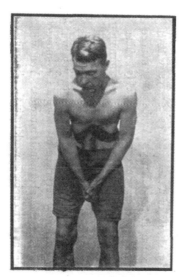 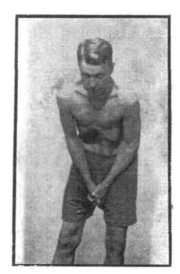

47. DAKSHINA AND VAMANA NAULI

Figure 4.13. Hari performing dakshina and vamana nauli, *Hatha Yoga (Illustrated),* by Swami Sivananda, Divine Life Society, 1939, page 160. Photographer unknown.

Swami Yogeshwaranand called vamana rechaka pranayama *wack-rechak pranayama* in his letter to Hari, and included a slight variation that would activate the ida nadi.

> Wack-rechak-Pranayam (Left exhaling) Sit in sukhasan. Exhale from the left nostril. Contract the udar (stomach) and raise the intestines of the left part of the body, so that it may stand like a sole, it should not move. Retain bahya (outer) kumbhak for some time and then inhale.
> This decreases fat of the stomach and keeps the bowels clean.[175]

His description of dakshina rechaka pranayama is the same, but with the sides reversed: he began by exhaling out the right nostril and raising the intestines on the right side of the body.[176] This would activate the *pingala nadi* (the psychic nerve related to the right nostril, warming, masculine energy).

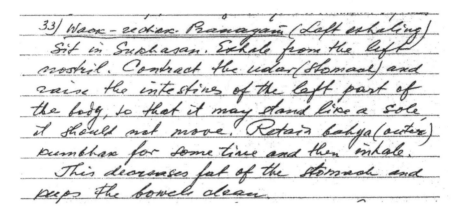

Figure 4.14. Letter from Swami Yogeshwaranand describing wack-rechak pranayama, undated.

Agni Pradipta Pranayama

Agni means "fire," and *pradipta* means "inflamed" or "burning." The element of fire represents heat as well as light. This pranayama produces tremendous heat in the body, and one will sweat during the practice. This means that it is beneficial for the removal of impurities, and it warms the body when it becomes too cold in the winter. Imagine meditating in a cave where the glacial headwaters form the Ganges River, high in the Himalayas. When we sit to meditate, our bodies can become cold in winter climates, because it involves little movement. This pranayama, as described to Hari by Swami Yogeshwaranand, can help to regain comfort and warmth in the body.

> Sit in Padmasan. Close the right nostril and inhale from the left. Fill the air down to the Muladhar, so that no portion be empty up to the kanth (throat). Retain kumbhak forcefully so that chest and face may become reddish. Be cautious, do not do much in the first time. Increase gradually the period of kumbhak. If you feel restlessness, then exhale from the right nostril gradually. Do not let the air go beyond kanth (throat), otherwise it may create unconsciousness.[177]

To prevent the "air" or prana from going upward beyond the throat, one could apply jalandhara and jihva bandhas. One possible reason for Hari's interest in agni pradipta could be the notable benefits. Swami Yogeshwaranand offered further clarification to this pranayama in several letters to Hari.

Charities, fasts and other meritorious deeds are not equal to even one-sixteenth part of this pranayama.[178]

While doing Agnipradipta Prana[yama], your abdomen should not be expanded too much. The expansion should be slight.[179]

Please do not strain or over strain your physical body.[180]

Chaturmukh Pranayama

Chatur means "four," and *mukh* means "face." Lord Brahma, the Creator, has four faces. Each face represents one of the four Vedas, the *Rik, Yajur, Atharva,* and *Sama Vedas*—the most ancient yogic texts known.

As explained earlier, jalandhara bandha puts a slight pressure on the carotid sinus, stimulating the sinus nerve and nerve impulses traveling to the brain. This is calming and possibly creates a trance-like state. The chaturmukh pranayama from Swami Yogeshwaranand is similar to jalandhara bandha in that pressure is put on the carotid sinus, but in this pranayama, this is done in four different directions.

The head moves in four directions (left, right, down, and up), each direction having a different effect on the nadis and the flow of prana. It is a method of breathing through the ida, pingala, and sushumna nadis without using the hand and fingers. One turns the head to the left, creating a slight pressure on the left side of the neck while extending the blood vessels along the right side. Repeat this to the right. Then, while looking straight ahead, lower the chin and then raise it, creating slight pressure on the front and back of the neck. There should be some force to the breath in order to create sound during the breathing. I notice when my head turns to the left, I can hear the breath more in my left ear than the right, and vice versa.

Here is Swami Yogeshwaranand's description of this pranayama for Hari.

Sit in kamal asan [the lotus pose], keep the body erect, turn [the face] toward the left shoulder. Inhale and then exhale immediately, without kumbhak. Try to exhale from the left nostril without the help of your fingers or hand. Now turn the face toward the right shoulder, inhale from both nostrils and exhale immediately from the right nostril without the help of fingers. While inhaling and exhaling, there should be some noise. Now turn the face down toward [the] Adams apple. Inhale forcefully from both nostrils, then keeping the face in the same position exhale with a force. Now turning the face ... up toward the sky, inhale and exhale. Repeat it 10–15 times and increase number according to your convenience. It is good for strengthen[ing] nerves and neck muscles. Gives peace to the mind. Purifies sounds of Ida and Pingala (nadis).[181]

Hridaya Stambha Pranayama

Hridaya stambha pranayama means "heart-stopping pranayama." This is a very advanced pranayama and not to be taken lightly, nor practiced without the strict guidance of a guru.

Hari mastered this technique, as reported in the 1937 Second Annual Report of the Divine Life Society, Latvian Branch.[182]

A renowned yogi named Deshbandhu intrigued medical professionals with his ability to stop his heart as in hridaya stambha pranayama. He could also stop the radial pulse in one wrist only, similar to how it is done using *nadi avarodha pranayama* (described below). Medical studies were conducted, and as far as they were concerned, the only plausible explanation was nerve control, as discussed earlier, but I will repeat it here because it is so important.[183]

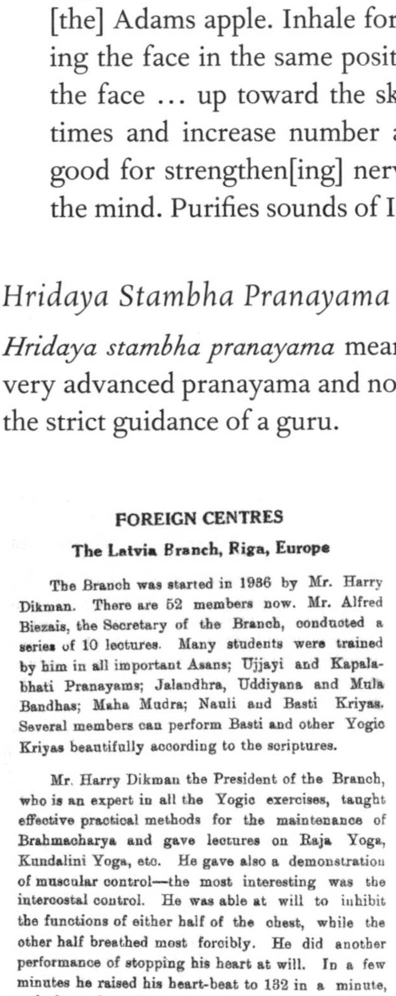

FOREIGN CENTRES

The Latvia Branch, Riga, Europe

The Branch was started in 1986 by Mr. Harry Dikman. There are 52 members now. Mr. Alfred Biezais, the Secretary of the Branch, conducted a series of 10 lectures. Many students were trained by him in all important Asans; Ujjayi and Kapalabhati Pranayams; Jalandhra, Uddiyana and Mula Bandhas; Maha Mudra; Nauli and Basti Kriyas. Several members can perform Basti and other Yogic Kriyas beautifully according to the scriptures.

Mr. Harry Dikman the President of the Branch, who is an expert in all the Yogic exercises, taught effective practical methods for the maintenance of Brahmacharya and gave lectures on Raja Yoga, Kundalini Yoga, etc. He gave also a demonstration of muscular control—the most interesting was the intercostal control. He was able at will to inhibit the functions of either half of the chest, while the other half breathed most forcibly. He did another performance of stopping his heart at will. In a few minutes he raised his heart-beat to 132 in a minute, and after a few minutes slowed it down to 21 beats in a minute. He suspended the action of his heart completely for four seconds.

Figure 4.15. Article describing Hari's demonstration at a meeting of the Latvian Yoga Society, at which he controlled and stopped his heartbeat, 1937.

Pranayama ... is, in effect, a process of bringing under control the Vagus nerve, over which, normally, we have no control. One can understand the importance of this control when one knows that all the vital forces are more or less under the control of the Vagus nerve and its centre: and when this is achieved by Yoga, there is said to be nothing in nature that cannot be brought under the control of the performer and all the forces of nature will obey him as his slaves.[184]

Paramhansa Yogananda could slow his heartbeat and completely stop the heart. Faye Wright, a devoted disciple of Paramhansa Yogananda, whom he later named Daya Mata, wrote to Hari about this in 1947.

Paramhansa wrote to you on May 8th answering the various questions listed in your letter to me. No doubt you have received the letter by this time. If not, another copy will be mailed to you. Paramhansaji is spending much more time in seclusion, writing and meditating. He is withdrawing from organizational activities as much as possible in order to devote more time to his writings, etc.

Paramhansaji has demonstrated many times the heart and muscle control of the body and doctors have examined him during such demonstrations, noting that the heart beat or pulse beat completely disappears, then returns at the will of Paramhansaji. Other times he has demonstrated slowing the heart down so that there are about six pulse beats a minute, sometimes more and sometimes less. He has also demonstrated withdrawing the current from the eyes so that when anything is quickly passed before them they are perfectly controlled and there is no sudden blinking of the eyes which is a natural reaction to quick movements near the eyes. You will be interested to learn, too, that Paramhansaji has trained a group of young disciples (boys) in the art of Hatha Yoga which they perform with remarkable mastery.

-2-

Thank you for your kind comments about my and other disciples' faithful service to the cause of Self-Realization Fellowship. It is little we can do in return for the manifold blessings we receive from God and the gurus. We have dedicated our lives to this search for God, and to serving Him through our works, and we rejoice that He is pleased to permit us this wonderful opportunity to so dedicate our lives, in the inspiring presence of one so holy as our Master.

With kindest regards,

Faye Wright

Figure 4.16. Letter from Faye Wright, later known as Sri Daya Mata, of Self-Realization Fellowship, July 11, 1947.

Paramhansaji has demonstrated many times the heart and muscle control of the body, and doctors have examined him during such demonstrations, noting that the heart beat or pulse beat completely disappears, then returns at the will of Paramhansaji. Other times he has demonstrated slowing the heart down so that there are about six pulse beats a minute.[185]

Dr. Swami Gitananda Giri was also adept at this practice, and he was adamant that it be done by experienced practitioners only. My dear friend William Phillips, a direct disciple of Swami Gitananda, said that he watched his guru perform this several times and that it was rather frightening! Swami Gitananda would lie down in *savasana* (corpse pose) and with a combination of jalandhara and mula bandhas, he would completely expel the air from his lungs, and his heartbeat stopped instantly.[186]

So why stop our heartbeat? Brother Bhaktananda from the Self-Realization Fellowship told Hari, "The only reason for learning how to control and stop the breath and heartbeat is that when they cease, one enters superconsciousness, and experiences the presence of God." He also reminded Hari that, "one practices spiritual techniques to learn to withdraw the life force from the senses at will. When one can do this, the techniques are no longer necessary."[187]

Paramhansa Yogananda wrote about this too.

The ultimate purpose of this lesson is not merely control of the heartbeat, but breath and heart control in order to focus the entire attention on God and thus enjoy ecstasy produced by contact with Him. Never do this exercise merely to control the heart, or for the demonstration-loving public. For that will divert your mind to the physical plane and overwork the heart. Control of the heart is useful when you are in deep Samadhi—in the ecstacy of the Joy or Divine Light. God appears to man as Cosmic Light, Cosmic Will, Cosmic Devotion, Cosmic Ever-New Bliss, Cosmic Vibration and Cosmic Love.[188]

Swami Sivananda suggested that he should focus more on raja yoga (meditation) than on achieving feats of hatha yoga such as stopping the breath or slowing the heartbeat, since "they are not really Yoga in the true spiritual sense of the term."[189] They can become distractions from the true goal: union with the Divine within. Hari was well guided by his teachers to stay on track.

- 3 -

```
far as possible.
       Kindly let thy sadhana tend more towards Raja Yoga than
towards Hatha Yoga alone. The stopping of breath, slowing of
heart-beat etc. are acheivements no doubt but they are not
really Yoga in the true spiritual sense of the term. That is
far more sacred a thing than mere yogic kriyas. To live on
little food and to sustain oneself upon the Cosmic Energy
will come to one at the proper time. When one progresses
in deep meditation he will spontaneously again remain
absorbed for days together with food or water. The meditator
gets mysterious sustenence from deep meditation itself.

       May God inspire you and bless you with sure success in
Sadhana.

                    With kind regards, Prem and OM,
```

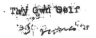

Figure 4.17. Letter from Swami Sivananda suggesting Hari focus more on meditation than on slowing his heartbeat, August 27, 1946.

Again, we are reminded that the siddhis, or powers, that we acquire as we advance in our yoga skill are not for show or for feeding the ego. No—they are to help us to know God. That is the ultimate goal of yoga: union with our highest Self. The pure, joyful bliss that we experience when we are able to withdraw from the distracting, outward-going senses and into the silence of the heart is truly what the effort is all about.

Please do not ever try hridaya stambha pranayama without the guidance of an adept teacher or your guru. It can be dangerous if done incorrectly. In his book *First Steps to Higher Yoga*, Swami Yogeshwaranand tells quite a story of practicing this pranayama without a guru or someone at his side. He lost consciousness through the process, and when he awoke, he was bleeding from his head. The story is worth reading.[190]

In the letter to Hari, Swami Yogeshwaranand warned him to be careful and not let the air pass toward *brahmarandhra*, the top of Brahma's canal, the place at the crown of the head where there is a soft spot in infants. This is very important. If you are not at a certain level of adeptness, you will not even comprehend what this warning means, let alone understand how to prevent it. Yoga practices reveal themselves in layers, as our understanding deepens through experience. If you don't understand something, you are not ready for it.

> Sit in Swastikasan, keep your backbone, chest, and neck straight. Press the right nostril with a forefinger and inhale from the left. Fill the air in the lungs. Now try to stop the heart beat by the pressure of the inside air. It is possible only when the air is filled so much that the chest may swell like a gnat. Now increase the pressure of the air by the will power and try to stop the heart beat. Be careful that the air may not pass toward brahmrandra [brahmarandhra], otherwise it will make unconsciousness instantly. By practicing it gradually, the heart beat slows down and stops eventually. This exercise must be done in the presence of the teacher, so that if it creates unconsciousness, he may treat it. In this pranayama, haste and hurry should be avoided. One should not try to stop the heart beat on the first day. It is attained after a long time. While doing the above, it should also [be] taken care that the air may not go toward the head. If it happens so, then exhale immediately. Hurry and impatience can do a lot of harm, it could even break the arteries and could damage the lungs. [If done properly,] it purifies the blood, develops control over breath and heart.[191]

Nadi Avarodha Pranayama

This is an advanced technique that the yogi Deshbandhu demonstrated for the Bombay Medical Union, showing his complete control over the flow of prana.[192] The purpose is to stop the pulse in a specific area of the body. *Avarodha* means "to block" or "to detain." So, in Deshbandhu's demonstration, using his mind, visualization, and nerve control, he directed the prana to his right arm and detained it there until the pulse stopped. This is an impressive demonstration of controlling prana and can be used in any area of the body. Only those with the utmost concentration of the mind and successful nerve control can achieve this. If the mind wanders at all, the energy will not remain contained. Swami Yogeshwaranand described to Hari his method.

Sit in padmasan. Close the right nostril and inhale from the left, make your hands in fists and put them on the knees. Now move the filled air by the force of your will power toward the right arm. Keep trying until the arm swells and pulse begins to stop. Afterwards do kumbhak and try to stop it completely. Until the pulse is … stopped, inhale briefly and transfer the air into the arm and retain kumbhak and again inhale briefly. Repeat it. When the air is filled in the arm, circulation of blood stops and the pulse does not beat. This pranayama could be done by standing also.[193]

Pranava Dhvanyatmaka Pranayama

Pranava is the sacred word *Om*. *Dhvan* refers to sound. *Atma* is the God within. To me, this pranayama is all about listening to the sacred Om, the sound of God within.

The *Mandukya Upanishad* refers to Om as "all." "OM. This eternal Word is all: what was, what is and what shall be, and what beyond is in eternity. All is OM."[194]

God is All. In a letter to Hari, Paramhansa Yogananda described the fullness of God so beautifully, it really touched my heart: "God is cosmic sound, cosmic light, cosmic vibration, cosmic love, cosmic ever-new joy, cosmic peace, cosmic wisdom, and cosmic ever-new bliss. These are the different expressions of God felt by the Yogi during ecstasy. The Yogis say that when the ears are closed and one hears the cosmic sound … [and] concentrates deeply upon that sound, he begins to develop omnipresence."[195]

Swami Sivananda Saraswati of Rishikesh explained to Hari, "Om is not only saying 'Yes'; but Om being a Great Mantra that pervades the three states of Consciousness and passing beyond, too, enables the affirmations to sink into the Subconscious and the Karana Shareera, too. Great Will Power is developed."[196]

The *Mandukya Upanishad* speaks of the four conditions of Om. First we envision the Om spelled Aum, representing all sound vibrations encompassed in the one sound of Om.

The *A* represents the waking state of outward-moving consciousness. Through the senses, we experience our manifested world. The *U* represents the dreaming state of inner-moving consciousness, where we enjoy the subtle inner elements. The *M* represents the sleeping state of silent consciousness, where we enjoy silent peace. Finally, the silence following the sounds of Om represents *Atman*, the awakened supreme consciousness.[197]

I first learned this pranayama without making any oral sound. Sit in va-jrasana (the "thunderbolt pose," with the spine very straight, so the kundal-ini can move up through the sushumna) with hands in *chin mudra* (tip of the index finger touching the tip of the thumb, palms facing downward). Breathe in, filling the lower, then middle, then upper lungs. Perform jalandhara and mula bandhas during kumbhaka. Release the bandhas when ready to exhale. Hear the inner sound of *A* as you empty the lower lungs, *U* as you empty the middle lungs and *M* as you empty the upper lungs.

The *A* energizes the prana from the toes to the lower abdomen, the *U* from there to the heart, and the *M* in everything above the heart. Repeat as often as you like, and then savor the deliciousness of the silence of the Om in its fullness. The bliss is indescribable.

Hari and Swami Yogeshwaranand communicated back and forth about this pranayama. It is a lovely technique. A soft Om sound is created during a gradual exhalation in this version from Swami Yogeshwaranand.

Sit in Kamalasan [the lotus pose]. Fill the air up to muladhar. Now parting the lips a little bit, produce the noise of Om. Exhale gradu-ally and deep, without breaking it. Concentrate on this produced sound and close your eyes. Increase the number of this exercise. Om should [be] pronounced—"O" for 40 seconds, "M" for 20 sec-onds. One forgets the world for hours when one concentrates on this sound. One gets peace and pleasure of mind and heart.

While exhaling, prana is raised from muladhara and up through the chakras just in front of [the] spinal column turn by turn and reaches the ajna chakra. The "gross prana" goes out through nos-trils and the subtle portion goes to sushumna.

When exhaling, add the nasal sound of "M" of AUM (ॐ) & try to listen [to] it & let your mind be allowed to be absorbed in it. Always, even at the time of inhalation, allow the breath to enter slowly, with perfect mastery, and take the prana together with the mental sound of AUM to muldahara & fix it there. [While inhaling] the course of "gross prana" goes through nostrils to lungs. Its subtle form or portion goes to vishu[d]dha chakra and then to the remain-ing chakras turn by turn to muladhara.[198]

Swami Sivananda added that when the kundalini is raised to a particular chakra at the commencement of a pranayama practice, it need not be brought down during rechaka or exhalation. On the final exhalation at the conclusion of the practice, one can gradually "will" her back down to muladhara. He also noted that some tantrik schools take the kundalini up and down with each pranayama.[199]

Vibhaga Pranayama

Dr. Swami Gitananda Giri taught *vibhaga pranayama* (sectional breathing) using *hasta* (hand) *mudras* to enhance the effects of the sectional breathing into the lower, middle, and upper lungs. These mudras actually control the physiological functions of the respiratory center at the medulla oblongata, known as the *aprakasha bindu*.[200]

Be aware that if you force a deep, full inhalation, you will indeed fill all three areas of the lungs, but if you simply breathe and watch, you will notice the subtleties as each area specifically receives the breath by using the hand mudras.

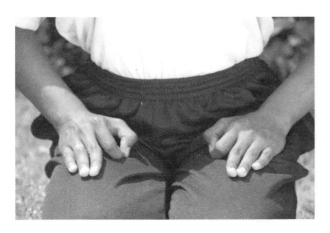

Figure 4.18.
Chin mudra.
Photo courtesy of
Yogacharya Dr.
Ananda Balayogi
Bhavanani.

To initiate breathing into the lower lungs, or *adham pranayama*, we use the *chin mudra*. Sit in vajrasana. Place the tips of the index fingers to the tips of the thumbs. Turn the palms down and place them near the hip creases at the top of each thigh. The remaining three fingers point slightly inward on the top of the thighs. This mudra is the "gesture of consciousness." Focus the mind on the *A* in Aum.

Now observe the breath as it enters and exits the lungs. You will notice the most receptive area for the breath is the lower lungs.

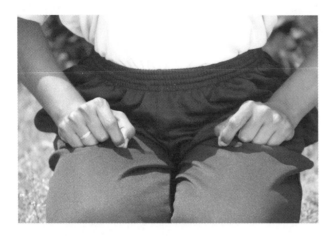

Figure 4.19. Chinmaya mudra. Photo courtesy of Yogacharya Dr. Ananda Balayogi Bhavanani.

To breathe into the intercostal or middle area of the lungs, known as *madhyam pranayama,* use the *chinmaya mudra.* Place the tips of the index fingers to the tips of the thumbs. Curl the remaining fingers into the palms of the hands, as if you were making a fist. Turn the palms down and place them near the hip creases at the top of each thigh. The chinmaya mudra represents "binding into the consciousness," the *U* in Aum.

Now observe the breath as it enters and exits the lungs. You will notice the most receptive area for the breath is the midchest area of the lungs. You can actually feel the ribcage expand.

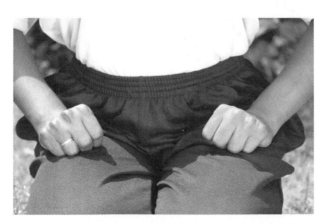

Figure 4.20. Adhi mudra. Photo courtesy of Yogacharya Dr. Ananda Balayogi Bhavanani.

For breathing into the upper lungs, known as *adhyam pranayama,* we use the *adhi mudra.* Place the thumbs into the palms of each hand and curl the fingers around the thumbs. Turn the palms down and place them near the hip creases at the top of each thigh. The adhi mudra represents "uniting with the highest," the *M* in Aum.

Observe the breath as it enters and exits the lungs. You will notice the most receptive area for the breath is the upper area of the lungs, beneath the collarbones.

To breathe into all three sections of the lungs, as in dirga or mahat yoga pranayama, we use *Brahma mudra* or *mahat yoga mudra* (gesture of grand integration). In Sanskrit, one of the oldest meanings of Brahma is "breath."

As in adhi mudra, you place the thumbs into the palms of each hand and curl the fingers around the thumbs. Then bring both hands at the navel, with the fingernails pointing upward.

Observe the breath as it enters and exits the lungs. Notice that all three segments of the lungs are open and receptive. First the lower lungs inflate, then the middle, and lastly the upper lungs. Brahma mudra brings it all together in complete union. It is the fullness of Om.

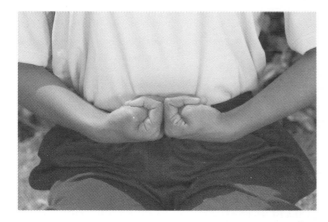

Figure 4.21.
Brahma mudra.
Photo courtesy of
Yogacharya Dr.
Ananda Balayogi
Bhavanani.

The yoga tradition teaches that the lower lungs feed the lower limbs with prana. The middle of the lungs feed the torso with prana, where our vital organs reside. The upper lungs feed the upper limbs, the head, and the brain with prana.

We can utilize the hasta mudras even further to control individual sections on either side of the lungs using *shunya mudra. Shunya* means "void," so using this mudra shuts down a specific section and concentrates the prana in another. For example, we can breathe predominantly into the upper left lung by putting the left hand into adhi mudra and the right hand into shunya mudra.

Shunya mudra is formed with the hand fully open and the palm facing upward. Put the right hand into shunya mudra and place it at the hip crease on the right thigh. Place the left hand in adhi mudra, palm facing down. Observe the breath as it enters and exits the lungs. Notice that the upper left lung is receiving the breath.

Shunya mudra can be used to individually isolate the three segments of the lungs on one side or to fully expand one lung by using Brahma mudra on the side we wish to inflate and shunya mudra on the side we wish to shut down.

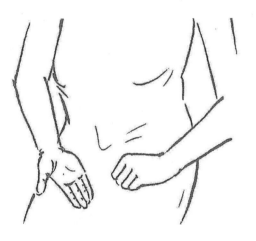

Figure 4.22.
Shunya mudra.
Drawing courtesy of
Yogacharya Dr. Ananda
Balayogi
Bhavanani.

One can gain even further control over the lungs by cross-breathing with these mudras. Putting the left hand in adhi mudra and the right hand in chin mudra will inflate the upper left lung and the lower right lung. Change and put the right hand in adhi mudra and the left hand in chin mudra. This will inflate the upper right lung and the lower left lung.

As with all yogic practices, the mind should be fully engaged in the process. Where the mind goes, the prana follows, so if the mind is wandering, the prana is not as concentrated as it could be.[201]

At times it is a great challenge to decide if a technique is a pranayama or a meditation. I make the classification based on this: if one is controlling or regulating the breath during the practice, then it is a pranayama (control of the prana). If one is allowing the breath to simply "be," without intentionally regulating the inhalation, exhalation, or retention, then I classify it as a meditation.

The remaining three techniques I have chosen to discuss are beautiful and tremendously beneficial for leading one's mind into meditation. I use the breath control to begin the process of reining in the mind, and then gradually I let go of controlling the breath and move into the bliss of meditation, allowing the breath to simply be.

Sarva Dvara Baddha Pranayama

Sarva means "all," *dvara* means "door or gate," and *baddha* means "bound." So sarva dvara baddha is a pranayama in which all the doors or gates from which prana can escape are closed. This pranayama uses yoni (or *shanmukhi*) mudra to close the gates of the senses and open the gate to the sushumna. The index fingers cover the eyes, the middle fingers press the nostrils, the ring fingers rest on the top lip, the baby fingers rest on the bottom lip, and the thumbs block the ears.

Swami Yogeshwaranand sketched out a brief description of the technique for Hari.

> Sit in Padmasan. Inhale and fill the air from muladhar up to the kanth (throat). Do kumbhak. Close the holes of ears with the thumbs, [eyes with the index fingers,] both nostrils with the middle fingers, and lips with the ring and little fingers. Concentrate in the centre of the eye brows. Retain kumbhak as long as you can and then [loosen] your [fingers] from the nostrils on exhale.[202]

The full technique is to breathe in, visualizing the prana flowing from the root chakra to the throat chakra. Retain the breath and apply shanmukhi mudra while concentrating on the ajna chakra. When ready, release the pressure of the middle fingers on the nostrils to allow for a slow, controlled exhalation. Release the power of the senses with the breath through both nostrils.

This pranayama will help lead one to pratyahara. When we withdraw from the senses and the outward-moving consciousness, we awaken the inward-moving consciousness and the divine light of the third eye. Awakening the third eye gives us knowledge of the Self, but as long as our attention is drawn outward through the senses, we are distracted away from this higher wisdom.

Sapta Vyahriti Pranayama

Mantras are sacred words of power. *Mantra* actually means "mind instrument," or a tool to protect one from the lower mind (which is the busy, ever-thinking mind). A mantra achieves this by creating more subtle thought waves and raising the vibration of our thought waves to a higher level, freeing us from the usual jibberish that goes on in one's mind. There is a quieter mind waiting beyond the thinking mind.

Sapta means "seven." *Vyahriti* means "statements" or "words." There are seven powerful mystical utterances, which are the names for each of the seven *lokas,* or worlds of existence. One combines the breathing with the repetition of these names, or mantras. This pranayama creates a very calm and sattvic mind, enabling deep *samyama* (concentration, meditation, and samadhi combined).

- *Om bhu* (earth or physical realm)
- *Om bhuvaha* (sky or astral realm)
- *Om svaha* (heaven or celestial realm, where the body goes at death)
- *Om maha* (cosmic realm—the abode of sages and enlightened beings)
- *Om janaha* (bliss realm, where we come to know Atman)
- *Om tapaha* (realm of discipline and strength where we come to know the Paramatman)
- *Om satyam* (realm of the ultimate Truth)

All seven are repeated mentally once during the long inhalation, and all are repeated mentally twice during the longer exhalation. It is a common practice to have your exhalation twice as long as your inhalation, as described by Swami Yogeshwaranand.

Sit in virasan. Inhale from the both nostrils gradually and do jap of 7 vyahritis while inhaling. While exhaling take so much time that these seven vyahriti could be repeated twice. Seven vyahritis are as follows. 1) om bhuh 2) om bhuvaha 3) om swah 4) om mah 5) om janah 6) om tapah 7) om satyamah.[203]

When greater control is achieved, the seven lokas can also be repeated four times during kumbhaka. With a one-second count per mantra, you would inhale for 7, hold for 28, and exhale for 14. This is a 1:4:2 ratio of inhalation, retention, and exhalation.

There is a variation of this pranayama using the short-form Gayatri mantra. The Gayatri mantra is very sacred and comes from the *Rik Veda*. You will recognize that it includes the first three lokas, or worlds, which relate to our physical existence. These are followed by the twenty-four syllable Gayatri verse calling on the divine sun, God-within, to illuminate our minds so we may know the Truth.

Repeat the short-form Gayatri mantra once during the inhalation, two to four times during kumbhaka (depending on your comfort level), and twice while exhaling. If you are not comfortable with the breath retention, then repeat the mantra on inhalation and exhalation, skipping the kumbhaka. Do not strain or you will lose the beautiful essence of the mantra. You must be able to savor the mantra comfortably, without struggle.

The short-form Gayatri mantra is this.

Om bhu bhuvaha svaha
Tat savitur varenyam,
Bhargo devasya dhimahi,
Dhiyo yonaha prachodayat

A third variation is to repeat the long-form Gayatri mantra once during the inhalation, two to four times during kumbhaka (depending on your comfort level), and twice during exhalation. If you are not comfortable with the breath retention, then only repeat the mantra on inhalation and exhalation. It is important that you are comfortable enough so you can savor the mantra. I am strongly attracted to this sacred, long-form Gayatri mantra, which includes all seven lokas. It is absolutely wonderful.

The long-form Gayatri mantra includes all seven lokas, addressing not only the three related to our physical world, but also those related to the spiritual worlds.

Om bhu
Om bhuvaha
Om svaha
Om maha

Om janaha
Om tapaha
Om satyam
Om tat savitur varenyam,
Bhargo devasya dhimahi,
Dhiyo yonaha prachodayat

Doing sapta vyahriti pranayama with the long-form Gayatri mantra at a 1:2:2 ratio means about 15 seconds for inhalation, 30 seconds kumbhaka, and 30 seconds for exhalation. This means one breath every 75 seconds.

Any variation on this pranayama is very absorbing, with every second being immersed in the sacred sounds. It is an absolutely beautiful and delicious practice.

Kevala Pranayama

I am placing *kevala* last among the pranyamas, because to achieve it you must master comfort in breath retention as well as absorption in meditation.

Sahita kumbhaka is any intended suspension of breath. All of the above pranayama have either no breath retention or an intentional one. As one gains control over the breath through pranayama, we are able to experience *kevala kumbhaka*, a natural, unintended suspension of the breath. This will often occur during times of deep concentration and meditation, if only for a few seconds. It is none other than the pause between the inhalation and exhalation, an absolute stillness of breath or natural stoppage, without effort. It occurs when the right and left nostrils (pingala and ida nadis) come into balance and the prana can move into the sushumna.[204]

The mind and the breath are so intimately connected that when we regulate the breath and slow it down, the mind will also slow down. If we hold the breath long enough, we will pass out, and the mind moves into unconsciousness. That is not the goal, but it demonstrates my point. When we regulate the breath as we do in pranayama, we are automatically regulating our thoughts. Thinking slows down and concentration becomes attainable. Longer pauses occur between the thoughts and between inhalation and exhalation. The complete, effortless, natural stoppage of breath means a complete stoppage of thoughts. According to Patanjali in his second sutra, "Yoga chitta vritti nirodha"—yoga is the suspension of the activities of the mind.

Swami Sivananda of Rishikesh told Hari, "This sudden cessation of Prana at that particular, crucial, psychological moment becomes of immense help to the Yogi in arresting the mind, which is already assuming the mood to Dharana. Hence, Kevala Kumbhak is an invaluable aid to Dhyana."[205]

The *Hatha Yoga Pradipika* states that mastery of this pranayama will rouse the kundalini, thus freeing the sushumna of all obstacles.[206] Here is Swami Yogeshwaranand's explanation of this pranayama:

> Kevali Pranayam. Sitting in posture of swastik asan, stop breathing without performing rechak or purak. In fact, there is no difference between stambh vritti (stopping) and kevali. One who could perform sahit kumbhaka with purak and rechak can perform kevali at ease.[207]

Watch and notice these lovely pauses as they appear for you. Enjoy the stillness at the top of the inhalation before exhalation and at the bottom of exhalation before inhalation. The slower and longer the breath, the less difference there is between movement and stillness. It is like the pause after the wave comes into the shore and before it heads back out to sea and like the pause out in the sea before the wave returns to the shore. The pauses at dawn before the start of day and at dusk before the darkness of night are both sacred times for pranayama practice. Stillness in breath equals stillness in the mind, and this stillness is where we can finally hear guidance from the Divine Will, the higher mind.

I know how important pranayama was to Hari. He practiced it regularly and encouraged me to do so as well. The practice will be met by many obstacles as we gently nudge up against the blockages in the nadis. These blockages manifest themselves in all sorts of ways—a stuffy nostril that will not open up, anxiety arising during kumbhaka, or impatience and annoyance while sitting. Working with breath retention can activate the sympathetic nervous system, resulting in fear. If you try to "just get through it," the practice will become frustrating. If you are gentle and patient with each obstacle as it arises, practice can become beautiful.

In the words of Ganga White, adopt the attitude "I get to do my yoga!" instead of "I have to do my yoga."[208] This pathway is a gift.

Chapter Five

MUDRAS
AND BANDHAS

WHEN WE CONSIDER THE EIGHT LIMBS OF YOGA of Patanjali's *Yoga Sutras*—yama, niyama, asana, pranayama, pratyahara, dharana, dhyana, and samadhi—we see that there is no specific limb for mudras and bandhas, yet they play a large role in yoga sadhana and the raising of the kundalini shakti.

According to the *Hatha Yoga Pradipika*, there are ten mudras and bandhas of great importance: *maha mudra, maha bandha, maha vedha, khechari, uddiyana bandha, mula bandha, jalandhara bandha, viparitakarani, vajroli,* and *shakti chalani*.[209] The jalandhara, mula, and uddiyana bandhas are essential not only to pranayama but also to the practice of the above mudras.

Asanas and pranayama work effectively with the gross physical body in preparation for the mudras and bandhas, which work on the energy body—the subtle body. Once asana and pranayama are perfected, they are uniquely combined to create mudras. Mudras are seals and bandhas are locks, which work together with pranayama, altering the normal nerve impulses, giving us control over the motor and sensory nerves,[210] such as the impulse of fear when we hold our breath for a long time. Ultimately, mudras and bandhas help to direct the prana into the sushumna, activate the kundalini, and raise her energy up through the chakras.

As described in the last chapter, on pranayama, the three main band-has—mula bandha, jalandhara bandha, and uddiyana bandha—are essential in joining prana and apana and then moving them into the sushumna. The jalandhara bandha moves the prana downward, the mula bandha moves apana upward, and when they join, the uddiyana prevents the co-joined prana from escaping. Prana is thus able to be drawn up through the chakras via the sushumna.[211] In this chapter, we will look at the other mudras discussed in the *Hatha Yoga Pradipika*.

Maha Mudra

According to the *Hatha Yoga Pradipika, maha mudra* destroys death and other sufferings from the *kleshas* (obstacles to enlightenment).[212] Hari taught me two ways to do this mudra. This first method starts with a ratio of 1:2:2 for inhalation, retention, and exhalation and later advances to a 1:4:2 ratio. Begin by sitting as in *janu sirsasana*, with the right heel pressing into the perineum to activate mula bandha and the left leg extended forward. In-hale with a slightly closed glottis, as in ujjayi pranayama. Retain the breath and lean forward, grasping the toes with both hands. Apply jalandhara and mula bandhas, as well as a slight uddiyana bandha, and focus on the ajna chakra. When ready to exhale, sit up straight, release the bandhas and exhale slowly—never fast. Repeat three times on each side, up to a maximum of forty times.[213] Be sure to do the same number of repetitions on each side.

Jalandhara bandha energetically presses the prana downward, and mula bandha pushes apana upward. As they join, the prana moves from ida and pingala into the sushumna with the support of uddiyana bandha. Having a straight spine as you lean forward is beneficial for the opening of the sush-umna. The *Hatha Yoga Pradipika* says the kundalini will stretch out like a snake that has been hit by a stick.[214]

Swami Narayanananda suggested it was best to grab the toes before in-halation and to exhale while holding the toes. He suggested practicing one, two, or three times on each side, alternating left and right sides each time.[215] He also said, "You have to concentrate your mind and [fix] the gaze between the eyebrows."[216]

Hari called the second technique *kriya maha mudra*. He said it was very powerful. Sit with the right heel folded into the perineum. Bend the left leg and draw the knee to the chest, keeping the foot on the floor. Pull the knee in tight as you inhale with ujjayi. Retain the breath and straighten the left leg out, bending forward over the leg. Hold as long as is comfortable. Rise up and pull the left leg into the chest again and exhale. Repeat on the opposite side. Then draw both knees tightly into the chest and inhale with ujjayi. Retain the breath and straighten both legs out, folding over them as in *paschimottanasana* (seated forward bend). Hold as long as is comfortable, then rise up and draw both knees tight into the chest again and exhale. Sit with a straight spine and concentrate on the ajna chakra.[217]

Madhavananda, an engineer and yogi from Bombay, said maha mudra and maha bheda mudra "are just wonderful to win over death and keep body young." He also suggested they are necessary after doing pranayama to help with blood circulation after sitting with crossed legs.[218]

Maha Bandha

This is similar to sitting in a half lotus position, but the left heel is pressed into the perineum. Place the right foot upon the left thigh. Inhale with ujjayi pranayama and retain the breath with all three bandhas. Concentrate on the sushumna. Having restrained the breath as long as possible, release the bandhas and exhale slowly. Repeat on the other side, with the right heel in the perineum and the left foot on the right thigh. Do three times on each side.[219]

Swami Sivananda advised Hari that in the process of kumbhaka during maha bandha, the belly is drawn upward, as in the slight uddiyana bandha that occurs naturally when the other bandhas are applied. During exhalation, the belly relaxes outward, and at the very end of exhalation, the belly is to be slightly drawn in again to make the exhalation complete.[220]

Hari gave three options for the placement of hands during maha bandha. Dhyana mudra has the hands in the lap, palms up, with the right hand resting in the left palm. Chin mudra is done with the thumb and index finger joined and the palms facing down, resting on the knees. Jnana mudra is done with the thumb and index finger joined and palms facing up while resting on the knees. There is a calming effect when the thumb and index finger join, which also symbolizes the joining of the *Jiva-Atman* (individual soul) and *Param-Atman* (Supreme Spirit).[221]

Swami Narayanananda affirmed that the inhalation and exhalation is through both nostrils but did not suggest ujjayi. He confirmed that while retaining the breath, the hands should be kept on the knees, and that this mudra should be repeated on each side up to three times.[222] He also suggested one should concentrate the mind on the kundalini shakti at the entrance of the sushumna nadi. "Think that the whole shakti has come to a point and ready to enter the sushumna."[223]

The *Hatha Yoga Pradipika* says that some avoid using jalandhara bandha here and instead press the tongue firmly against the upper palate in jihva bandha. This mudra prevents the prana from flowing through the numerous nadis, uniting ida and pingala nadis with the sushumna. (The prana enters the sushumna.) This mudra frees one from death and enables the mind to remain fixed at ajna chakra between the eyebrows.[224]

Maha Vedha

Traditionally, this mudra is done seated in the half lotus position, as in maha bandha. Hari suggested we sit in the full lotus, padmasana. The locked feet press the heels against ida and pingala nadis and make it much easier to bounce the body. Inhale with either ujjayi pranayama or surya bheda. The mind should be concentrated on either the muladhara or ajna chakra. Apply the bandhas during the breath retention. Now, place the palms on the ground on either side of you and raise the body off the ground, and then gently strike the ground with the buttocks, up to eleven times. Be careful not to hit the tailbone, only the fleshy areas of the buttocks. Then set the body down again, release the bandhas and exhale. Repeat a minimum of three times, increasing gradually up to eleven repetitions. Changing the position of the legs is good for physical reasons, but otherwise it is not necessary.[225]

This mudra causes the prana to leave ida and pingala and go into the sushumna, which leads to immortality. The body assumes a trance-like state. This mudra bestows great siddhis when practiced. Aging is held at bay, since wrinkles do not appear, hair does not turn gray prematurely, and tremors do not occur. Keeping the body healthy and vital is of great importance to a yogi, and therefore this mudra is highly esteemed.[226]

Alternatively, one can sit in the half lotus posture, as done in maha bandha. Swami Vishnu Tirth described this technique.

> The term Maha Vedha literally means great piercing. It is one of the ten chief mudras of Hatha Yoga. It is so named perhaps be-cause it is a combination of Padmasan, Sidhasan, Maha bandha and

Shakti-chalan. Like Sidhasan, your "stan" [or place—in this case, the perineum] is pressed by the heel of one foot, as for Maha bandha. The other foot is placed on the thigh of the first, as is done for Padmasan. For Maha Vedha, having seated in Maha bandha posture, the body is raised up and let fall alternately giving strokes on the heel or tossing the body to and fro for the purpose, and thus the kundalini is stimulated to activity.[227]

Do this first with the left heel in the perineum and right foot on the left thigh. Then change, with the right heel in the perineum and left foot on the right thigh. Repeat a minimum of three times on each side.

These three mudras are meant to be done together to move the prana into the sushumna, activate the kundalini, and manifest the siddhis. The *Hatha Yoga Pradipika* clearly states that maha mudra and maha bandha have no value without maha vedha.[228] It is worth noting that these mudras can be done by applying only the jalandhara bandha in the early stages. Later, when one is comfortable enough, all three bandhas (jalandhara, mula, and uddiyana) can be applied at once.[229]

Khechari Mudra

Kha means *akasha*, "space," and *chari* means "to move." The purpose is to stimulate the *soma nectar*, also known as *amrita*, that drips from the *soma chakra*, which lies above the roof of the mouth, between the ajna and sahasrara chakras. Sometimes it is called the *bindu chakra*. Preserving the soma nectar diverts it into the nadi system of the subtle body, which frees one from karma, disease, and death. Namadeva Acharya describes this process in his book *Chakra Mantras: Liberate Your Spiritual Genius through Chanting*.

Looking like a full moon when completely active this chakra has the function of speeding our journey back toward that place from which we have come. It is a major player in the achievement of immortality by the Ego-Mind Personality.

This chakra contains the etheric liquid called the *amrita* or nectar of immortality. In its active state, the chakra drops liquid down into the spine where it then is carried into the nadi system, the subtle body equivalent of veins and arteries.[230]

This nectar is normally dripping constantly and being consumed by the "sun," which lies in the area of the solar plexus—a triangle created between the navel and the two nipples. Curling the tongue into the space at the back of the throat creates a great heat in the body and causes the nectar to flow.[231] The yogi who captures this nectar with the mind concentrated on kundalini is said to cognize the Divine, and this cognition becomes word, or sweetness of speech, from the vishuddhi chakra. What a beautiful purification! One also becomes free from all diseases, sexual desires are sublimated, and siddhis are acquired.

In this mudra, the tongue is lengthened enough so that it can be folded back into the gullet and curled upward into the hole in the skull at the back of the throat. This closes the place where the three paths meet (nasal passage, pharynx, and trachea, or ida, pingala, and sushumna). This space is known as *vyoma chakra*.[232] The eyes are fastened upon the point between the eyebrows.

This is a controversial mudra, because it takes some time to lengthen the tongue naturally by "milking" it with the fingers. Many are too impatient, so they hasten the process by gradually cutting the frenulum under the tongue, a hair's breadth at a time. If this is done too quickly, one can end up with a speech impediment, or no speech at all! This method of lengthening the tongue is not recommended, because it is a dangerous procedure.

Swami Vishnudevananda said this mudra brings an artificial type of samadhi called *jada samadhi*, or inert samadhi. It cannot bring the highest experience or destroy desires. It is a way of trying to stop the prana without purification.[233] It is nevertheless a highly regarded mudra, with thirty verses of the *Hatha Yoga Pradipika* devoted to explaining the practice and its benefits (3:32–54 and 4:38, 44–49). Its benefits are considerable: approximately half an hour of khechari mudra saves a yogi from poisons, disease, old age, and death. Hari believed this mudra was critical to arrest the loss of and increase the absorption of the amrita nectar. We agreed, however, that there were much safer techniques of achieving the goal of this mudra, such as *amritpan khechari*.

Amritpan Khechari

Madhavananda described this alternative to the khechari mudra technique, *amritpan khechari*. *Amritam* is "nectar of immortality." The name of this technique means "to drink the nectar of immortality." It takes the aspirant into deeper and profoundly subtler regions, beyond the intellectual and analytical layer.[234]

Sit in a comfortable asana with closed eyes. Curl back the tongue to the best of your ability, as in khechari. Inhale from the manipura chakra to vishuddhi chakra in spinal passage, then exhale, making a hissing sound, like that of a cobra—with force—from the vishuddhi to the *lalana chakra* (an esoteric chakra above the soft palate at the back of the throat, and just below the ears, near the glottis). The mouth is closed, and the tongue is curled back the whole time. Repeat eleven times.[235] It is quite easy to make the hissing sound with the tongue curled back. This variation, known as amritpan khechari mudra, can be used as a substitute for khechari mudra at any time, with or without the hissing.

A little story comes to mind here. I was greatly impacted by Hari's behavior toward me as a young twenty-two-year-old. He was so humble, respectful, and kind to me. (It was easy to love him as a guru and not to question his directives. I would have washed his feet and drunk the water if he asked me to, but of course, he never would have asked such a thing! He was a shining example of a true yogi.)

After Hari passed away, I went to see an eighty-year-old yoga master in California, near San Francisco. He was astonishingly adept at his asanas, and I thought I could learn hatha yoga from him. After a few classes, he asked me to stay late one day to discuss something. He pulled out all the certificates he had been awarded for mastering yoga to show me how highly regarded he was. Then he tried to kiss me, claiming he wanted to taste my amrita nectar. At that moment, he revealed to me that no matter how well he had mastered his beautiful asanas, he had clearly not mastered his desires or his ego. Remember: always be discriminating. Not all "masters" are equal. That was the last yoga class I took with him.

Viparitakarani Mudra

Viparitakarani mudra is another way to capture the nectar from the soma chakra before it is consumed by the sun and causes the body to become old. The position is a half-shoulderstand, but of course, as mentioned earlier regarding mudras, it isn't so much the physical action that is important, but rather the energetic result.

In this mudra, the sun—the solar plexus—has reversed positions with the plexus for the moon above the palate. This reversal prevents the flow of the ambrosial nectar from the moon from dripping into the sun.

Lie on your back. Raise the legs up, as in *sarvangasana*, "shoulderstand," and rest the hips in the hands. The toes should be directly above the eyes. The body should not be straight, but rather angled at the hips, as they rest on the hands. The chest is not pressing against the chin, as it is in sarvangasana, so there is no restriction of the throat, allowing the prana to flow freely. You should be completely comfortable in this pose. Breathe and relax. Become aware of the reversed flow of prana. Practice this daily and gray hair will disappear, according to the *Hatha Yoga Pradipika*, indicating that the aging process is being arrested.

Hari added kumbhaka to this mudra. After inhalation, retain the breath and apply either amritpan khechari mudra or jihva bandha by pressing the tongue against the upper palate and sealing the back of the throat. This prevents the nectar from falling down through the ida and pingala into the sun. Mula and uddiyana bandhas can also be applied.[236] During this breath retention, one can visualize the flow of prana progressively from the manipura chakra at the solar plexus to the anahata, vishuddhi, ajna, soma, and sahasrara chakras. Exhale slowly and feel the flow of energy going to the crown of the head.

Swami Vishnudevananda advised Hari not to practice this mudra in the evening hours.[237] Madhavananda says that viparitakarani is helpful for complete physical rejuvenation, a correct and balanced flow of hormones secretion, and mental strength.[238] It is not known if this nectar from the soma chakra is a hormonal secretion, but it is understood by yogis to be a psychic or energetic secretion. Swami Sivananda of Rishikesh said amrita is not a physical substance—it is the subtle shakti in the prana.[239] Some things are not clearly understood until our consciousness is ready to receive it.

Vajroli Mudra

Vajra means "thunderbolt" in Sanskrit. *Vajroli mudra* stimulates the genitals with prana-activated blood. In this mudra, there is a constriction of the urethral muscles—the same muscles used to cut off the flow of urine—combined with uddiyana bandha. This mudra strongly influences the nadis that supply the sex organs with spiritual energy. After some practice, a man can retain the energy from the semen even when ejaculating, and women can preserve the secretions from orgasm. The belief is that this preserved energy can be used for health and spiritual growth.

Generally, as human beings, we live completely diverted by our senses. It takes many years to understand that the pleasures of the senses are drawing us away from our beautiful true Self within. They create such diversion. Brahmacharya teaches us to moderate these pleasures so we gain control over them, rather than allowing the senses to control us. Pratyahara helps us to draw our attention inward and away from them. Through these practices, we are eventually able to have a peaceful mind and successful meditations.

We dwell at a lower vibratory level when the kundalini is dormant at the base of the spine. At this level, the sexual energy is focused on the purpose of procreation. When kundalini is activated, our vibratory level becomes finer, and we move beyond the basic human needs of the three lower chakras and into the spiritual chakras, where we begin to align with our spiritual nature. Here the sexual energy can be transformed for spiritual purposes, but only when one is ready. Vajroli mudra is one of the yogic techniques used by celibates to transform this energy (see Chapter 2, Hari and Brahmacharya, page 41).

Suppression of sexual energy does not work—sexual energy must be transformed, not suppressed, otherwise it will find another outlet for expression, and that is usually not a positive event. Yoga practices transform the energies of our lower nature and enable us to reach the goal of yoga—union with our true Self, the Spirit within.

Shaktichalani Mudra

Shakti is a name for kundalini, and *chalani* means "to manipulate, shake, churn, or rotate." *Shaktichalani* thus means "to move the shakti" or " to move kundalini." This term is used for many different practices in which the shakti is rotated, churned, or manipulated. In essence, it is any exercise for moving the kundalini shakti. With the above mudras, we attempt to channel the prana into the sushumna and awaken the kundalini; now we want to move her.

Technique one: One interpretation of the method described in the *Hatha Yoga Pradipika* is surya bheda pranayama or other pranayamas that "manipulate" the shakti.[240] Heat is generated when we inhale through the pingala nadi on the right, which helps to activate the kundalini. The ida and pingala nadis (left and right nostrils) are manipulated when we move back and forth between them. Sit in vajrasana or siddhasana. Inhale through the sun (pingala nadi) and retain the breath according to your comfort. Exhale through the moon (ida nadi). Use a ratio of 1:4:2. Manipulate the shakti in this manner for an hour and a half at dawn and at dusk.

Technique two: Bhastrika pranayama is one of the most powerful ways to raise the kundalini. Sit in siddhasana or padmasana. Hold the feet firmly with the hands and perform rapid inhalations and exhalations successively. The inhalation and exhalation should have an equal force, as in a blacksmith's bellows. After ten or twenty repetitions, or whatever is comfortable for you, inhale and hold the breath with bandha traya (jalandhara, uddiyana, and mula bandhas). Bounce the body up and down, as in maha vedha, so the prana moves up the sushumna to brahmarandhra (the spot at the crown of the head where there is a soft spot in infants). Then exhale and contract uddiyana bandha to continue drawing the energy upward.[241]

Technique three: Arthur Avalon wrote in *The Serpent Power* that "Shakti-calana is the movement of the abdominal muscle from left to right and right to left; the object being to arouse Kundalini by this spiraline movement."[242] While seated in siddhasana, inhale deeply and join prana and apana. Pull the rectus abdominis muscles from side to side to create a churning of those muscles (see dakshina and vamana rechaka pranayama in chapter 4 for more detail). Contract the anus in ashvini mudra repeatedly until the prana enters the sushumna. Breath retention and the mantra *Hum Hamsah* cause the kundalini to rise upward to the sahasrara chakra.[243]

Technique four: Swami Venkatesananda offered a more subtle variation of shaktichalani. "Inhalation through the right nostril, a brief retention followed by exhalation out the left nostril. Then movement of the abdomen from right to left and left to right, which is dynamic nauli kriya but not the rotary movement. The movement is 'experienced' more within and less observable externally than the nauli kriya. [Repeat] by left nostril. The purak-kumbhak-rechaka can be repeated every few minutes."[244]

This nauli technique can be done seated or standing. After exhalation, the breath is held out while the shakti is manipulated by drawing the rectus abdominis back and forth, similar to what was described in madhya, vamana, and dakshina rechaka pranayamas, but with less force.

Technique five: Madhavananda offered a technique of shaktichalani that is a rotation of consciousness rather than a physical rotation. Sit in padmasana or siddhasana. Close the eyes, resting your hands on the knees. Inhale the breath from muladhara chakra to *bindu chakra*. (The bindu chakra is at the back of the head, directly behind the ajna chakra. Some say this is the source of the soma nectar.) Raise the head and close the seven gates (two eyes, two ears, two nostrils, and the mouth) with your hands, as in yoni mudra. Retain the breath and mentally lower your consciousness back to the muladhara chakra in the spinal passage, and then raise your consciousness up through the front passage of the spine. Rotate your consciousness like this as many times as you can during one breath retention. Come back to the bindu chakra and exhale, lowering your consciousness down the spinal passage to the muladhara chakra. Repeat mentally "muladhara" three times and start the second round. Repeat this complete cycle five times.[245]

Madhavananda said, "It is something like a child—he first learns to stand and manipulate balance at one place. The next step is to learn to start walking. Now he can make this balance dynamic—he moves, yet maintains balance. In the same way here, we rotate our consciousness."[246]

Order of Practice: Abhyasa Krama

Swami Vishnudevananda advised Hari to do his sadhana practice in this order: "First asana should be practised, ending in Savasan. Secondly, [uddiyana] and [nauli] should be practiced. Then comes pranayama. This is done by starting with sukha poorvat [sukha purvak], Ujjayi, and Bastrika, etc. Then Mahamudra, mahabhanda [sic] and Mahaveda should be practiced. These are the abhyas kramas."[247]

Swami Shivananda Saraswati of Assam advised Hari of a different order to perform the bandhas and mudras: first mula bandha, then maha bandha, maha mudra, then shaktichalani, and lastly maha vedha.[248]

Practices vary from school to school, lineage to lineage, and student to student. It is simply the way that the guru has found works the best from his or her perspective.

These next mudras are important for moving inward. They are helpful for pratyahara, dharana, dhyana, and samadhi, the last four limbs of Patanjali's yoga.

Yoni or Shanmukhi Mudra

Yoni mudra is a technique we use to block out the senses in order to go inward. Our senses are constantly drawing us outward through sounds we hear, things we see, scents we smell, and so forth. This mudra will lead us to a state of pratyahara and eventually to meditation. It is also called shanmukhi mudra, a name that describes more clearly what the process looks like.

Swami Sivananda said that yoni mudra enables one "to develop intense concentration, inward, free from external distractions. Gradual steady practice gives spiritual vision. This is meant by 'seen'. Kuthastha [supreme changeless soul] and other subtle points of Sukshma Sarira [astral body] cannot be seen by the fleshy eye."[249]

Shan means "six," and *mukhi* means "face," "mouth," or "gate," so we are blocking six "gates" of the face through which we lose prana through the wandering senses. (Some say there are seven gates, when both nostrils are counted, as described in technique five of shaktichalani mudra.)[250]

With our thumbs we block the ears, the index fingers gently cover the eyes, middle fingers block the nostrils, the ring fingers close the upper lips and baby fingers close the lower lips. The fingers over the nose will seal the nostrils only when one is holding the breath. When inhaling or exhaling, they are relaxed, but still held in place.

Swami Venkatesananda described a beautiful technique of combining yoni mudra with the hamsa mantra on inhalation and kumbhaka, while the soham mantra is repeated on exhalation. He began by noting that the mantras do not go as high as the sahasrara chakra.

No special Mantra has been mentioned for the Sahasrara. In fact, it is not regarded as a Chakra at all, it being the culmination of the dhyana itself, and that psychic abode of all the shaktis dwelling ordinarily in all the six lower chakras. It is unusual to meditate upon the lotus feet of the Satguru or the Supreme Siva in that chakra, if it is regarded as such. The Paduka Panchakam which you will find in THE SERPENT POWER describes this.

When, with Yoni Mudra you have taken the shakti to the Ajna, the Yoni Mudra itself may be abandoned and, with the hands dropped on the lap, meditate; and during this meditation, visualise the consciousness linking the Ajna with the lotus feet of the Guru in the sahasrara. When this is achieved, then with the further inhalation and exhalation, it is easy to feel the power flowing up and down this channel, i.e., the grace of the Guru flowing into the Ajna. The Mantra used in this is one's Ishta Mantra or Soham or Om.

The "Hamsah" mantra is associated with the ascent of the shakti, which itself takes place with every new inhalation. The "Soham" mantra is used only when the shakti descends, in the Yoni Mudra practice. The shakti descends to the Ajna before going further down. If the explanation concerning the sahasrara is clear, then you will realise that the sadhaka of his own accord is not in a position to take the shakti beyond the Ajna, only divine grace can do so. Hence, the shakti for our practical purposes is at the Ajna, imbibing the Grace of Guru. The descent commences therefore from the Ajna.

Even the "walking stick" does not cover the Sahasrara! (I have requested a friend in Sydney to send you a diagram). Sahasrara is beyond; its nature, etc., are not within the powers of intellect and speech. In physiological terms, the psychic channel perhaps includes the pineal and the pituitary glands and perhaps the mid-brain before descending along the spinal column."[251]

Some texts do not include the kumbhaka, but Swami Venkatesananda assured Hari that his Gurudev Swami Sivananda of Rishikesh recommended kumbhaka, because it seemed to enhance the powers of concentration facilitated by yoni mudra.

The texts do not mention kumbhaka. But Gurudev recommended kumbhaka, which does seem to enhance the powers of concentration facilitated by the yoni mudra. The mantra hamsah is to be repeated during the kumbhaka.... While descending from the sahasrara Padma, we use "soham," and it is uttered just once during the recaka; in the same way, the mantra "hamsah" is uttered only once during the [puraka] or when the recaka is complete and there is external kumbhaka during the ascent to the sahasrara.[252]

Sometimes yoni mudra is practiced with the Pranava Om sound. Inhaling through both nostrils, press the middle fingers to close the nostrils and hold the breath for as long as is comfortable, then exhale out the mouth, saying one long Om for the duration of the exhalation. Repeat this process over and over, immersing yourself in Om vibrations.

Swami Yogeshwaranand suggested Hari inhale through the mouth in *kaki* (crow's beak) mudra. This is done by pursing the lips as though you were going to whistle through them. The kaki mudra helps to "reduce the internal superfluous heat created during this technique, which can be detrimental to your health."[253]

Breathe in through the pursed lips. Close the mouth and do kumbhaka. Press the inhaled air toward the muladhara chakra and contract the mula bandha upward. Mentally say Om, using the mental power of thoughts to consider that kundalini has illuminated and light is traveling upward to the *sahasrara dala* (head), piercing through and illuminating all the chakras. Perceive the light passing through the spinal cord, illuminating the spine. Sometimes the light stops traveling after reaching two or three chakras. If it does so, contract mula bandha again.[254] With mental effort, try to throw or transmit the light upward toward sahasrara. After feeling the exertion of kumbhaka, exhale through the nose only. Take a complete rest, so you will be fully prepared to do a second practice if you wish. The time to be spent in one practice depends upon the strength and energy of the body. You can repeat it if your body allows it.[255]

Swami Kriyananda explained to Hari, "The senses become naturally disconnected one by one, the deeper one goes into meditation. Touch is the first to go. As one becomes accustomed to the process, he can consciously withdraw the energy from the senses one by one, and remain just as disconnected from the body as he chooses to be."[256]

Yoni or shanmukhi mudra is also used in the practice of bhramari pranayama, as described in chapter 4, "Pranayama." This practice will help to calm the mind and take one to a state of pratyahara. When we are able to block the five senses, we go inward and open ourselves up to the sixth sense. The spiritual light of true knowledge then begins to become known.

Shambhavi Mudra

The *Hatha Yoga Pradipika* tells us that the yogi who practices *shambhavi mudra,* or any of the other mudras, will acquire various siddhis.[257] It is often refered to as "eyebrow gazing." Shambhu is a name for Shiva, who has his third eye open. Shambhavi is the feminine form of the name Shambhu, as if the feminine Shakti is being drawn to the third eye to meet with Shiva. The *Hatha Yoga Pradipika* says this mudra is guarded like a respectable woman and approached by few.[258] A preparatory exercise for shambhavi mudra is *tratak* (candle gazing). While gazing at a candle flame, the yogi tries not to blink. This helps concentration and limits intruding thoughts. It prepares the eyes for staring blankly for an extended length of time without blinking and trains the mind to not become attached to what it "sees."

For shambhavi mudra, sit in a comfortable asana. Keep the spine straight and rest your hands on the knees. Soften the eyes and stare ahead blankly, seeing nothing. Hold the gaze steady, without blinking. When you feel ready, turn the eyes upward toward the space between the eyebrows, the ajna chakra. Do not force them—keep the action gentle. Continue to sit in this fashion as long as is comfortable, reining in the mind whenever you catch it wandering. If your eyes become tired, you can close them for a bit, but you should maintain the focus toward the ajna chakra in the dark space surrounding your closed eyes. When the eyes are rested, open them and repeat the process. Upon completion of the practice, rub your hands together and place the warm palms over your eyes to help relax the muscles around the eyes.

Swami Sivananda of Rishikesh said to Hari that he may notice "lights" when he concentrates on the ajna chakra.

> Let the lights come but pay no heed to them. Fix your entire attention on the Lotus and especially on the bija OM [the seed sound Om]. This is the key to Atma Gyana [knowledge of the God within]. The lights may mislead you. They are just encouraging signs reassuring the Yogi that he is progressing well in Yoga. Beyond that they have no purpose. When the mind gets merged in the Ajna, then you will enjoy an indescribable bliss; you will then be one with the Light of lights, enveloping the entire universe. When this Atmic Jyotis [light of the Atman] appears, you will have no extraneous thoughts. You will be perfectly calm and blissful.[259]

```
      Concentration on the Ajna Chakra:  Let the lights come:  but
pay no heed to them.  Fix your entire attention on the Lotus and
especially on the Bija OM.  This is the key to Atma Gyana.  The
lights may mislead you.  They are just encouraging signs reassuring
the Yogi that he is progressing well in Yoga.  Beyond that they
have no purpose.  When the mind gets merged in the Ajna, then you
will enjoy an indescribable bliss:  you will then be one with the
Light of lights, enveloping the entire universe.  When this Atmic
Jyotis appears, you will have no extraneous thoughts.  You will
be perfectly calm and blissful.
```

Figure 5.1. Letter from Swami Sivananda regarding shambhavi mudra, April 7, 1948.

Swami Yogeshwaranand suggested that this mudra helps one to acquire knowledge of the causal body.

> Sit straight by any Asana on which you have a mastery. Look straight with open eyes without any movements of lids, without any aim in

front. Meditate on LING (KARAN) (causal) body situated in the heart.
The main idea is to keep eyes open and meditate on [the] heart for
acquiring knowledge of [the] causal body. It is a definite practice.[260]

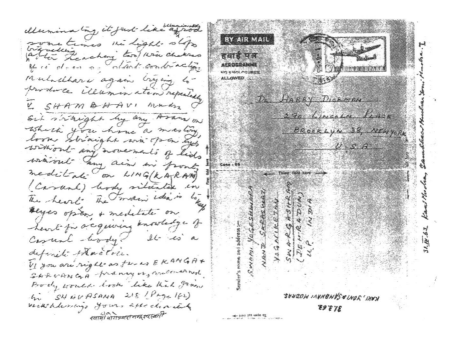

Figure 5.2. Letter from Swami Yogeshwaranand explaining shambhavi mudra,
March 31, 1963.

Why is acquiring knowledge of the causal body important? It is said
we have three bodies. The physical body, or *sthula sharira*, is made of molecules—muscles, bones, blood, and so forth. This physical body is brought
to life through prana entering the body. Without prana, the physical body is
lifeless. The subtle or astral body is the *sukshma sharira* or *linga sharira*. As
breath flows in the physical body, prana flows through the astral body. The
astral body is a replica of the physical body, with prana flowing through the
chakras and nadis just as information or nerve impulses flow through nerves
and ganglia in the physical body.

The third body is the causal body, the *karana sharira*. This causal body
is the "seed" body, which carries the seeds of our learnings from one lifetime to the next; these reside in the unconscious mind. If we accomplished

asana in a past life, we may be extremely flexible in this lifetime. Or, if we become a master at playing the piano at a very young age, it is a sign that this knowledge was carried forward from a past life. There are many more subtle things we have learned in the past, and, when the environment is right, they are "remembered."

This is how we have déjà vu moments of remembering. Erich Schiffmann says that when we meet people and we feel we have known them before, it is because we have! Our spirit within "recognizes" them, even if our mind does not—we can feel that we know them.

Swami Narayanananda said, "Kundalini Shakti is not a mere blind energy. It is a conscious energy. It is the cause of all mind Powers. All the powers of the mind belong to the Kundalini Shakti. So, Kundalini Shakti by Its infinite powers retains multifarious thought impressions in the causal state."[261] Spiritual knowledge comes to us in many ways and removes the veils of ignorance.

Madhavananda described a beautiful shambhavi mudra technique.

Sit in asana with the eyes closed. Go to the Muladhara Chakra and inhale, raising your consciousness in spinal passage up to the Sahasrara Chakra, and then with retention stay there. Try to open like a lotus flower. Then, with exhalation descend back down to the Muladhara. Imagine the green stem of the lotus coming down the sushumna and in Muladhara there is the root of the stem. Now stay in the Muladhara Chakra with meditation for small time. Repeat if time.[262]

This visualization with the mudra reminds me of an amazing experience I had when Namadeva Acharya initiated me into the long form of the Gayatri mantra. I settled into the chair beside Namadeva, and he started to say the sacred mantra to my left ear, adding my chosen *bija* mantra at the end of each repetition. He said it over and over again. I have no idea how long he said it, as time disappeared. In the midst of the mantra, I felt something like a green beanstalk (for lack of a better description) growing from my feet upward through my body and out my arms and ears, eyes, and head. Immediately, the green turned to gold, and it was as though every nadi in my body was filled and overflowing with vibrant gold! When it was over, I was completely blissed out. I have marveled over the amazing joy I experienced ever since!

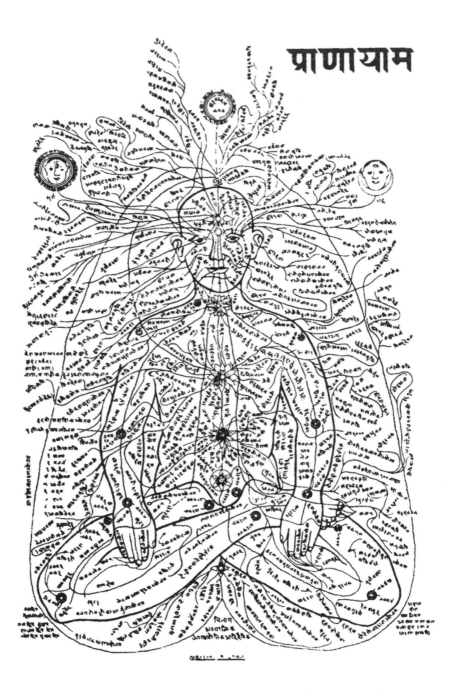

Figure 5.3. Classic drawing of the nadis. Circa nineteenth-century Tibet (attributed to the prophet Ratnasara).

Mudras in Pranatasana

Dr. Francisco Luid (Swami Tirthananda Saraswati) taught us three very important mudras at the 2005 International Yoga Teachers Congress in Barcelona, Spain: the mudras for emotional and psychic balance and the mudra for humility. I find them to be very useful to follow at the end of my practices.

As we deepen our yoga practices, we may find emotions begin to rise from the svadhisthana chakra. As we begin to purify our hearts, the emotions can rise up and be somewhat overwhelming. This mudra will help us to stay balanced through the process. Kneel on the floor and fold forward into child's pose *(pranatasana)*. Place your hands, with palms open, under your face, so your face rests in the palms of your hands. This is *pushpaputa mudra,* the mudra for emotional balance.[263]

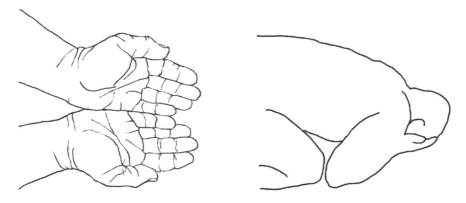

Figure 5.4. Pushpaputa mudra: gesture of offering a handful of flowers to the Divine. The face is placed into the palms of the hands while kneeling in child's pose. Drawing by Jo C. Willems.

When we purify our minds and move into the psychic realm of the higher chakras, we may find ourselves feeling skeptical or somewhat unstable. Kneel into pranatasana (child's pose) and make a triangle with your thumbs and index fingers touching. Place the palms down on the floor in front of you and put your third eye into the triangular space you have created. This is *trimurti mudra* (also called *surya prana mudra*), the mudra for psychic balance. This mudra helps us find balance as we move through the process of opening the third eye. You can use this to balance any psychic disturbances.[264]

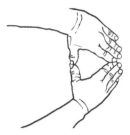

Figure 5.5. Trimurti mudra: having three forms (balance within the cosmic dance of Brahma, Vishnu, and Shiva). This mudra is also known as surya prana mudra, the gesture of perceiving the solar energy. The mid-brow area of the forehead rests on the triangle created by the hands. Drawing by Jo C. Willems.

The third mudra from Dr. Francisco Luid is *saanjali mudra,* the mudra for humility. I suggest all yogis should practice this mudra regularly, as the ego is the greatest enemy on the path, claiming for its own all progress and victory in yoga, when in truth victory belongs to the soul.

Kneel into pranatasana (child's pose) and extend the arms overhead with hands in *namaskara mudra* (prayer position). The ajna chakra rests on the floor. Offer yourself as a vehicle of transmission for the True knowledge to be shared with others. Let your thoughts be humble and your actions be for the good of all.[265]

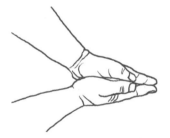

Figure 5.6. Saanjali mudra: gesture of offering one's own self. Drawing by Jo C. Willems.

There are many more mudras than the ones I have explained here. There are hand mudras and all kinds of various full-body mudras. It is important to remember that they are powerful techniques reserved for those who have prepared themselves through the previous stages of yoga. As mentioned earlier, they are not just physical poses; they are a way of working with the pranic energy, and in order to do them correctly, one must be prepared and be of healthy body and mind, have cleansed the nadis, be living the yamas and niyamas, and be guided by a skilled and experienced teacher.

Chapter Six

PRATYAHARA
AND DHARANA

THERE ARE EIGHT LIMBS in Patanjali's ashtanga yoga (*asht* means "eight," *anga* means "limbs"). The first limbs—yama, niyamas, asana, and pranayama—are considered yoga of the outer limbs, or *bahiranga yoga*. Hari referred to dharana, dhyana, and samadhi as *antaranga yoga,* or yoga of the inner limbs. The debate is where does pratyahara belong? Patanjali included pratyahara with the inner limbs, but Yajnavalkya (a seventh-century sage and philosopher of Vedic India) considered pratyahara the last stage of *bahiranga yoga,* yoga of the outer limbs. Hari agreed with Yajnavalkya.[266]

I have come to view pratyahara like a very important bridge between the outer and inner stages of yoga. The more we are able to withdraw from the outward-going activity of the senses, the more we are able to enter into the inner stages of yoga.

Hari mastered many of the physical practices of hatha yoga, but when I was with him, these were not the focus of his teachings. We spent much more time on philosophy and practicing the inner stages of yoga—dharana, dhyana, and samadhi. This progression from hatha yoga to raja yoga is to be expected. Swami Shivananda Saraswati of Assam offered an explanation.

As far as I remember, in my previous letter, I wrote you about the different stages of human mind. Thus there are the lower mind or restless mind, the concentrated mind, the aspiring mind, the pure mind, the intuition mind, the Divine mind, and the Super mind. Hatha yoga can help us only up to the level of concentrated mind and aspiring mind.... Then we have to work for purifying our mind, and this process for purifying the mind [is the] chief aim of Raja yoga, Jnana yoga, Bhakti yoga, and Karma yoga, etc.[267]

How do we purify the mind? The yamas and niyamas are the essential tools, as explained by Swami Sivananda of Rishikesh.

Side by side with instructions of practical Yogic processes, place always stress upon the great importance of Sadachara [right conduct], Yama and Niyama. Inspire the students with the noble idealism. Spur them on to strive for a life of lofty virtue, active goodness, and selflessness. You must stress the need for self-purification and self-mastery. But the true inner Yoga is the transformation of the essential nature of man. The lower human nature should gradually give place to an illumined divine nature through a process of spiritualization of the entire being of man. This should be brought home in an effective manner, yet with great sympathy, understanding and insight. The aim is to attain divine consciousness.[268]

The Chakras as Transmitters of Energy

This speaks to me of how the seven chakras relate to the stages of the human mind, of which there are also seven. If we are spirits expressing ourselves through form, then the chakras are transmitters of human energy or consciousness at any given moment during our development as yogis.

The *muladhara chakra* is concerned with survival and a sense of belonging. Our basic needs of food, clothing, and shelter must be met, or we will be preoccupied with them, and this will be reflected in our behavior. We must establish roots for a solid foundation. This chakra relates to the restless mind.

With ample food and a roof over our heads, we can become creative. The *svadhisthana chakra* is a center of creativity and procreation. We are generally very focused when creating art or music, writing, and engaging in sex. Sensual pleasures distract us unless they are restrained. This chakra relates to a concentrated mind.

The *manipura chakra,* in the solar plexus area, is where our prana, or life force, is accumulated and stored. It is a center of power and the will to achieve our goals. The aspiring mind relates to this chakra.

These are the three lower chakras, which relate to our physical presence in the material world. According to Swami Shivananda Saraswati of Assam (quoted above), this is as far as hatha yoga can take us. Since hatha yoga is a physical practice, we must change our sadhana from physical to spiritual in order to move into the spiritual chakras. Here is where raja yoga, jnana yoga, bhakti yoga, and karma yoga become important pathways. Through these yogas, we are able to move toward understanding the spirit within and to achieve Oneness.

The *anahata chakra,* or the heart center, is a special place. It is widely understood that the soul resides in the region of the heart. The soul is pure and loving and benevolent. The *Chandogya Upanishad* speaks of this region beautifully.

> There is a Spirit that is mind and life, light and truth and vast spaces. He contains all works and desires and all perfumes and all tastes. He enfolds the whole universe, and in silence is loving to all. This is the Spirit that is in my heart, smaller than a grain of rice, or a grain of barley, or a grain of mustard-seed.... This is the Spirit that is in my heart, greater than the earth, greater than the sky, greater than heaven itself, greater than all these worlds.[269]

The heart center is a center of choice; it is where we choose to dwell in the lower, earth-related chakras or to move into the spiritual realm of the higher chakras. The more we get to know who we really are, the more we will be inspired to know our spiritual selves, and the more the higher chakras will be awakened. The heart center is known as the "unstruck sound," or silence. This is where we hear the inner sounds of the spirit. The pure mind relates to this chakra. The more pure our mind is, the more pure our intentions become, and the more we are able to comprehend the spirit.

The *vishuddha chakra,* at the throat, reflects the power of one's voice. We can make someone's day or completely destroy it just by something we say. The more we purify the heart center, the kinder our words will be. Our voice powerfully reflects our consciousness.

For many, sound is the first expression of God.

In the beginning was the Word, and the Word was with God, and the Word was God.[270]

OM. This eternal Word is all; what was, what is and what shall be, and what beyond is in eternity. All is Om.[271]

The throat chakra relates to hearing the intuition mind. The more we delve into the realm of the higher chakras and the more our hearts open, the more we awaken the intuitive mind and are able to experience it.

The *ajna chakra* resides in the space between the eyebrows, about an inch inside the brain cavity. Here, in our meditations behind those closed eyes, we connect with the Divine. This relates to the Divine mind.

Once we reach the ajna chakra and are able to cognize the Divine, we lose our individuality and move into union, Oneness, with the Divine at the *sahasrara chakra*. This is a superconscious state, a state of samadhi, and it relates to the Super mind.

Pratyahara

Pratyahara is a process of withdrawing our consciousness from the senses so it can turn inward for concentration. The senses draw us outward, away from the spirit within, so unless we withdraw contact with them, our minds will constantly be roaming about, away from inner wisdom. Hari told me to watch my thoughts as though I were watching television. If I imagine I am watching the subtitles of a foreign film, it helps me to be uninvolved in the thoughts. I am simply watching.

Hari asked many yogis about this limb of yoga. Swami Thapovanam from Uttarkashi, India, attempted to shed some clarity on it.

Sense-control and pratyahara are not one and the same thing. They are different things. Sense-control means mastery of the senses and not withdrawal or inaction of the senses. Pratyahara means withdrawal of the senses from their respective objects. Control of the horses does not mean the withdrawal of them from all their activities. To lead them through proper paths according to our will is their control. Suppose a young man sees a young woman. He may have a look at her beautiful figure just as he sees a beautiful dove or deer. No need of withdrawing his eye-organ from her. As it is Adharma (sin) and as he is master of his senses, he will have no[t] any sexual desire upon her. If the vision itself of a certain thing (for instance, ugly and immoral cinema, etc.) is harmful, he will not even go to see and enjoy it. Briefly saying, this is sense-control. Pratyahara is quite a different thing. It is practiced by yogic sadhakas through Pranayama, sitting on a suitable posture, according to the instructions of yoga shastra [sacred books] and also perfect yogins. Pratyahara is practiced and used for attaining perfect and long Samadhi. Pratyahara is not intended as a sadhana to sense-control or mind-control.[272]

Pratyahara is the withdrawal of the senses from their respective objects—the eyes from all forms, the ears from all sounds, etc. Just like a tortoise at will withdraws his limbs from outside, a yogi who has control over his Prana by long and successful practice of Pranayama can withdraw his senses from the objects. But this is very difficult for ordinary yogins. Therefore this too is not an easy path available for all.[273]

Even without the practice of Pratyahara, one can get the highest concentration of mind and Samadhi by devotion and wisdom also. These are all different paths to attain concentration, Truth-realization, and the highest peace of mind.[274]

There is no question that Hari mastered this limb of yoga. He showed me a photo of himself taken after his brother had pushed pins through his cheeks to demonstrate the deep state of pratyahara he had achieved. No disturbances from the senses arose. As always, Hari was humble. He didn't have the photo taken to show off and feed his ego, he simply needed to show his progress to his teachers so he could receive further instruction.

Hari explained that if you can draw the life force through the chakras to the brain and disconnect it from the senses, this is perfect pratyahara. If the energy is stabilized in the brain (and not in any of the chakras), it gives all the internal organs a rest. In this state, one gains so much control that it is possible to stop the heart.[275]

Here is a very simple pratyahara technique Hari taught me. Sit in siddhasana. The eyes may be half-closed or fully closed (leaving the eyes open demonstrates even greater ability to withdraw from the senses). Let the mind run on aimlessly. Do not try to control it. Let all thoughts come

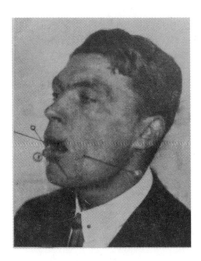

Figure 6.1. Hari in pratyahara.
Photographer and date unknown.

in, regardless of whether they are good or bad—simply watch them come and go. Do not become involved with the thoughts; just watch them. If you want to add a mantra, repeat *Om Sakshi*, "witness of source (or mind)." We learn how something works by watching it. Watching how the mind works helps us to understand it, which leads us to understand how to control it. Hari felt it was important to do this every day, and over many months of daily practice, the negative thoughts will lessen and those that remain will be more positive, until complete control is gained.[276]

Swami Sivananda of Rishikesh encouraged Hari to practice it regularly: "make a firm habit of practicing pratyahara several times during your daily activities. Do deliberate pratyahara amidst the din and distractions and try to keep the mind steadily fixed to some work. Also just before you commence Dhyana [meditation] withdraw yourself completely. Turn the mind fully inward and commence meditation."[277]

Swami Vishnudevananda suggested Hari draw the rays of the mind inward, away from external objects.

When the thought is shut up from external objects, naturally you can direct the energy, and this is conserved for the control of the mind. The Prana or the vital energy is spent during thinking, willing, and action. Mind has to use Prana for all its actions, and when this pranic energy shuts away from the mind, automatically the mind stops functioning. Mind produces thoughts through the help of the Prana, and when this pranic energy, which is spent by the mind for thinking, are brought to a stand still, the Yogi has reached the stage of pratyahara and concentration. So when all the rays of the mind are turned toward itself, it means that the energy spent by the mind by thinking, etc., is utilized for concentration. When the Prana stops, naturally mind also stops, as both are interconnected.

Hatha Yogins try to control the Prana in order to control the mind, and Raja Yogins try to control the mind to control its power—the Prana—which causes distraction of the mind. In Raja Yoga it is called Chitta Vritti Nirodha and in Hatha Yoga it is called Prana Nirodha.[278]

Nirodha means "restraint," "prevention," or "control." We are trying to restrain or control the thought waves and also preventing the loss of prana through the senses.

Sage Yajnavalkya described a technique of concentration, a process of withdrawing the mind and prana gradually, step by step, from one part of the body at a time. Swami Sivananda shared this technique with Hari.

One starts at the big toes of the feet and progresses upward by a series of successive acts of such concentration-cum-withdrawal, through the several occult centres of the body, leading finally to the crown of the head. The eighteen parts mentioned by Sage Yajnavalkya are given below. By this process the mind and Prana are totally drawn away from the entire body and finally centered in the top of the head where the practitioner dives into deep meditation.

1. Great toes
2. Ankles
3. Middle of shanks
4. Part above shanks & below knees
5. Centres of knees
6. Centres of thighs
7. Anus
8. Centre of body (just below waist)
9. Genitals
10. Navel
11. Heart
12. Pit of the throat
13. Root of the palate
14. Root of nose
15. Eye-balls
16. Centre of eye-brows

17. Forehead
18. Crown of head

It is when the senses are active that the mind becomes outgoing.... The senses are made active by the play of Prana. With the withdrawal of Prana, the different parts of the body are rendered quiescent and their activity inhibited. Here in this technique the effective withdrawal of Prana is achieved by the withdrawal of the mind. It is not so much a process of Pranayam, but the making use of the interconnection between the Prana and mind that this withdrawal of Prana is [affected]....

The mind is firmly withdrawn after a short spell of deep concentration upon a particular part. Automatically—together with the ingoing mind—the Prana too gets withdrawn. Prana follows the mind.

Thus, stage by stage, the Prana is withdrawn from the big toe upwards right up until it reaches the region of the crown of the head by which time the meditator is, as it were, oblivious of the body. In this state the meditation proceeds undisturbed and becomes very effective. This is one of the processes to enter into undisturbed and intense Dhyana.

Sit upon your Dhyana Asana. Create the right mood and Bhav [positive attitude toward God] by little chanting of Pranava Mantra (OM). Next negate the entire phenomenal universe, including this earth. When you reach the state where you are only aware of the body, then commence this process of withdrawal. Closing your eyes first direct your entire mind upon the two big toes. Concentrate there. Then gradually draw up the mind from the region of the toes to the next point, viz. the ankles. Now concentrate here. Then withdraw yourself to the third point i.e. middle of the shanks. Concentrate here. Next withdraw into the fourth part, and so on. After a few days progress, depending upon the interest and the earnestness with which you do it, you will be able to go through the entire series of 18 parts and reach the seat of meditation on the crown of the head with a short time after taking up your seat in the meditation Asan.[279]

This process described above is not unlike yoga nidra (yoga sleep). The big difference is that in yoga nidra we are lying down in savasana (corpse pose) rather than sitting up. When I studied and lived in the Sivananda Ashrams of Swami Vishnudevananda's, no yoga class was finished without going through the yoga nidra process. I would go deeply into a state of pratyahara, experiencing the bliss of sense withdrawal. You could use the technique described above while lying in savasana.

Of course, these techniques are much more effective if we can listen to a recording of the steps, so we don't have to "think" our way through them. In fact, it is nearly impossible to guide yourself though the process of yoga nidra. In one letter to Hari, Swami Sivananda told him he would mail him gramophone records that he made to record some lectures, mantras, and kirtan. He certainly went out of his way to ensure that his correspondence students were well taught. "I will send you the Gramophone records. Let us try. We can nicely pack the records here, but the Customs authorities will open the parcel on the way and damage the contents to careless re-packing."[280]

Dharana

Dharana is concentration. If we can concentrate the mind, our energy is concentrated as well—it is not fractured and dissipated. The practice of pratyahara helps us to be able to concentrate more fully. This ability to concentrate leads us to dhyana, or meditation.

Hari taught me the following twenty kriya yoga practices related to the stages of pratyahara, dharana, and dhyana. Oddly, in my notes, they are written down in reverse order, as though he dictated them to me from last to first. The techniques build on each other, so they are intended to be done as one complete practice and should not be broken up. The process takes a long time to complete, however, so one must work through them a little at a time. For example, learn the first kriya and practice it daily for a week. Then learn the second kriya and do the first and second together for a week. Then learn the third kriya, and practice all three for a week. Once all the kriyas are learned, the entire practice can be done as one.

The first nine are pratyahara kriyas, followed by ten dharana kriyas and lastly one dhyana kriya. These make up an incredibly powerful practice.[281]

1. Viparitakarani Mudra

Go into viparitakarani mudra (the half-shoulderstand pose) so the body is inverted. Close the eyes. Curl the tongue back into the throat in amritpan

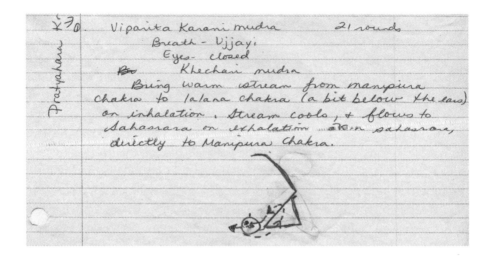

Figure 6.2. Drawing in author's notes on viparitakarani kriya, taken while studying with Hari, Concentration p. 4, 1979.

khechari mudra to stimulate the flow of the amrita nectar. Using ujjayi breath, inhale and visualize bringing a warm stream of the amrita nectar through the sushumna from the manipura chakra to anahata chakra, vishuddhi chakra, and lalana chakra. Hold the breath briefly and allow the nectar to cool, then, using ujjayi, exhale this cool stream of nectar to the ajna chakra, then to the bindu (the posterior fontanel at the back of the head) and to the sahasrara chakra at the crown of the head. From sahasrara, move right back down to the manipura chakra for the next inhalation to repeat the process, increasing the flow of nectar. Repeat this twenty-one times.

Arohan and Awarohan

There are two psychic passages that are integral to many of the following kriyas. *Arohan* is the ascending psychic pathway, and *awarohan* is the descending one. Arohan begins at the muladhara chakra and proceeds up the front of the body to svadhisthana, manipura, anahata, vishuddhi, and across the throat to bindu, the fontanel at the back of the head. Awarohan descends from the bindu to ajna, to vishuddhi, and down the back of the body to anahata, manipura, svadhisthana, and muladhara. As we breathe in this fashion, we feel the sensation of the energy rising up the front of the body and descending down the back of the body with the breath. The flow of consciousness is elliptical.

In most of the kriyas, your head moves from chakra to chakra as the chakra names are repeated and your consciousness moves to each chakra. Muladhara and bindu are both repeated three times, whereas svadhisthana, manipura, anahata, vishuddhi, and ajna are repeated once each.

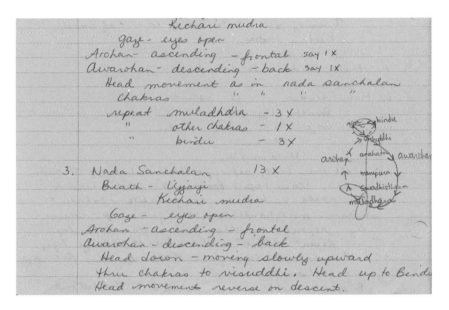

Figure 6.3. Drawing in author's notes on arohan-awarohan, taken while studying with Hari, Concentration p. 3b, 1979.

2. CHAKRA ANUSANDHANA

Anusandhana means "to investigate." *Chakra anusandhana* is a beginner's exercise to investigate or learn the true location of the chakras and bindu. In this sense, "learning" the location means to gain an inner knowledge of their locations rather than a simplistic idea of where they are. Chakras are not just spots along the back of the spine; they are energy centers that radiate through the front of the body, too.

Sit in a meditation pose like siddhasana with eyes closed and breathe normally. The head is erect at the start, though it moves as your consciousness passes through the chakras. Be sure to give each area your attention—you can mentally repeat the name of each chakra as you pass through the area. Lower your head to direct your gaze toward the muladhara chakra. Inhale and move your consciousness, ascending up the front of the body from the muladhara chakra to svadhisthana, manipura, anahata, vishuddhi, and across to bindu at the back of the head. At vishuddhi, the head is first in a neutral position and then the chin rises as consciousness moves to bindu. Then exhale in reverse, from bindu to ajna, then vishuddhi, and down the back of the body through anahata, manipura, and svadhisthana to muladhara, where your head is lowered again. Repeat the process nine times, without straining, but merely noticing each chakra.

3. NADA SANCHALAN

Nada means "sound," and here we have a rotation of sound consciousness. This process builds on chakra anusandhana. During inhalation, visualize the prana ascending (arohan) up the front of the body and, during exhalation, the prana descending (awarohan) down the back of the body.

To begin, sit in a comfortable seated pose like siddhasana or padmasana. The eyes are open. As you breathe, use ujjayi breath with the tongue rolled back in amritpan khechari mudra. Lower the chin to look at muladhara chakra. Repeat (mentally) "muladhara" three times, then inhale up the frontal part of the body, repeating the names of each chakra, moving the consciousness from muladhara to svadhisthana, manipura, anahata, and vishuddhi. As the mind moves up though each chakra the head moves up with them. At vishuddhi the head is in a neutral position, and then the chin rises as consciousness moves to bindu. Hold the breath and repeat mentally "bindu, bindu, bindu." Let this repetition of "bindu" burst into an extended "Om" while exhaling down the back of the body, taking your consciousness to ajna, vishuddhi, anahata, manipura, svadhisthana, and muladhara. The head movement follows the chakras as you bring your attention to them. Repeat this process thirteen times.

4. PAVANA SANCHALANA

Pavana (or *pawana*) relates to the movement of wind or air. Here we have a rotation of breath consciousness. Begin as in the previous practice. After mentally repeating "muladhara" three times, say "arohan" mentally and inhale up the frontal part of the body, repeating the names of each chakra as you move your consciousness from muladhara to svadhisthana, manipura, anahata, and vishuddhi. As the mind moves up though each chakra, the head moves up with them. When consciousness is at the bindu chakra, hold the breath and mentally repeat "bindu, bindu, bindu." Say "awarohan" mentally and exhale down the back of the body, taking your consciousness to ajna, vishuddhi, anahata, manipura, svadhisthana, to muladhara. The eyes gradually close on the way down so they are fully closed at the muladhara chakra. The head movement also follows the chakras on the way down. Repeat this process forty-nine times.

5. SHABDA SANCHALANA

Shadba means "word" or "sound." *Sanchalana* means "rotation." Here we practice a rotation of word consciousness. Again, begin as in nada sanchalan. Lower the chin to look at muladhara chakra. Repeat "muladhara" three times mentally, then listen for the inner sound "So" as you inhale and ascend up the frontal part of the body and move your consciousness from muladhara to svadhisthana, manipura, anahata, and vishuddhi. As the mind moves up though each chakra, the head moves up with them. At vishuddhi, the head is in a neutral position, and then the chin rises as consciousness moves to bindu. Hold the breath and repeat mentally "bindu, bindu, bindu." As you exhale, descending (awarohan) down the back of the body, listen for the inner sound of "Ham," taking your consciousness to ajna, vishuddhi, anahata, manipura, svadhisthana, to muladhara. The eyes gradually close on the way down, so they are fully closed at the muladhara chakra. The head movement also follows the chakras on the way down. Repeat "muladhara" mentally three times. Repeat this process fifty-nine times.

6. MAHA MUDRA

Maha is "great," and *mudra* is "seal." This technique is done in the maha mudra position as described earlier. In this technique you use ujjayi breath and amritpan khechari mudra. When the head rises at the bindu, the eyes gaze in shambhavi mudra toward the ajna chakra.

Sit on the left heel and stretch out the right leg. Lower the head and engage mula bandha and repeat "muladhara" three times. Inhale with mula bandha, ujjayi, and khechari mudra up the front passage (arohan) to bindu, raising the head as before. Retaining the breath, bend forward and grab the right foot with the hands while performing shambhavi mudra (gazing to the third eye) and repeat mentally "bindu, bindu, bindu." Be sure to draw your torso toward the extended leg. Exhale, descending (awarohan) the back passage, and release shambhavi mudra and mula bandha. Sit upright. Repeat four times with the right leg extended, then four times with the left leg extended, then four times with both legs extended, for a total of twelve times.

7. Maha Bheda

Maha is "great," and *bheda* is "separating." Sit in siddhasana, with the lower foot pressing into the muladhara chakra. Lower the head and engage mula bandha and mentally repeat "muladhara" three times. Inhale with ujjayi and amritpan khechari mudra up the front passage (arohan) to bindu, raising the head as before. Retain the breath and mentally repeat "bindu" three times. Exhale, descending (awarohan) the back passage. Retain the breath out and perform jalandhara bandha, uddiyana bandha, and mula bandha as long as is comfortable. Release the three bandhas and repeat "muladhara" mentally three times. Repeat this process twelve times.

8. Manduki Kriya

Manduki means "frog," and *kriya* is "spiritual action or work." This kriya is said to be intoxicating! Sit in a kneeling position, with knees wide and toes touching behind the buttocks (as in mandukasana). Gaze at the tip of the nose (nasikagra drishti). Concentrate on muladhara chakra to activate the earth element and the sense of smell. Perform amritpan khechari mudra and breathe in through both nostrils, taking the breath to the ajna chakra, then exhale, taking the breath out through each respective nostril. The flow of breath resembles a cone shape from the entry at each nostril and joining at the ajna chakra, then back out again. It is very important to have no strain during the breathing. Become aware of any subtle scents you smell, such as sandalwood, which is said to be the scent of the astral body. Repeat until you feel the intoxicating effects, or up to three minutes.

9. Tadan Kriya

Tadan means "to beat." This kriya is very similar to maha vedha mudra. Sit in padmasana (lotus pose), or if you cannot sit in this pose, sit in ardha (half) padmasana or ardha siddhasana. Inhale using ujjayi and amritpan khechari mudra taking the breath mentally to muladhara chakra. Retain the breath and engage mula bandha. Press your hands down beside the buttocks to lift them off the floor. Gently beat the muladhara chakra by beating your buttocks up and down, up to eleven times. Set them back down and exhale slowly. Start with a few rounds and gradually increase up to seven times.

This is the last of the nine pratyahara kriyas, and we move into the ten dharana kriyas.

10. Naumukhi Mudra

This mudra closes the nine gates, or openings, where we can lose prana. To close the nine gates (two eyes, two ears, two nostrils, mouth, anus, and sex organ), we use three mudras. Shanmukhi mudra closes the ears with the thumbs, the eyes with the index fingers, the nostrils with the middle fingers, and the lips with the ring and baby fingers placed on the upper and lower lips. Mula bandha closes the anus, and vajroli mudra closes the sexual gate. (Vajroli mudra is a muscular contraction to draw the urethra upward and inward, similar to that used to stop yourself from urinating.)

During this process, visualize roots going down at muladhara chakra and a stem rising up the spine all the way to vishuddhi chakra. Visualize at the top of the stem, above vishuddhi chakra, a trident that will pierce the bindu.

Sit in siddhasana. Become aware of muladhara chakra and feel its roots extending downward into the earth. Repeat "muladhara" mentally three times. Inhale, using ujjayi and amritpan khechari mudra, up the arohan (frontal passage) from muladhara chakra through each chakra to vishuddhi, and raise the head as your consciousness moves to bindu. Retain the breath and close the nine gates with your mudras. Hold your inner gaze at the ajna chakra and imagine a stem coming up the spine from its roots at muladhara chakra up to vishuddhi chakra. The trident above vishuddhi chakra pierces the bindu chakra. Repeat mentally "bindu bedhan, bindu bhedan, bindu bhedan" and try to feel the electrical sensation as it is pierced. Release the mudras to open the nine gates and exhale down the awarohan (back passage) from bindu to muladhara chakra. Repeat "muladhara" mentally three times. Repeat this process five times.

11. Shakti Chalani

Chalani means "to churn," and this kriya facilitates the rotation of shakti (kundalini energy). To begin, sit in a comfortable seated pose like siddhasana or padmasana. The eyes are closed, with an inner gaze toward the ajna chakra. Lower the chin to look at muladhara chakra. Repeat mentally "muladhara" three times, then using ujjayi breath with amritpan khechari mudra, inhale up the arohan of the body, moving the consciousness from muladhara to svadhisthana, manipura, anahata, and to vishuddhi, and then raise the head as consciousness moves to bindu. Hold the breath and visualize a thin green serpent with its tail in its mouth, filling the arohan and awarohan passageways and forming a figure 8. With its tail in its mouth at bindu, it forms a closed circuit in the passageway. Watch and see if the serpent will move through the passageway. When ready to exhale, with ujjayi, descend down the back of the body taking your consciousness from bindu to ajna, vishuddhi, anahata, manipura, svadhisthana, and to muladhara. Your head movement, as usual, follows the chakras as you bring your attention to them. When you return to muladhara, repeat mentally "muladhara" three times. Repeat the process five times.

12. Shambhavi

Although we have discussed shambhavi mudra before, in which the drishti (focus) is to the third eye, this is different and a most beautiful technique. To begin, sit in a comfortable seated pose like siddhasana or padmasana. The eyes are closed, with an inner gaze toward the ajna chakra. Visualize a pink lotus flower at the sahasrara chakra at crown of the head, in the form of a flower bud. The green stem of the lotus flower goes down the spine in a straight line all the way to muladhara, where its roots are planted into the earth below.

Inhale using ujjayi breath and amritpan khechari mudra, observing the energy traveling up the lotus stem in the spine, like a caterpillar, from muladhara to sahasrara. Retain the breath at sahasrara; the caterpillar kisses the closed lotus, and it slowly opens in all its glory. Try to see all the details of your lotus flower. Throughout this, retain the breath comfortably. When ready to exhale, close the lotus flower back into a bud and, using ujjayi breath, exhale the descending energy down the stem of the lotus flower in the spine from sahasrara to ajna to vishuddhi, and so forth, to its roots at muladhara. Repeat this process eleven times.

13. Amrit Pan

The flowing of the amrita nectar. The visualization will be as in viparita-karani mudra, the first kriya described above, except we do this sitting. Sit in siddhasana or padmasana. Close the eyes and breathe in ujjayi with the tongue curled back into the throat in amritpan khechari mudra. With each inhalation, bring a warm stream of the amrita nectar through the sushumna from the manipura chakra to anahata chakra, vishuddhi chakra, and lalana chakra. Hold the breath briefly while the nectar cools, then exhale this stream of cool nectar to the ajna chakra, to the bindu, and to sahasrara chakra at the crown of the head. From sahasrara, move right back down to the manipura chakra for the next inhalation to repeat the process, increasing the flow of nectar. Repeat this nine times.

14. Chakra Bhedan

This is a process to pierce the chakras. You must be able to "see" the chakras. Try to see the "light" in the ajna chakra first. When that becomes easy, try to see the light in another chakra. When this is successful, the light in the ajna will change, because it is a reflection from the other chakras.[282]

The breathing is ujjayi; with closed eyes, gaze to ajna chakra. Curl the tongue back into the throat in amritpan khechari mudra. Inhale and draw the energy up the front arohan passage from muladhara chakra to svadhisthana, manipura, anahata, and vishuddhi chakras. Exhale from vishuddhi to bindu to ajna, across the throat at vishuddhi, and down the awarohan back passage to anahata, manipura, and svadhisthana. Start the next inhalation at svadhisthana; go down to muladhara and then up the frontal passage to svadhisthana, manipura, anahata, and vishuddhi. Exhale to bindu, ajna, and vishuddhi, and descend down the back passage to svadhisthana, as described above. Continue the process fifty-nine times. You can name each chakra during the process, as you try to see its light.

15. Sushumna Darshan

This technique is to increase our ability to visualize the chakras in their locations along the sushumna. In your mind's eye, draw the basic *yantra* (mystical diagram) of each chakra. Sit in siddhasana or padmasana. Bring your attention to the muladhara chakra at the base of the spine. Think the color red and imagine drawing the yantra. Draw a circle. Within the circle, draw a square, and within the square, draw an inverted triangle. Draw four petals around the circle.

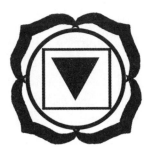

Figure 6.4. Muladhara chakra.
Drawing by Jo C. Willems

Move your awareness to the svadhisthana chakra in the pelvis. Think the color orange. Draw a circle, and inside the lower half of the circle, draw a crescent moon (in the shape of a smile). Draw six petals around the circle.

Figure 6.5. Svadhisthana chakra.
Drawing by Jo C. Willems

Move your awareness to the manipura chakra, in the region of the navel, and think the color yellow. Draw a circle, and within the circle, draw an inverted triangle. Draw ten petals around the circle.

Figure 6.6. Manipura chakra.
Drawing by Jo C. Willems.

Move your awareness to the anahata chakra, at the region of the heart. Think the color green. Draw a circle. Within the circle, draw a triangle, and over that, draw an inverted triangle. Draw twelve petals around the circle.

Figure 6.7. Anahata chakra.
Drawing by Jo C. Willems.

Bring your awareness to the vishuddhi chakra, at the throat. Think the color blue. Draw a circle, and within that, draw an inverted triangle. Within the inverted triangle draw a smaller circle. Draw sixteen petals around the outer circle.

Figure 6.8. Vishuddhi chakra.
Drawing by Jo C. Willems.

Move your awareness to the ajna chakra, between the eyebrows, and think the color indigo or the color of a ripe plum. Draw a circle and place an inverted triangle within the circle. Write Om within that triangle. Draw two large petals, one on either side of the circle.

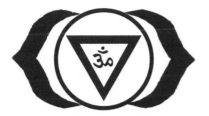

Figure 6.9. Ajna chakra.
Drawing by Jo C. Willems.

Move your awareness to the bindu. Draw a circle. Within the circle near the bottom, draw a crescent moon. Draw a dot above the crescent moon (as in the Om symbol).

Figure 6.10. Bindu chakra.
Drawing by Jo C. Willems.

Move your awareness to the sahasrara chakra. Think the color white or violet. Draw a circle, then a triangle within the circle. Draw one thousand petals around the circle. Now see all the chakras along the pathway of the sushumna.

Figure 6.11. Sahasrara.
Drawing by Jo C. Willems.

16. Prana Ahuti

This is an offering of prana from God. After visualizing and feeling each chakra location, we are infused with prana. Sit in siddhasana or padmasana. Imagine the hand of God resting gently on your head as prana rains down upon you and flows down through the chakras from the sahasrara to muladhara. All sorts of sensations may be experienced here, such as jerking motions, a cool feeling, warmth, heat, or jolts of electric shudders up the spine. Simply notice these responses. You need only do this once.

17. Utthan Kriya

Utthan means "to rise up from the ground," so this is the raising of the kundalini from the muladhara chakra. Sit in siddhasana or padmasana with the eyes closed. Bring your consciousness to the muladhara chakra. Visualize the *lingam* (a symbol representing Shiva) within muladhara chakra with the kundalini coiled three and a half times around it. Imagine the serpent uncoiling and moving up into the sushumna. Notice how far it can move upward before it returns to the muladhara. Be attentive to any sensations that may occur as the serpent moves.

18. Svarupa Darshan

This practice facilitates seeing one's own form. Sit in siddhasana or padmasana. The breath should be natural and the body kept very, very still. Observe the breath in its natural ebb and flow. Do not try to control it, just observe it. The body will eventually become stiff, without movement. Visualize the form of your body so still.

19. Linga Sanchalan

The *linga sharira* is the astral body, so this is the rotation or movement of the astral body. Continue from the last kriya, sitting in siddhasana or padmasana. Keep the breathing normal and the eyes closed. With this still, unmoving body, inhale and feel the expansion of the astral body. On the exhalation, feel the contraction of the astral body. Observe the expansion and contraction of the astral body. The contraction is important. Eventually you will contract the astral body until it comes to one single point of light, like a small, luminous golden egg without rays. Now we move into the final stage, the dhyana kriya.

20. DHYANA

Continue from the last kriya, with the still body, until the astral body has contracted to a small, luminous golden egg. Observe this golden egg. As you breathe, it will begin to expand and become larger and larger, until it eventually fills your physical and astral bodies. Your form is a glowing light. It is neither physical nor astral; it is the causal body.

Swami Yogeshwaranand said that pratyahara is the control of the senses and that dharana is the control of the mind. Both are different steps of sadhana, leading us toward deeper stages of dhyana and, ultimately, to samadhi.[283]

Chapter Seven

DHYANA

HARI WAS A VERY DEDICATED MEDITATOR and spent most of his spare time in meditation. He said, "Prana follows the mind, and the mind follows prana. So where we center the mind, the prana collects."[284] He recorded his meditation times regularly in a little notebook and calculated daily the minutes he spent meditating.

We meditated in the morning facing east and in the evening facing north. The scriptures are not clear on why meditation was to be done in this way, but Hari suggested it had to do with the movement of the sun. Hari also said one should never face the north when sleeping.[285]

One evening Hari came to my room and invited me to meditate with him. I had eaten too much that night and so declined. To this day I cannot believe I said no to him. What wisdom was he going to share with me? What transference of energy or knowledge did I miss? What special memories would I have of that meditation? It still feels like such a foolishly missed opportunity.

There are numerous meditations throughout the letters written to Hari. First, though, I want to share with you a tidbit from Swami Vishnu Tirth regarding *bandha traya* for meditation.

Bandha Traya with Siddhasana for Meditation

Bandha traya the practice of applying all three bandhas, or locks, during the process of pranayama. Jalandhara bandha is the throat lock, in which we lower the chin toward the jugular notch. Mula bandha is the root lock, in which we draw up on the pelvic floor, and uddiyana bandha draws the navel area upward. These are described in more detail in the section "The Bandhas" in chapter 4, but here they come naturally and automatic.

Swami Vishnu Tirth regarded bandha traya in meditation essential for the raising of the kundalini. He drew this from the text *Bhawartha Dipika*, fondly known as "Jnaneshwari." Apparently this text was spontaneous wisdom received by the author Shri Jnanadeva around 1290 AD, and it was written down in Marathi (the official language of the state of Maharashtra, India) as he spoke it.

> By pressing hard with the heel the mid part of both the holes of Apan [the perineum], thus opening the Muladhara door. He applies the three bandhas, thus uniting pran and apan and clearing the passage for Prana Shakti to ascend up. The Kundalini Power, being aroused, rises up through the central passage of the spine from the lowest, Muladhara, up to the Ajna plexus [the mid-brow] and makes the cloud like Sahasrara shower with nectar, which flows down to the lowest plexus Muladhara.... Then the aspirant experiences meditation and the objective consciousness of the object of meditation.[286]

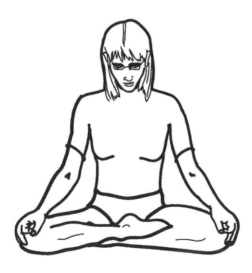

Figure 7.1. Siddhasana with a natural bandha traya applied. Drawing by Brieanne Mikuska.

Swami Vishnu Tirth said:

From the above, it is clear that an aspirant has to sit in Sidhasan with the 3 bandhas on. Kundalini should, by this practice, rise up to sahasrara to make it shower nectar and bathe the whole system by it. Thereby the requisite meditation would ensue. No doubt Uddiyan must be a steady one.....[287]

Automatically, or naturally, the lower part of the abdomen below the navel would tend to be drawn in … without much effort on the part of the sadhaka. When in meditation, the lower part of the abdomen should be drawn in instead of bulging out. That would help meditation. However, if you apply effort for Jalandhar and Uddiyan, your meditation would suffer. Therefore, the three Bandhas should naturally and easily follow the sitting posture.[288]

He further clarified this to Hari:

When a person sits on sidhasan with his chin touching the chest, [the] head naturally appears somewhat sunken between the shoulders. No effort for it is necessary. Jalandhar bandha helps meditation, and [allowing the] head [to] lower down toward the front is a part of the sidhasan.[289]

To sum this up: think of the three bandhas as part of siddhasana; without them, the pose is not complete. While sitting in siddhasana, hold the spine erect, gently lengthening in the neck and relaxing the shoulders. Allow the chin to lower slightly toward the jugular notch, to a natural resting place. This gentle lengthening of the neck supports the cervical spine so the lowering of the chin does not compromise the erect spine. The right heel presses into the perineum, stimulating a slight mula bandha effect, while the left leg rests on the right thigh. The lower part of the abdomen, below the navel, will naturally tend to be drawn in, without effort, stabilizing the body and the erect spine. A gentle uddiyana bandha will then follow, to offer support to the mid-spine. (See "Controlled Lower Abdomen" in chapter 4).

The natural flow of the prana vayu is upward, and the apana vayu moves downward. Applying jalandhara bandha, we change the direction of prana, moving it downward, against its natural course. With mula bandha, we force the apana upward. This is to help us conquer nature, the forces of *prakriti,* causing the union of prana and apana to occur in the mid-region of the body, where the *samana vayu* rests (a balancing force, midway between prana and apana). Uddiyana bandha prevents these conjoined forces of prana from escaping by compressing it from all sides. Then the prana can move into the sushumna.[290] Kundalini should thereby be aroused or awakened, and meditation will come without exertion.[291]

In trying this myself, I do indeed find that a gentle bandha traya comes automatically in siddhasana. It is worth trying for some of these meditations.

Sivoham Meditation

I want to begin these meditations with one Hari taught me, which is meant to join these forces of prana. He learned it from Gajanan Maharaj, who lived in or near Poona, India. Hari didn't name it, but I call it "Sivoham Meditation." In siddhasana or your comfortable meditation seat, focus the eyes to the tip of the nose *(nasagra drishti).* The tongue is curled back into the modified khechari mudra (amritpan khechari)—the tongue is positive, the palate is negative, so this mudra creates a current of energy movement. The apana will not draw upward unless the tongue is back. Four mantras are repeated mentally—not over and over, as in japa, but the mantra is said, and then the meaning is pondered. It is then said again, and the meaning is again pondered.

> *Sudhoham* comes from *suddha,* which means "purity," and *aham* means "I am."
> *Budoham* comes from *Buddha,* which means "enlightenment."
> *Muktoham* comes from *mukta,* which means "free."
> *Sivoham* comes from *Siva.* Siva is a name for God.[292]

As you meditate, mentally repeat the word *Sudhoham.* Ponder its meaning for several minutes—I am purity.

Mentally repeat *Budhoham.* Ponder its meaning for several minutes—I am all enlightenment.

Mentally repeat *Muktoham.* Ponder its meaning for several minutes—I am free.

Now add the mantra *Sivoham*. Repeat it mentally while you ponder the meaning—I am Siva; I am God.

Continue with the process pondering the meanings of these mantras.

Upanishad Mantra Meditation

This beautiful meditation was sent to Hari from Swami Shivapremananda not long after his brother passed away in 1975. It includes powerful mantras from the Upanishads that awaken the spirit within. Ponder their meaning and the sensations they bring to you as you meditate.

The first mantra is *Idam prana ayam atma Brahma*, "consciousness of prana awakens in me the consciousness of my atma, which is one with God." The second mantra, *Idam prana sarva bhuteshu gudah*, "through the experience of prana, I experience the spiritual essence, which is in all as it is within me." The third mantra, *Idam prana pragnanam iti Brahma*, "the experience of prana awakens in me the transcendental consciousness of God." The meditation concludes with the Poorna Shanti mantra.

Sit in a meditative posture. Breathing is free. Gradually the mind is absorbed in experiencing the puraka and rechaka (pranas). As a consequence of concentration, the breath becomes slow.

For five minutes experience the cool air inside the upper nostrils and the warm air in the lower [nostrils]. Continue to feel the breath [and] contemplate on the unity of the cosmic prana (puraka) and individual prana (rechaka). Puraka represents peace, infinity, purnam [fullness], transcendence. Rechaka represents spiritual freedom, expansion of consciousness, diffusion of the individual breath. Contemplate on these qualities for some time, feeling the breath.

For one or two minutes breathe freely, feeling relaxed with eyes closed. Once more the mind is absorbed again in experiencing the prana inside the nostrils. Mentally and slowly repeat "Idam prana ayam atma Brahma" for five minutes, feeling the breath. Contemplate for the next five minutes on the meaning—consciousness of prana awakens in me the consciousness of my atma, which is one with God—feeling the breath.

Breathe freely, feeling relaxed for two minutes. Breath is slow and deep again. Inhaling, move the mind upward and backward along the convex outline of a new moon in the middle of the head, the forward point being the nostrils and the backward point inside the back of the head. Exhaling, move the mind from the back upward and forward along the lower line of the convex moon. Feel the breath thus for five minutes.

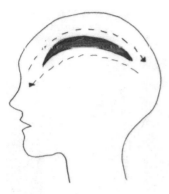

Figure 7.2. Upanishad Meditation from Swami Shivapremananda, part 2: inhaling over and exhaling under the convex moon. Drawing from author's notes.

Continuing, mentally repeat slowly "Idam prana sarva bhuteshu gudah," for five minutes. For the next five minutes contemplate on the meaning—through the experience of prana I experience the spiritual essence, which is in all as it is within me—feeling the same movement.

Relax for two minutes, breathing freely, with eyes closed in the same posture. Breath is deep again. Feel only the inhalation, the sensation of prana moving up to the top of the head and in the Sahasrara chakra, in the shape of the lower half of the moon. [Give] no attention to exhalation. Constantly maintain the sensation [of the prana flowing up and into the Sahasrara chakra], renewing it every time by feeling the puraka, for ten minutes.

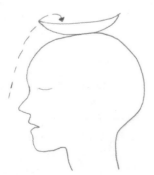

Figure 7.3. Upanishad Meditation from Swami Shivapremananda, part 3: filling the lower half of the moon. Drawing from author's notes.

For the next five minutes mentally repeat, "Idam prana prag-nanam iti Brahma," feeling the prana inside the top of the head. Continue this feeling and contemplate on the meaning for another five minutes—experience of prana awakens in me the transcendental consciousness of God.[293]

Conclude with the verbal repetition of *Om* and the *Purnam adah shanti* mantra, as follows:

Om poornamadah poornamidam
poornaat poornamudachyate
poornasya poornamaadaaya
poornamevaavashishyate
om shanti shanti shanti.

This mantra means: That (Brahman) is full; this (all of creation) is also full; from Brahman comes creation; even though creation comes from the fullness of Brahman, Brahman always remains full. In other words, Brahman remains unaffected and remains full and complete, no matter what is taken from it.

London, 19 May 1975

Revered Hari Maharaj,

Om Namo Narayanaya.

Thank you for your letter of March 4. Please excuse my long delay in answering it. I was away in India for four weeks and, returning here, have been constantly on the move in England, conducting spiritual retreats and seminars for yoga teachers. Tomorrow again I am leaving on an eight-week lecture tour of Belgium, Holland, West Germany, Switzerland and Italy. Will return to England for four weeks to conduct three more seminars, and will arrive in New York by the middle of August. I shall depart for Buenos Aires on Sep 20. Will be staying at Spring Valley, near Nayak, NY.

I am sorry to know that your brother passed away. Life is indeed transitory and one has to accept every day as it comes.

Here are a few simple lessons. I already gave you an indication on a slip of paper.

Sit in a meditative posture. Breathing is free. Gradually the mind is absorbed in experiencing the puraka and rechaka pranas. As a consequence of concentration the breath becomes slow. For five minutes experience the cool air inside the upper nostrils and the warm air in the lower. Continuing to feel the breath contemplate on the unity of the cosmic prana (puraka) and individual prana (rechaka). Puraka represents peace, infinity, purnam, transcendence. Rechaka spiritual freedom, expansion of consciousness, diffusion of individual breath. Contemplate on these qualities for some time, feeling the breath.

Figure 7.4. Letter from Swami Shivapremananda on Upanishad mantra meditation, sent to Hari not long after his brother passed away, May 1975.

Meditation for Healing the Sick

This meditation technique was written for Hari by Swami Sivananda of Rishikesh, while Hari was living in a DP camp after the Second World War. One of his companions was sick and in need of surgery. Swami Sivananda was an ayurvedic doctor in India and was often found treating the poorest and most ill patients for free. He created the Sivananda Charitable Hospital and offered free medical relief camps. All services continue to be offered for free by medical doctors doing karma yoga. The hospital is a magnet for ill people. When I was in India with my family, ill people were lined up on the bridge outside the Sivananda Ashram on the Ganges River.

In his letter, Swami Sivananda expressed his great pleasure that Hari and his friends in the DP camp practice yoga together, in spite of their living conditions.

> It is most encouraging to find that living in circumstances and sur-
> roundings that would have sent most people to the mental hospital,
> there is a Yogi-family steadfastly devoted to the Holy Yoga. Indeed,
> the Great Founders and Teachers of Yoga would consider it a great
> victory to the Yoga itself; their satisfaction is surely a great achieve-
> ment for you both. [294]

As one who never missed an opportunity to help those in need, Swami Sivananda taught Hari this meditation technique so he could direct his healing energy to others around him.

> *Meditation and sick persons:* Meditation can work wonders in healing
> the sick. Meditation by the sick person himself is, of course, produc-
> tive of miracle. It is, however, possible for a third person to do it for
> the sufferer. Often, even if the sufferer knows the art, he might find
> himself in a position where he may not be able to apply it on account
> of acute suffering. The method is this:
>
> Have a brief wash, if you find this would clear the mind. Chant
> OM OM OM. If you can find a little secluded place, do a few rounds
> of Bhastrika and a few rounds of Sukh-Purvak Pranayama. Feel, as
> you inhale, that the Lord's Healing Power is flowing into you, and,
> during Kumbhak, is filling your entire being. [Doing] SOHAM Japa
> for a little while will help you, too, to raise your own consciousness
> to a high level.

Then approach the patient. Sit by the bedside. Remain calm, serene, and meditative. It is better not to let the mind be disturbed by any thoughts, especially of the disease. Now, with open eyes, concentrate on the heart of the sick person. Feel, feel, and feel intensely the Presence of the Anamaya *(diseaseless)* Atman there. Feel that the Atman which is in you is in him, too. Connect the two: merge one in the other: meditate now deeply.

After this process is over, feel for a few minutes that the Lord's Healing Power has filled the patient and that he is better. Now, cheer him up with consoling words. You will find the patient yielding rapidly to this treatment. After the treatment is over, go again into meditation and re-charge yourself with His Healing Power....

All enquiries into the condition of the patient, etc. should be well in advance of the above process. For Sri Akulis, kindly give the enclosed Prasad and ask him to apply it on the Trikute [third eye]. The Lord will guide him. If he submits to the operation, please treat him in accordance with the above method before he undergoes the operation. Treat the doctor, too, by feeling the Presence of the All-Merciful Healing Lord in Him.[295]

Chakra Meditation

This meditation, from Swami Vishnudevananda, is based on three letters from Swami Vishnudevananda.[296] What is so wonderful about it is the detail that Swami Vishnudevananda included to give Hari a clear image of the chakra yantras, even by means of little hand-drawn sketches. He had all the letters of the Sanskrit alphabet written out for each chakra petal, which I have removed, simply because I do not think they are necessary for introducing this meditation. I have slightly edited these descriptions to make them flow a little more smoothly.

The sahasrara chakra is not included in this meditation. There is no yantra, no god or goddess, no mantra for this chakra, as it is beyond the *tattvas* (elements), beyond the senses, beyond the activity of the mind, beyond the manifested gods and goddesses, and merged into the One.

The well-known book *Kundalini Yoga for the West*, by the German-born Swami Sivananda Radha (founder of the Yasodhara Ashram in British Columbia), does not have a chapter for the sahasrara chakra. She mentions it, but the book is devoted to understanding the six chakras below it.[297]

The sahasrara is a thousand-petaled lotus flower, representing the culmination of the energy of all the other six chakras when they are opened. When the power is achieved over the six chakras and the granthi knots are untied, the sahasrara opens for the passage of the kundalini shakti. There is complete Oneness with Brahman, and the door to pure consciousness and immortality is opened.

As explained earlier, in a letter from Swami Venkatesananda (in the section "Yoni or Shanmukhi Mudra" in chapter 5), the sahasrara is not regarded as a chakra at all. It is the psychic abode of shaktis from the six chakras. According to Arthur Avalon's book *The Serpent Power*, the sahasrara is the highest seat of the jiva, or soul. Once communication is established between the soul at the sahasrara and the other psychic centers, specific nadis can bring information down from the sahasrara to the ajna chakra and the others.[298] I interpret that this is how we tap into the divine consciousness—the divine will.

At the end of this meditation, I have added a method for including the sahasrara after completing the meditations for each of the six chakras, for those who wish to use it.

> The lotus represents the saint who is in the world but out of the world. Even though the lotus comes from mud, it is very pure and beautiful. So also the saint ... even while living in the world, is also pure and holy.
>
> Meditation is done on all the chakras beginning from Mooladhara upwards to Sahasrara. Meditate first on the lotus and the petals. Then meditate on the shape within the lotus, which may be a square, triangle, moon, or other shape. Meditate on the Bija Mantra for each chakra. Meditate on the Deva and Devi [god and goddess] for each chakra. They represent the powers of each chakra to overcome obstacles and difficulties. If there is a Lingam there, meditate on that too (There is a lingam at the Mooladhara, Anahata, and Ajna chakras, where the granthis are). Meditate on the tattva or element for each chakra to gain power over it. Then start over again. Do this process for each chakra. It should take about half an hour for each.
>
> 1) Mooladhara Chakra
> Mooladhara Chakra has 4 red petals with 4 Sanskrit letters. Within the 4 petals is a yellow square representing the four directions on earth. Meditate on the earth Bija mantra LAM within this square, which represents the Prithivi or Earth.

Svayambu Linga (Siva Lingam) is in the Mooladhara Chakra. It is within the Triangle or Trikona. This Linga represents Lord Siva. The Kundalini is coiled around the Svayambu Linga with her head resting in a slight depression at the top, shutting the Brahma Dvara or opening to the Sushumna. Meditate on this.

Brahma is the Lord of the Mooladhara. He is seated on the back of a beautiful swan. Meditate on the color red, his four faces, and his four lustrous arms. In his four hands he holds the following things: The staff (Danda), gourd (Kamandalu or holy vessel), the rosary (Rudraksha beads or Aksha Sutra) and Abhaya Mudra (gesture or mudra for dispelling fear).

Meditate on Dakini Devi, the presiding Divinity of the Mooladhara. She has four arms and shines with beauty. Her eyes are brilliant red. She is resplendent like the lustre of many suns rising all at the same time. She is the carrier of the revelation of the ever pure Intelligence. In her two right hands she carries a spear (Shoola) and a staff (Katvanga) surmounted by a human skull. In her two left hands the Sword and drinking cup. By meditating on her form, the Yogi acquires knowledge of the earth [element]. [299]

2) Svadishtana

The Svadishtana chakra sits at the root of the genitals in the Sushumna. It has 6 petals of a vermillion colour with 6 Sanskrit letters. The colour of the letters are of shining lightning and within it is the white shining water region of Varuna, the God of water tattva, shaped as a half moon. Inside the half moon, seated on a Makara or crocodile is the Bija of water "Vam," which is as stainless and white as the autumnal moon. Meditate upon the white Varuana Bija VAM within the lotus.

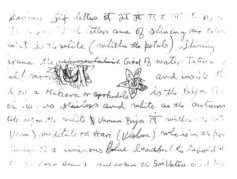

Figure 7.5. Letter from Swami Vishnudevananda describing how to meditate on the chakras, sketch of svadhisthana chakra, March 20, 1956.

Meditate on Hari (Vishnu) who is the pride of early youth. His body is luminous blue and beautiful to behold. He is dressed in yellow raiment, has four arms, and wears the Sri Vatsu and Kaustubha Gem. He is seated on Garuda the eagle.

Here is where Rakini Devi always dwells. She is of the colour of a blue lotus. She is dressed in celestial raiments and ornaments, and she is exalted with the drinking of Ambrosia or Nectar, which drops from Sahasrara. In her hands are a spear, a lotus, a drum, and a sharp battle axe, and she is seated on a double lotus.

3) Manipura

The Manipura Chakra is of the colour of the rain cloud and has ten petals with 10 Sanskrit letters. The colour of the letters are lustrous blue with a Bindu or dot above each letter. In the centre of this lotus is the red region of Fire, which is triangular in shape, and within the triangle is the Fire Bija mantra, RAM, which is red in colour and seated on a ram. Above the ram is Rudra (Siva as an elder), seated on a bull, and his whole body is smeared with basma or white ash.

On a red lotus in the centre of the chakra is the Shakti Lakini. She is blue, has three faces with three eyes in each. [One of the eyes on each face is the third eye.] In her two arms [she holds] the vajra or thunderbolt and Shakti weapon of fire. In the other arms she shows the mudras for dispelling fear and granting boons. Meditating on this chakra gives one the power over Fire.

4) Anahata

Anahata Chakra is of the colour of the Bandhuka flower (Red) and on its twelve petals are twelve Sanskrit letters. Each letter is a vermillion colour. In the centre is a hexagonal Vayu Mandala of a

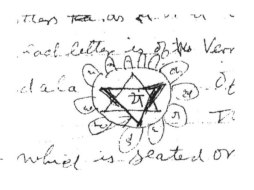

Figure 7.6. Letter from Swami Vishnudevananda describing how to meditate on the chakras, sketch of anahata chakra, March 20, 1956.

smoky colour. The Vayu Bija is YAM, which is seated on a black antelope.

The Devata is Isha of three eyes. His two arms are extended with the mudras for granting boons and dispelling fears.

Devi Dakini is seated on a red lotus, and she is four armed and carries the noose, the skull, and makes the sign of Vara ... [granting boons] ... and Abhaya ... dispelling fear. Her colour is of golden hue, and [she is] dressed in yellow.... In the middle of the mandala is Siva in the form of a Bana Linga with the crescent moon and bindu on his head. He is also of golden colour.

5) Vishuddha Chakra

Vishuddha chakra is at the base of the throat with sixteen petals of smoky purple hue. Its filaments are ruddy and the sixteen vowels are red colour with a bindu above each letter. Inside is the Chandra Mandala and within that the Bija HAM. The Ham Bija is pure white and is seated on a white elephant. It is Akasha Tattva, ether or space.

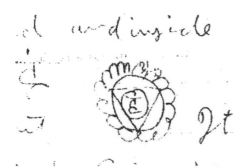

Figure 7.7. Letter from Swami Vishnudevananda describing how to meditate on the chakras, sketch of vishuddha chakra, March 20, 1956.

The Devata is Sada Siva seated on a lion skin which is placed on the back of a bull. Here Sada Siva is like Ardha Nareesvara (half the body is male and half is female) so half the body is snow colour and half is gold. He has five faces, each with three eyes, and ten arms. In his hands he holds the sula (trident), the tampa (battle axe), kadga (sword), vajra (thunderbolt), dahara (fire weapon), pasha (noose) and he makes the mudra to dispel fear. He is smeared with ashes, wearing a tiger skin and a garland of snakes.

Shakti Sakini is within the chakra, white in colour, also with five faces but with four arms. Each face has three eyes. She is clothed in yellow and carrying in each hand a bow, an arrow, a noose and a goad. [A goad is used to train elephants. This represents our elephant mind, or ego. If the goad can train the largest of land animals, it surely can train our minds.]

6) Ajna Chakra

The Ajna chakra has two petals and is white, and the two letters Ham and Kshàm are on these petals. They are also white. Within the centre of the triangle is OM, the Bija Mantra, the first word of the Vedas. Above this is the seat of mind.

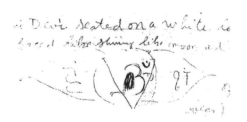

Figure 7.8. Letter from Swami Vishnudevananda describing how to meditate on the chakras, sketch of ajna chakra, March 20, 1956.

Also within the triangle within the lotus is the Itara Linga, a form of Siva, which is brilliant like lightning. This form of Siva enables one to cross kala or time.

The presiding Deity is Hakini Devi, seated on a white lotus, and she herself is white. She has six faces, shining like the moon, and three eyes in each. She has six arms, holding a rudraksha rosary, a human skull, a small drum, a book, and she makes the mudras to dispel fear and to give boons.[300]

Here I include an optional sahasrara opening meditation that I developed: as all six chakras are now awakened, observe the sensation of the crown chakra opening. A thousand white petals open to the heavens, with white, radiant energy flowing upward. Feel the universal energy flowing through you and from you. Enjoy and embrace this sensation as your individual energy immerses itself into the One, just as a drop of rain merges with the ocean.

To conclude the meditation, bring your awareness back to the body and mind. Visualize the petals of each chakra gently closing, starting at the sahasrara and moving down, one at a time, to the ajna, vishuddhi, anahata, manipura, svadhisthana, and muladhara. Slowly open your eyes, then lightly tap your feet on the ground to reconnect you to this earthly plane.

Heart Meditation

When we meditate, we may focus on an external object, such as a candle, a deity, or the sound of Om. And often we feel a deep oneness with our Source. These two aspects of meditation can be joined by meditating on the heart, which can be a beautiful experience. The heart may be the object, but it is the Spirit that lies within it that we want so deeply to connect to, so that we not only see the beauty of our true Self but also see the true Self within others. The heart will guide us to our "inner guru," the *sat guru*, or the true guru that we so desperately long to know. Swami Vishnudevananda explained it to Hari.

> Dive deep in the chakra of the heart. This means when you withdraw the senses from the object and turn inward. The knowledge [that] comes from within that is from the Consciousness of Chit. Consciousness is Sat, Chit & Anand. When the rays of the mind are focused and stilled, the knowledge comes from within itself. This is the Vedantic way. A devotee prays, and he also gets the knowledge from within. This is called intuition. This power of Intuition will come only through His Grace.
>
> In the Spiritual Path, without the Grace of God and teacher, one cannot completely get success. Every moment of our sadhana, many obstacles are awaiting. We have to transcend these obstacles one by one and march on to our goal. Much of our knowledge acquired in our previous births [is] lying in subconscious state of mind. This will also be brought to the conscious mind by meditating and purifying.[301]

With this idea of diving into the heart, the following meditation is a beautiful practice based on what we feel. The author of the letter this comes from is not identified.

> The higher objects of concentration are not external objects such as light, sound, etc., but subjective realities like "I-feeling" (Aham), pure "I-sense" (maha atma—Great Self), etc., which are to be thoroughly grasped by philosophical method to enable one to have a grasp of them for concentration. In the matter of practice we gladly give you the following hints:

The locality for concentration is within the chest where the reflexes of pleasure and pain are felt. It is not to be located by anatomical notions, but by *feeling*. After localizing this "Heart of hearts," the sense of locality is to be got rid of by concentrating the attention on *feeling* only.

Entering into this "Heart," imagine pure limitless space as clearly as you are able to do so. A few days practice will, it is expected, enable you to realize it.

Then think yourself as pervading that space, as if that space is your body. To be more explicit, as you feel yourself pervading your body by the "I-feeling," equally so during concentration you will have to pervade the space by your "I-feeling." The rationale is that by this practice our limited and gross "I-feeling" may be gotten rid of (at least loosened) so that we may proceed toward our limitless personality.

You may, while concentrating, repeat (mentally) the syllable *OM*, which helps to quiet the mind. The meaning of the syllable [Oneness with God] is what you are practicing, and by that syllable, recollect the pursuit of Yoga.

When you have realized this *"Dhyana,"* then try to stay in it without any other thought. It will be possible to do so by constant mindfulness (Smriti) and watch. After practicing for some time, you may let us know your experience and difficulties.[302]

The author added some practical guidelines to go along with the meditation, including how to make time for it.

Needless to say that you should practice "Yama" and "Niyama" as far as practicable in your position of life. You need not be afraid of re-incarnation. We are doing it from time without beginning, and a few more incarnations will not make much difference. By this practice and the study of Yoga philosophy, it is hoped you will be reassured on that score.

As for what you write about your duties, etc., you take a common-sense view. We have nothing to say on that point. Where there is a will, there is a way. We can, if we are determined, make time for doing what we really love and wish to do. Our other pursuits are thereby automatically regulated.[303]

When we move into the emotional realm of the heart chakra, I highly recommend following the meditation along with the mudra for emotional balance described at the end of chapter 5. As we begin to purify our hearts, the emotions can rise up and be somewhat overwhelming. This mudra will help us to stay balanced through the process.

Guhya Chakra Meditation

Guhya means "mystical" or "hidden." The *guhya chakra* (also spelled *guha*) is also called the *Brahma chakra*. Some authorities name it the "guru" or "master" chakra. It is difficult to locate the exact position of this chakra, so Swami Vishnu Tirth tried to shed some light on its anatomical location for Hari. In addition, a drawing by Tarachand Garg provides a good visual for this description (see fig. 7.10).

> [The] brain consists of innumerable centers of knowledge connected with both afferent and efferent nervous systems. [These chakras] cannot be called plexuses like the lower ones. Guha chakra may be located in the middle. On both sides of the brain (cerebrum) there are two channels as if to serve as drainage, called lateral ventricles, therein flows through them a fluid named cerebral fluid. The front parts of both [ventricles] converge at one point just behind the mid-eyebrow and empty their contents into the third ventricle, from which the fluid flows down from the back exit into the fourth ventricle and down through the spine. The brain is situated above the roof of the third ventricle. Thus you can picture your brain in your mind and try to fix your attention on the Ajna chakra in the area where the lateral ventricles meet. That should take your mind to the requisite center of the brain as directed by your thoughts, desires, or meditative piece of knowledge. If the mind is thoughtless, vacant, and still, it will be directed to the centre or guha chakra.[304]

To practice this meditation, sit in siddhasana or your most comfortable meditation seat. Lower the chin slightly, and let the three bandhas naturally come into place. Swami Vishnu Tirth, acknowledging the difficulty of finding the location of the guhya chakra, said that it could "be imagined to be between the two side ventricles within the brain" (this was edited significantly for flow):

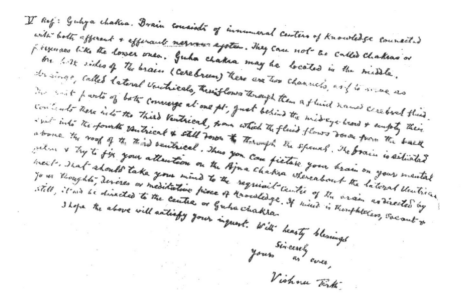

Figure 7.9. Letter from Swami Vishnu Tirth explaining the guhya chakra, May 16, 1966.

When you fix your mind there [on the guhya chakra] for a while, you will feel somewhat intoxicated and hear a sound like that of a bee humming. There are different methods of this meditiation according to different schools. You may, if you like, picture in your mind a red bee there, but I advise meditating without any such imagery. You will then see light—either dim or bright—sometimes a full moon with a starry sky and, at other times, a dazzling sun becomes visible. These visions appear of their own accord, without any effort, during the calm meditation.[305]

Continue the practice for as long as is comfortable.

Shunya Dhyana

Shunya means "void" or "emptiness." Achieving this emptiness of thought is a great challenge for most of us. This meditation from Swami Shivananda Saraswati of Assam was full of encouragement as he explaind to Hari the challenges of this meditation in our efforts to reach the Infinite. I love his explanation of how thinking is limiting.

It is an unavoidable stage for all who practice Shunya Dhyana when the Sadhaka has to fight out [the] advent of thought from without during Dhyana. To succeed in keeping your mind free from all thoughts, i.e., to make your mind Shunya, you should try to concentrate your mind a bit more. Don't get disheartened by initial failure, because it happened with us when we practiced it, and it happens with all who try to do it. Repeat the process time and again till you become the master of your mind. Regarding this, we have the instruction in the Gita.... Get yourself above mundane desire and try and try and try again. When you will succeed, you will be the master of your mind.

There are stages of Dhyana on the Infinite. At first think of the ocean or the sky as boundless and limitless. From psychological points of view, to think is to think within limit, however extensive that limit might be. Mind being limited, you cannot think of the unlimited or the Infinite. But as you will make progress, you will have the experience that gradually you will lose your separate identity, and a complete fusion between you and the Infinity will be established. You will merge yourself in profound oneness. At that time of realizing perfect oneness, you will have no sensation of the presence of any sort of idea or thought or anything else.[306]

He continued in another letter:

One may practice Shunya Dhyana for three months or more without practicing any other kind of Dhyana, or one may practice Shunya Dhyana and Dhyana of Infinite Space simultaneously, i.e., sometimes Shunya Dhyana, sometimes other kind of Dhyana. So, it depends on the liking of the sadhaks. [The] Sadhak should mind only that he shall have to control his mind, he shall have to make his mind thoughtless or he shall have to make his mind fully concentrated in one subject of thought or Dhyana.

Dhyana is mental activity. So you need not always see the Sky. Concentrate on your mental Sky. Think and feel that you are one with the Sky, you are one with the Infinite.

[The] preliminary stage of Dhyana is the direct method of Pratyahar. Naturally [the] mind will go hither and thither, and [the] sadhak will try to fix his mind on [the] object of Dhyana. It is called

"Obhyas" or repeated effort or attempt to concentrate the mind in one thought or in one object.[307]

The shunya meditation can be practiced thus: sit in a comfortable position with a straight spine. Close your eyes. Think of the ocean or the sky as boundless and limitless. Begin to merge yourself into the profound oneness.

Behind those closed eyes, become aware of a vast, limitless space. There are no boundaries to that space. Begin to lose your separate identity and feel a complete fusion between you and the infinite space, just as the river merges with the ocean and becomes one with it.

When thoughts intrude, return again to the void. Perhaps envision the endless sky. Think and feel you are one with the sky, one with the Infinite. Just as each cloud eventually dissipates and becomes one with the vast and boundless sky, begin to lose your separate identity and feel a complete fusion between you and infinite space.

At that time of realizing perfect oneness, you will have no sensation of ideas or thoughts or anything else. Simply experience oneness with all.

Shambhavi Mudra Meditation

Shambhu is a name for Siva, and *Shambhavi* is a name for Parvati, his consort and the mother of Ganesha. Parvati suggested to Siva that all the knowledge he acquired during his meditations was useless unless he intended to share it with others, so Siva suggested that he share it all with Parvati, and she could write it down for him.

Swami Vishnu Tirth, one of Hari's most beloved teachers, enlightened Hari on many aspects of yoga, and when he didn't have time, he had his disciples write the letters. This is the case with *shambhavi mudra;* it was a practice that Hari pursued clarity on, as it is mentioned in so many yogic texts and is related to the void or space of the ajna chakra. The knowledge shared with Hari on this topic deserves to be noted.

Shambhavi mudra is described in chapter 4 of the *Hatha Yoga Pradipika* as directing the eyes upward, toward the space between the eyebrows.[308]

According to the *Advaya Tarak Upanishad* of Shukla Yajurveda, this position of the eyes is not practiced but comes automatically.

In the case of both internal and external introspection, when both the eyes are devoid of the power of shutting and opening, there occurs what is known as the mudra pertaining to Shambhu. By the residence therein of sages who have assumed that mudra, the Earth is rendered holy. At their look, all the worlds are sanctified. Whoever is afforded the opportunity of worshipping such great yogins also become liberated.[309]

Dr. Chandra Singh Yadav answered a letter of Hari's on behalf of Swami Vishnu Tirth and explained this further:

The difference between Shambhavi and Tratak is that whereas the eyes remain open in Shambhavi Mudra, the mind is introverted, and the eyes do not see the external objects, while in Tratak the external world is visualized.

This introversion of the mind is described in the Bhagavad Gita Chapter 5 Verses 27–28 as shutting out the thoughts of external sense enjoyments. One must:

- Have the eyes fixed on the space between the eye-brows (Ajna Chakra),
- have equalized the Prana and Apana breaths flowing within the nostrils (exhalation and inhalation),
- have brought his senses, mind, and reason under control,
- be intent on salvation and free from desire, fear, and anger etc.

Then such a contemplative soul is ever liberated.

The Ajna Chakra has been rightly incorporated in the Medulla through various nerve connections, mainly the optical and auditory nerves, which end in the pineal gland. They work in some mysterious way to rarefy the mind into higher subtler planes of stillness with a simultaneous inversion of optical vision, giving the outer eyes an expression of blankness and cessation of breath.

The quintessence of blankness is the state of vacancy and thoughtlessness of the mind, where no object of any kind should remain except a serene void where even the thought of attaining such a blank-ness has no room to exist. If one is able to keep one's mind free of all thinking for sufficiently long time, the mind would naturally, without effort, merge into pure consciousness of Samadhi (Trance), otherwise effort is necessary to achieve the stillness of mind. For the attainment of such a blessed state of mind, constant practice is very essential, for, the mind is very unsteady and difficult to curb.[310]

Tarachand Garg, another disciple of Swami Vishnu Tirth, who worked in the Department of Anatomy at Mahatma Gandhi Memorial College in Indore, India, continued to clarify the anatomical effects of this mudra:

> About your question regarding concentration on Ajna chakra, if we go through your literature, we find that a yogi should concentrate in the middle of eyebrows on the frontal bone. This is the correct position, because when a yogi concentrates ... two things happen—
>
> (1) When the eyes are focused in the middle of eyebrows, they are converged and look up-wards. The muscles responsible are supplied by [the] oculomotor nerve. The nucleus of this nerve is situated in the mid brain near the aqueduct of midbrain in close proximity to a nucleus called "nucleus of darkschewitsh." This is connected with the pineal body, as shown in the accompanying chart and diagram. The nucleus of [the] oculomotor nerve is also connected with the pineal body via the medial longitudinal bundle, through the posterior commissure of the brain. Therefore any activity of the nucleus of oculomotor nerve will have an effect on [the] pineal body. This gland is very important in Yoga and according to yogic texts, it is known as "Jnan Netra" or the third eye of knowledge. It means that when this is active, the person attains a higher spiritual knowledge. Mythologically it is therefore shown as a third eye on the forehead of Lord Shiva.
>
> (2) When we look at any point, the retina will also be stimulated and a sensation will be aroused which will reach the optic chaisma via the optic nerves and from here will go to the superior corpora quadrigemina through optic tract. This will have an effect on [the] pineal gland, as shown in the chart. Thus the pineal body will ultimately be affected.
>
> From the above, we find that concentration in the middle of eyebrows will have an effect on [the] pineal body. Now let us see the extent of [the] Ajna chakra.
>
> According to the Soubhagya Laxami Upanishad, this chakra has three parts which lie at—

1) The level of the roof of the mouth
2) The root of the nose
3) The level of middle of eyebrow

If we draw horizontal lines at these levels around the skull we find that they correspond to the levels of the

1) fourth ventricle and pituitary gland
2) aqueduct of the midbrain
3) third ventricle and pineal body, respectively

Further the same Upanishad mentions that:

At the first level, the yogi should meditate on Shunya, i.e.: voidness.

At the second level, the yogi should meditate on an ascending line of smoke resembling the shape of a needle.

At the third level, the yogi should meditate on a candle flame.

Each of these is indicative of the shape of the important structure at that level.

Void or shunya = zero—a round thing = pituitary
Needle = thin cylindrical = aqueduct
Candle flame = pineal gland

We also know that within this area lay the various nuclei of the motor nerves to eye and the optic nerve is also connected with this area. Thus you will see now that the practices prescribed by the shastras, as mentioned above, lead to an activity of this area and the pineal body also. As a result, the pineal body looks like a candle flame to the inner vision of a yogi.[311]

Based on the above information on shambhavi mudra, we may practice the meditation in the following way:

Sit in a comfortable position. Place your hands in jnana mudra with the tips of the index fingers touching the tips of the thumbs, palms turned upward, hands resting on knees. Begin by watching your breath, observing in the natural flow of breath; the length of inhalation and exhalation should be equal.

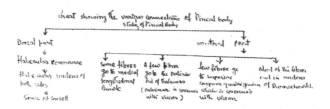

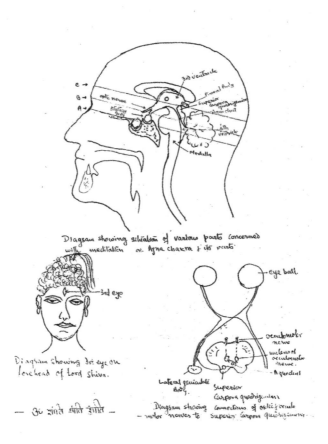

Figure 7.10. Diagram in letter from Tarachand Garg demonstrating how shambhavi mudra affects the pineal gland, pituitary gland, and the ajna chakra, December 25, 1957, p. 2.

Gently close your eyelids halfway and notice how your eyes naturally turn upward toward the ajna chakra. Observe the flow of breath. (If it is hard to relax with the eyelids half-open, then close the eyes for now, but practice holding them half-open a little every day.)

Begin to breathe in and out effortlessly through the third eye. As you inhale, feel the prana flow into the third eye, then through the brain and down the spine. As you exhale, watch the breath flow back up the spine, through the brain, and out the third eye. Just observe, without judgment. The more internal you become, the quieter the breath will be.

As you settle deeper into the silence, meditate on the shunya, the void, the nothingness. Notice how vast the space is behind the closed eyes. It may appear circular. It may appear completely boundless. Feel the calm within the void. Continue resting in this for about five minutes, or longer, if possible.

Within that void, notice a thin line of smoke ascending upward. It resembles the shape of a needle or the thin line of smoke ascending from a lit incense stick. Notice its movement upward, dissipating into the void. Simply notice. Relax into the calm space within and continue for about five minutes, or longer, if possible.

Within the void, notice a candle flame. Observe its light within the void. Sometimes it may appear dark surrounded by light, sometimes light surrounded by dark. Simply observe it as it appears for you. Allow yourself to relax into the radiant light within the void.

Continue the practice for as long as is comfortable.

I recommend following this practice with the mudra for psychic balance, as described at the end of the chapter 5.

Meditation on the Mantra *Hrim*

In a letter to Tarachand Garg, Hari asked about being initiated into Swami Vishnu Tirth's yoga path of awakening the kundalini. Tarachand was coming to the United States in 1959 to continue his anatomy studies at the University of Minnesota and was then going to New York to visit Hari. Tarachand told him, however, that Swamiji very rarely offered this *shakti pat diksha* (pronounced "deeksha") any longer. He had two disciples who did this for him, but, of course, they were in India, and Tarachand was not able to do it for them.[312]

In shakti pat diksha, the guru transmits the higher energy to a worthy disciple. Hari hoped Swami Vishnu Tirth could confer this energy to him. Swami Vishnu Tirth said he could not do it from a distance, nor could he come to the United States. But he did offer an alternative.

He suggested Hari adopt japa meditation of the mantra *hrim* (pronounced "hreem") for at least an hour daily. He had to abstain from beef, meat, fish, eggs, and alcohol. "The mantra Hrim carries with it some Shakti, and it may help you to some extent, though not to your full satisfaction."[313]

In my notes from the time I studied with Hari, I wrote the following explanation of the mantra hrim. *H* is for Siva, *R* is for Kali, *I* is for the individual soul, and *M* is the merger of them. Within this bija mantra lies the power to merge the masculine and feminine energies with the individual soul—that sounds like a powerful merger of Shakti to me!

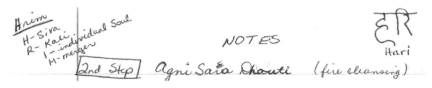

Figure 7.11. Hrim mantra from author's notes, 1979.

To do this meditation, we must know how to use japa mala beads. The mala has 108 beads, plus a *meru*, a larger bead with a tassle hanging from it. This is your starting point. Hold the string of beads in your right hand, over the middle finger, at the level of the heart, the anahata chakra. The index finger does not touch the beads, as it represents the ego mind. The lower part of the string of beads can be held in the left hand at the level of the navel, the manipura chakra. Starting at the first bead next to the meru, repeat your mantra and pull a bead to the right, using your thumb and middle finger. Each time you say your mantra, a bead is pulled to the right, one by one, until you have repeated the mantra 108 times. When you reach the meru bead again, pause and thank your guru and teachers for their guidance. Turn the beads around by flipping them onto the crook of the thumb, then tuck the middle finger under the string and flip them back over it. Avoid touching the index finger in the process. You will now be going in the opposite direction for the next round. Turning the beads around and going the other way represents release from the cycle of reincarnation.

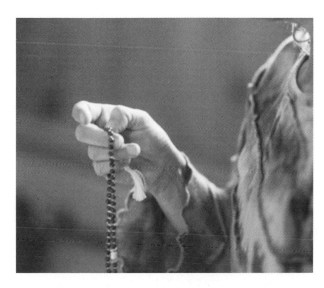

Figure 7.12.
Using mala beads.
Photo: Galen Scorer.

Here is a meditation on Hrim as told to Hari by Swami Vishnu Tirth; I have reconstructed it from instructions found in several letters from 1960 to 1966.

Sit in Siddhasana. Meditate on the meaning of each letter of the mantra.

H stands for Siva or Brahman.

R stands for his power or Shakti.

I (pronounced "e") means consciousness.

The nasal sound of *M* denotes merging of personal consciousness into the Divine.

The *H* should not be silent, but when pronounced together with the *R*, the emphasis will lie on the *R*. The *R* stands for force, as if the Divine force is taking you beyond body and mind.

Thus you will see the sound of the mantra will take one's consciousness bereft of [the body consciousness] to the divine consciousness.[314]

Awareness of self-consciousness is meant [as the] "I feeling." In the beginning it may be body-consciousness, but gradually every physical consciousness will be lost. Pure consciousness is undoubtably attributeless—free from all foreign excrements, and that is the nature of Atman (self). [The] seat of "I consciousness" for [this] practice is near the heart, a bit towards the right.[315]

Even if you cannot follow the meaning of each letter of the Mantra Hrim as suggested, simple mental repetition of the syllable "Hrim" without thinking of the meaning it implies, also helps the awakening of the Kundalini.[316]

Repeat the mantra Hrim using the japa mala beads 108 times. Pause at the meru ... and again meditate on the meaning of each letter in the mantra. Turn the mala beads around so you do not cross the meru, and going the opposite direction, repeat the mantra Hrim 108 times. Remind yourself of the intention of the mantra, "My personal consciousness merges with the Divine Consciousness."

Continue using the mala beads in this way for as many repetitions as you desire. When you are done, set down your mala beads and let stillness and blankness of mind come without any effort on your part. When the mind is withdrawn from thoughts, it comes to a standstill, but the consciousness of the Self is still there, undisturbed and free from external influences.

Feel in the senses that the Atman is not body, senses, or mind. Rather, meditate on the Self beyond body, senses, and mind. Fix the mind on Atman.

Merge your personal consciousness with the Divine Consciousness. Such a mind ultimately becomes merged in samadhi, and upon revival of consciousness, it will give self-realization.

Meditation on Nad

In chapter 4 of the *Hatha Yoga Pradipika*, meditation on *nad* (sound) the inner sounds is discussed as an effective way to attain *Laya*, or absorption into the Self (or absolving all else). The inner sounds resonate from the *akasha*, "spaces" or "inner voids" of the higher chakras, those in the spiritual or psychic realm, including the heart, vishuddha, and ajna chakras, depending on where the prana has risen to.[317]

The sounds mentioned in the *Hatha Yoga Pradipika* vary slightly from Swami Vishnu Tirth's letters, but I don't think that is important. We must remember that prana is energy, and how we experience its manifestation is interpreted through the mind. These sounds are personal for each of us and therefore difficult to describe. They are the sounds of our own inner vibrations, which are not heard via the ears, but rather through the ear of the heart. It will not be the same experience for everyone, though different people's experiences will definitely be similar.

The ten inner sounds that one may hear are described by Swami Vishnu Tirth: (1) *chin nada,* or the sound of a honey bee or crickets; (2) *chin-chin nada,* or the sound of a waterfall or ocean; (3) the chiming of a bell; (4) the blowing of a conch shell; (5) the music of string instrument; (6) the beating of a drum; (7) a flute; (8) the high pitch of drum beatings; (9) the sound of a bugle-like pipe instrument called *bheri;* (10) thunder.[318]

According to the *Hatha Yoga Pradipika,* there are four stages within which these sounds manifest. Each is related to where the prana is in the sushumna. Swami Vishnu Tirth says that as one progresses, the inner sounds become more audible. The eyeballs also automatically (without any voluntary effort) roll upward.[319]

The first stage is called *arambha avastha,* which means "the beginning stage." The sound can be heard when the *Brahma granthi* has been pierced so the prana can move into the sushumna. Prana moves upward through the sushumna to the shunya or void of the heart, where bliss arises in the anahata chakra. The unstruck sound of the heart can be heard, along with tinkling sounds, like that of ornaments striking together.

The second stage is *ghata avastha.* A *ghata* is a pot or a vessel, and now we are moving deeper into the vast world within the vessel of our being. When the *Vishnu granthi* is pierced, the prana unites (meaning the prana, apana, nada, bindu, the jiva atman, and the param atman) and enters the *ati shunya,* the void of the vishuddhi chakra in the throat area. One may hear the sounds of the kettledrum rising from within this void.

The third stage is *parichaya avastha.* This is a more intimate stage—we gain a much deeper understanding of the Self, beyond the physical. The prana moves up to the *maha shunya,* the void of the ajna chakra in the space between the eyebrows, the seat of all siddhis. Here the sound of the mardala drum is heard, and we move beyond the mind into the blissful state of atman that arises from these inner sounds.

The fourth state is *nishpatti avastha,* an ecstatic state when the prana can rise to the Brahmarandhra at the top of the sushumna. Shiva and Shakti unite. The *Rudra granthi* is broken in the ajna chakra, and the prana flows up to the brahmarandhra. Here the inner sound of the *vina,* a stringed instrument, is often heard. At this stage, one has attained raja yoga, where the duality of the jivatman and paramatman no longer exists.[320]

To move into this meditation, sit in siddhasana or your comfortable meditation pose. You do not need to fix your eyes at the mid-brow point.

You can simply close your eyes and keep your attention on the inner sounds, the nada.

In the beginning you can use yoni mudra (see that section in chapter 5) to block the senses from going outward. Close the eyes with the index fingers, the ears with the thumbs, the nose with the middle fingers (symbolically), and the mouth with the ring and baby fingers. This will help you to hear the sounds in the sushumna passage.[321] When your arms tire or your attention has moved inward, lower your hands to your knees in jnana mudra (described in the section "Maha Bandha" in chapter 5).

Direct your attention toward nada, the inner sound. You may begin by listening for the sounds in the inner right ear,[322] the ear of the heart, the ear of the soul. Listening here helps attune one to Om, the vibrational sound of the universe, the highest mantra, the music of the spheres.

As the sound of Om appears in the inner right ear, extend that sound gradually to the left ear and then to the whole body. Receive the Om into the whole being.

As your meditation deepens, listen for what other sounds arise—possibly chimes, flutes, or drums. Allow the mind to concentrate on the sounds. Allow yourself to merge with the sounds effortlessly. Simply observe the sounds as they appear. Do not strive to hear them. Relax into the inner, higher self. Let the sounds carry you there, to the consciousness of the True Self.

Continue the practice for as long as is comfortable. When you are ready, lower your chin slightly toward your chest so that when you open your eyes, you have a downward gaze to gently bring you back into the world of senses.

Mantra *diksha* (initiation) is traditionally given in the right ear because that is the positive side of the body. The right is God, and the left is our human form. Hearing the mantra in the right ear stimulates the right brain, which awakens the heart on the left side of the body.[323] There is a special correlation between the inner right ear and the superconscious experience.

As one receives Om into one's whole being, one also receives the guru's inner blessings as guidance. These things cannot be accomplished by tension or striving, but only by deep, upward relaxation into the inner, higher Self. Paramhansa Yogananda recommended chanting Om softly into the right ear of a person who is in the process of leaving the body.[324]

Vedic Trinity Meditation

Although I call this a meditation, it is also called Vedic Raja Yoga Pranayama, done with meditation on the Vedic Trinity. Swami Shivananda Saraswati of Assam named it a pranayama, but it is a pranayama with meditation, so I have chosen to include it here. (See "Kumbhak Pranayama" in chapter 4.)

Vedic Pranayama fixes equal importance on the three stages, i.e., Purak Kumbhak and Rechak, and [the] time fixed for each is equal. But it has to be done with meditation of the Vedic Trinity—namely, Brahma, Vishnu, and Shiva. Shiva, the symbol of the Absolute or the Supreme Soul (God of Jnanapanthi or Nirguna Brahma); Vishnu (The God of Supreme Love) happens to be the symbolic expression of the qualified god or Iswara; Brahma—is the Supreme Energy Incarnate, who shapes the Universe, [creates] everything and hence the God of Creation. Brahma has four faces on four sides, with which he [supervises] of controls his creation—the whole universe.

Vedic Pranayama locates these three gods at three important centres of the body, where they should be meditated upon—with pranayama. With Purak, Brahma must be meditated at the region of the navel, Vishnu at the heart with Kumbhak, and Shiva at the forehead with Rechak. A fleeting mind during pranayama is a natural loss; hence such meditation directly helps deeper concentration and concomitant benefits.

The Trinity have different colours; Brahma—fiery red, Vishnu—sky blue, and Shiva—Absolute White—or snow white rather. Here the colours are also symbolic—red for creation, sky blue for Infinity or God Consciousness, Whiteness for Absolute, where all colours or quality lose their entity and vanish.

The yogins find importance in the meditations of these three colours, thrice daily in the part that they have a direct bearing upon individual's health by balancing the activity of Vata, Pitta, and Kafa (air, bile, and mucus). Of course, [this] is the preliminary stage of Vedic Pranayama. There are also higher stages of it with Vedantic meditations, i.e., Brahma—Vabana.

What consists of Raj Yoga and Vedic Pranayama? Vedic Pranayama has given equal importance to the three phases; Rechak,

Purak, and Kumbhak, which Raj yoga pranayama stresses upon the Kumbhak only, its aim is to increase Kumbhak as far as possible.

Pranayama with meditation gradually concentrates the mind and dips it into sublimity. When alone, the practice of Raj Yoga should be started when Vedic pranayama is well practiced and [the] mind is somewhat under control. During its practice of Raj-Yoga, [the mind] should be completely free of any thought or even of the minutest vibration of it (Surya Brahma), since the aim of both pranayama is the achieve Samadhi. It is evident then why the maximum stress lies on stilling the mind [in] Vedic and Raj-yoga pranayama. So, the full value of pranayama lies in stilling the mind and realising of the Absolute. Thus the higher method[s] of pranayama have the only objective in the communion with the Supreme Consciousness.[325]

To experience this meditation, sit in a comfortable position with an erect spine.

Inhale for a count of six. Visualize Brahma at the region of the navel, with four heads facing the four directions. The color is fiery red, symbolizing creation. Engage the mind as you try to grasp the essence of Brahma as the Supreme Energy who shapes the Universe. He creates the whole universe and supervises his creation. All is a divine plan.

Retain the breath for a count of six. Visualize Vishnu at the heart region, sky blue for the vastness and infinity of God Consciousness. Vishnu is the ultimate protector, preserving all that is good in the Universe. Feel the Supreme Love that emanates from your heart.

Exhale for a count of six. Visualize Siva at the forehead, the Absolute Supreme Soul, without qualities. Siva is the transformative energy, removing all that is no longer needed, making way for the new. Pure white energy radiates from the area of the third eye, and all colors and all qualities vanish into the white light.

Repeat for up to thirty minutes with even, equal breaths. If a lower count is more comfortable, then decrease your count, as required, to be completely comfortable with the pranayama. Too much effort will distract the mind, resulting in a loss of prana. When you are ready, lower your chin slightly toward your chest, so that when you open your eyes, you have a downward gaze to gently bring you back into the world of senses.

Meditation Using Drishtis

Drishtis are where we focus our eyes and, therefore, our attention during meditation. During my time in Swami Vishnudevananda's ashram in the Bahamas, it was suggested to me that I should focus my eyes toward the ajna chakra, the space between the eyebrows, also known as the *bhrumadhya drishti*. The process helped me to quiet the mind, but I did not really understand why I was doing it. There is also another common drishti for meditation, the *nasikagra drishti*, that is, the tip of the nose. Sri Satyakam illuminated information about the drishtis as explained in the Bhagavad Gita.

> In Gita we get importance of both Nasikagra and Bhrumadhya Drishti. Bhrumadhya drishti generally helps us to meditate on Self, Vichara (self-discrimination) and topics regarding Jnana (knowledge) yoga. Nasikagra Drishti helps us generally to meditate on devotional topics, (Bhakti Yoga) such as Iswar Pranidhan and Japa. We should give preference in accordance with our taste and nature. Here bear in mind that you should not practice Bhrumadhya Drishti for a long time, which may be harmful.[326]

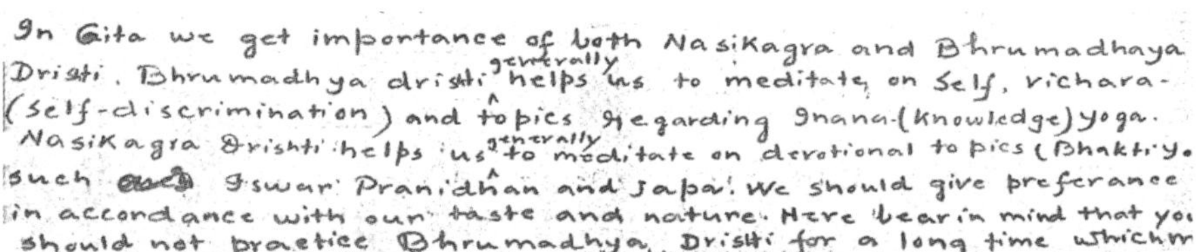

In Gita we get importance of both Nasikagra and Bhrumadhaya Drishti. Bhrumadhya dristi generally helps us to meditate on Self, vichara (self-discrimination) and topics Regarding Jnana (knowledge) yoga. Nasikagra Drishti helps us generally to meditate on devotional topics (Bhakty. Such as Iswar Pranidhan and Japa. We should give preferance in accordance with our taste and nature. Here bear in mind that you should not practice Bhrumadhya Dristi for a long time whichm be harmful.

Figure 7.13. Letter from Sri Satyakam, Amritan Yogapeeth, Jadarpur, India, undated.

These two drishtis support us according to how our personality is inclined—those ruled by their heads and those ruled by their hearts. If we are drawn to God through knowledge and jnana yoga, then we would use bhrumadhya drishti, holding our eyes gently upward toward the space between our eyebrows during meditation. If we are more inclined toward bhakti yoga, the path of love and devotion, we may focus our eyes in nasikagra drishti, a downward gaze toward the heart, represented by gently directing our eyes to the tip of the nose. The eyes can be open or closed.

Sometimes we may be led by our hearts but feel the need to balance that with higher knowledge, so we use bhrumadhya drishti. Or vice versa— when we are predominantly led by our heads and need to seek into our heart or deepen our practice of *iswara pranidhana* (surrender to the Divine), then we use nasikagra drishti.

Japa and Ajapa Meditation

Japa is the process of repeating a mantra continuously during meditation. The mind is purified by constant japa. It raises the vibrations of thought waves from rajasic to sattvic. Repeating the Lord's name uninterruptedly draws all the Divine qualities into the mind and heart. It relieves mental and emotional stresses while firmly grounding one in God's strength.

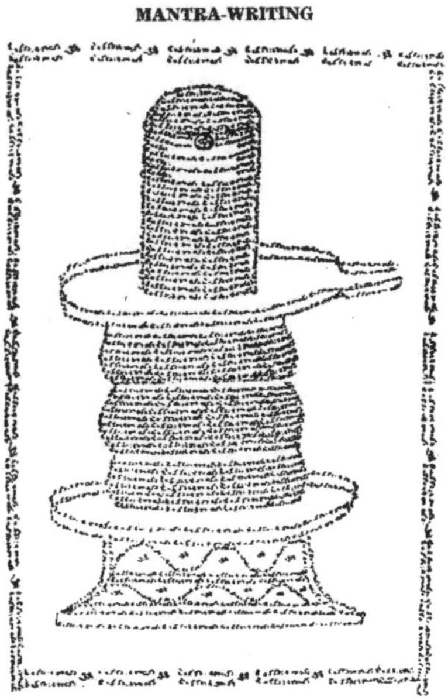

Swami Sivananda says japa gives a nicely refreshing and exhilarating spiritual bath. It wonderfully washes the subtle body (linga sharira or astral body).[327] Through japa alone, one can realize God in this life.[328] He says japa checks the force of the thought-current moving toward objects. It forces the mind to move toward God, toward the attainment of eternal bliss. It eventually helps to have darshan (direct perception) of God.[329]

There are several different forms of japa. Verbally repeating the mantra is called *vaikhari japa*. This helps to shut out all worldly sounds and is helpful if you become sleepy during your practice. When the mantra is whispered or hummed softly, it is called *upamsu japa*, and when a mantra is repeated silently, it is called *manasika japa*.

MANTRA-WRITING

Figure 7.14. Swami Sivananda's likhita japa of Om Namah Sivaya mantra. From *Japa Yoga* by Sri Swami Sivananda, eighth edition, Divine Life Society, 1978, 82.

Sandilya says in *Sandilya Upanishad:* "The Vaikhari Japa (loud pronunciation) gives the reward as stated in the Vedas; while the Upamsu Japa, whispering or humming, which cannot be heard by anyone, gives a reward a thousand times more than the Vaikhari; the Manasika Japa (mental Japa) gives a reward a crore times more than the Vaikhari Japa."[330]

When a mantra is written over and over again, it is called *likhita japa.* This develops tremendous power of concentration and spiritual benefits. Pictures can be drawn by writing a mantra in a continuous line during a meditation sitting, as Swami Sivananda of Rishikesh demonstrated in his book *Japa Yoga.*[331]

In mental repetition of japa, manasika japa, the mantra continuously revolves in the mind. This is the most powerful japa—and the most challenging—since we are so easily distracted when in silence. The lips should not move when we mentally repeat the mantra. This technique is said to give a hundred million times the benefits of vaikhari japa.

But there is another form of japa, known as *ajapa japa,* which is described in the *Gheranda Samhita.*

> The breath of every person in entering the body makes the sound of "Sah" and in coming out, that of "ham." These two sounds make So Ham "I am That" or Ham Sa "The Great Swan." Throughout a day and a night, there are twenty-one thousand and six hundred such respirations (that is, 15 respirations per minute). Every living being (Jiva) performs this japa unconsciously, but constantly. This is called Ajapa gayatri.[332]

Here is how Swami Shivananda Saraswati of Assam described the process for Hari:

> Through the breathing system, the Jiva [individual soul] is always uttering "He is I am, I am the Supreme Divinity." When we inhale, it is uttered "sho" and when exhaling, it is uttered "Hang." This natural Jap is Ajapajap. If a Sadhak, without doing anything, only [is] attentive to this system of Ajapajap, his mind will be concentrated.
>
> There is another kind of Ajapajap. When you inhale, you may draw air with the rhythm of Aum. After a long practice, it will be a habit even in sleeping state.[333]

Technique 1

To practice the ajapa gayatri meditation, sit in a comfortable position with an erect spine. Begin by watching the breath. Let it flow freely, without trying to control it. Simply notice the natural ebb and flow of the incoming and outgoing breath.

Begin to notice the natural pauses that occur after the inhalation and before the exhalation, and after the exhalation, before the inhalation. As you inhale, listen within for the sound of *So* riding on your breath. As you exhale, listen within for the sound of *Ham* riding on your breath. (*Ham* is pronounced as "hum.")

Continue observing the breath and listening to the mantra *So Ham* with each inhalation and exhalation. When your thoughts wander, bring them back to the mantra's meaning: "I am one with my Creator."

Technique 2

Hari taught me another ajapa gayatri technique from the natha yoga lineage. The higher technique is to concentrate on the ajna chakra with the eyes half-open. Notice, as you breathe, if you start with an inhalation or an exhalation. This is a subtle observation.

If you are not sure, then follow the method that appeals to you.

Ham Sa means "I am He," and *So Ham* means "He is I." It is not necessary to repeat the mantra, but always be aware of the sound and the meaning of it for union with God.

If you exhale first, use the mantra *Ham Sa.*

Exhale *Ham*—I go out with the breath to mix with the universe or God.

Inhale *Sa*—He comes in with the universe and becomes me within myself.

If you inhale first, then start with the mantra *So Ham.*

Inhale *So*—He comes in with the universe and becomes me within myself.

Exhale *Ham*—I go out with the breath to mix with the universe or God.

Repeat this mantra for a half-hour or so. Then sit with yoni mudra to continue the meditation, and listen for the inner sound in the right ear. Alternatively, you can systematically move your attention from the manipura to anahata and to ajna, holding your attention at each location. When you reach the ajna, you will automatically raise to sahasrara.[334]

Technique 3

Because the ajapa gayatri is such a sacred and beautiful mantra, there are many variations on the technique. Here is one last technique from Hari, one I also learned from yoga master Bill Phillips, and which merely integrates both mantras into one breath. Remember to observe the breath as it flows naturally, without controlling it in any way.

Inhale *Ham Sa.*
Exhale *So Ham.*
Inhale *So Ham.*
Exhale *Ham Sa.*

Visualize the prana moving up the back of the spine from muladhara to sahasrara on the inhalation, and back down the front of the spine on the exhalation. The breath follows the mantra, so as the mind slows down, so does the breath. The breath may actually stop for moments as in kevala kumbhaka (see the section "Kevala Pranayama" in chapter 4), in which there is no movement in thought or breath.

Ham Sa and So Ham are actually one, the inhalation and exhalation of ordinary life. The difference lies in the degree of development. Ham Sa is the uneven flow of prana and relates to the state of ignorance. So Ham is the even flow of prana and relates to the state of enlightenment and brings a natural state of samadhi. Prana in the form of Ham Sa moves through the right and left nadis, pingala and ida. Under the guidance of a guru, prana becomes So Ham and moves into the central nadi, sushumna, and kevala kumbhaka can occur.

Swami Muktananda said in his book *So'Ham Japa,* "When So'ham becomes active in prana-apana, the breath is suspended (kevala kumbhaka). When a man perceives hamsa as so'ham, he is emancipated from all bondage."[335]

Meditation on the Guru or the Ishta Devata

The guru is "a guide to the Spirit" and, generally, your spiritual teacher. A guru is designated a guru by his or her own personal guru; a guru is never self-named a guru.

Those who are fortunate enough to have found a guru will place a photograph of their guru on their meditation altar. This helps to remind them that their guru is a direct guide to the Spirit within.

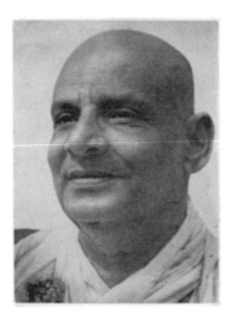

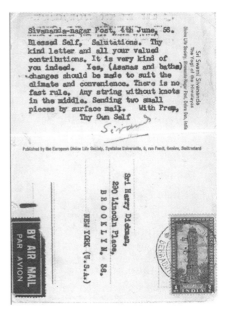

Figure 7.15. Postcard (front) from Swami Sivananda of Rishikesh, June 4, 1956.

Figure 7.16. Postcard (back) from Swami Sivananda of Rishikesh, June 4, 1956.

Those who do not have a guru can choose an *Ishta Devata*. Since everything is from and of God, then the Ishta Devata is the form of God that you

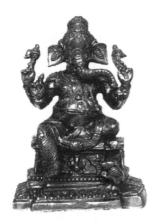

Figure 7.17. Statue of Ganesha as an Ishta Devata. Photo by author.

have personally chosen to remind you of God, the Atman within you. Generally a person is attracted to the specific qualities of a god or goddess, such as Ganesha, the remover of obstacles; Lakshmi, the bountiful provider; Siva, the great warrior; or Jesus, the son of God. The Ishta Devata becomes a vehicle for you to develop and strengthen your own divine qualities similar to the god.

It is not the photograph or the statue that are important; it is what those objects represent—God within. We start by meditating on the "name and form" to have something to concentrate on. The form stirs emotion within us as we feel love and gratitude for the teachings we receive from them. We entrust them with our need at the moment: how to remove an obstacle, how to interpret a passage of scripture, the healing for a loved one—these sorts of needs. As our meditation deepens, we move beyond the name and form into the deeper essence or truth of what they represent for us. They become the vehicle for us to connect to the Divine deep within. The last stage is complete union with your guru or Ishta Devata. There is no separation, only oneness, and all wisdom is revealed.

Sometimes this is referred to as "knower, knowledge, known." We think we know, but we know not. The real knower is the Atman within, whom we can come in contact with through our guru or Ishta Devata. The knowledge is the eternal truth that is realized or known during this process, known from the perspective of eternal truth. Our consciousness becomes one with that of our guru. Yoga master Erich Schiffmann teaches us to "get online with Big Mind, just like our computer connects to the server and we connect to the World Wide Web." It is a good analogy for when we get "online" with God through meditation.

Swami Sivananda of Rishikesh said, "To establish contact with one's own Guru or other yogis, one need not resort to astral travels. As a matter of fact, the relationship between an aspirant and a guiding yogi are transcendental; astral contacts are too low for this purpose. Put yourself in spiritual communion through meditation in Brahmamuhurta; you will inevitably be able to catch up the vibrations of Great Ones and myself. A few such sittings will convince you of the efficacy of this method."[336]

Paramhansa Yogananda told Hari, "Just as one dynamo [generator] spreads electricity in all the lights of this city, so the God-contacting devotee's spirit is spread to all those who are in tune with him. That is what I meant in the sentence, 'I am always with you in Spirit.' Those devotees who are in tune with their guru through unconditional devotion, obedience, and loyalty, feel the constant flow of their teacher's blessings."[337]

Hari's teachers from Self-Realization Fellowship said, "The blessings of the Master come to each soul in that degree that he is receptive. Let nothing rob you of the joy that conscious realization of His presence will bring. Night and day, God alone. Meditate deeply, and serve selflessly."[338]

I want to explain about the *Brahmamuhurta* mentioned above by Swami Sivananda. Although Brahmamuhurta is considered by some as the last hour before sunrise, Swami Sivananda suggested it is much longer.

The Brahmamuhurta is the last quarter of the night or the 2½ to 3 hours immediately preceding sun-rise. There is no special kind of meditation, but you should remember one or two points to benefit fully from it. When you sit for such meditation, commence with the earnest sankalpa [intention], "Now I will contact and receive the elevating spiritual currents generated by my Master in His meditation today". Then after having begun the Dhyan, put thyself in a fully receptive sattwic attitude and concentrate on the one you wish to contact. It is not necessary to synchronise timings of Himalayas and Germany. It is in relation to the meditator. All spiritual vibrations radiating from a given centre are permanently lodged in the Akashic medium. Later on you can contact and receive them at whatever time you meditate, putting thyself in the receptive state.[339]

With all of this in mind, Hari reminded me to meditate every chance I can—five minutes here and fifteen minutes there—and to record the minutes in a little notebook. It all adds up through the day and consistently takes one deeper to the Atman, on and off throughout the day.

To prepare for this meditation, sit in siddhasana or a comfortable meditation seat. Place a picture or statue of your guru or Ishta Devata on your altar so you can see the image clearly, and then take that image inward.

Imagine the guru or Istha Devata in a subtle form and offer worship mentally. Offer flowers, incense, or *prasad* (a spiritual offering of food) or anything that is spiritually meaningful as gifts. Set your sankalpa (intention), such as, "Now I will contact and receive the elevating spiritual currents generated by my guru or Ishta Devata."

Treat your guru in your meditation with immense adoration, love, and kindness, as you would do if you were really at his or her feet in the flesh.

You might repeat a mantra that conjures up the essence of your worship, such as *Om Gum Ganapatayei Namaha* or *Om Namah Sivaya*. Let the mantra fill your heart and mind, filling any space so no intruding thoughts can distract your mind away from your love and adoration. Be completely receptive, with a sattvic (pure) attitude.

What are the qualities within your guru that you wish to develop within you? Take those loving qualities and plant them, like seeds, within you. Water them daily in your meditations so that they flourish throughout your daily activities. Become one with those loving qualities.

When the mind wanders, return your thoughts to the image of the guru or Ishta Devata. Continue the practice for half an hour or as long as is comfortable.

Samyama

Samyama is the practice discussed in Patanjali's *Yoga Sutras* 3:1–6. The practices of the three inner stages of ashtanga yoga—dharana, dhyana, and samadhi (concentration, meditation, and contemplation)—blend one into the next.

Concentration is the practice of fixing the mind on an object. The object may be external, like the photo of your guru, or internal, like a chakra. The mind is held completely focused on this object, and the effect is that one's mental power is focused internally.

Meditation is a steady, continuous flow of attention toward the object of concentration. Each thought wave is related to the object, one after another, so there is no break in the flow. More and more knowledge is acquired as you focus your full attention continuously on the object.

Lastly, contemplation of the object is the practice in which one acquires complete understanding of the true nature or spirit of the object, in which the meditator becomes one with the object. There is no separation, no self-awareness. This is samadhi.

Through the process of samyama, the deeper knowledge of any manifested object is taken right to the Source. This is how yogis acquire siddhis and the power over anything—knower, knowledge, known.

Swami Sivananda of Rishikesh shared a technique of samyama to achieve control over the senses, or *indriyas*.

Meditation on the actual process of perception; of hearing, of feeling, [of seeing, of touching, of smelling]. The Yogi here delineates the various stages of sense-perception. By degrees, he reaches the Purusha, the real Perceiver! Once he knows the Purusha as the perceiver, hearer, etc., he has achieved perfection in this practice, and is able to acquire the fullest control over his indriyas.

He continued with the process of samyama on discrimination:

In short, the idea here is that the Yogi should not be led away by even the highest offers of enjoyment. Vedantic texts ridicule even the status of Brahma and Indra! Sri Sankaracharya defines Vairagya as dispassion or aversion toward even the position of Brahma, the Creator! The Yogi should discriminate between the real and the unreal. By doing Samyama on the power of discrimination itself, the Yogi acquires real intuitive knowledge of the method of distinguishing the real from the unreal and thus is in a position to brush aside the unreal, even if it be the position of the gods, and aim only at Final Liberation through knowledge of the Self.... A Yogi of powerful will can rouse his Inner Will Power by a mere thought. Through the intense and steady practice of Samyama on the powers of the mind and on the control of the mind, he masters this horse of great power. That is the secret of will and memory.[340]

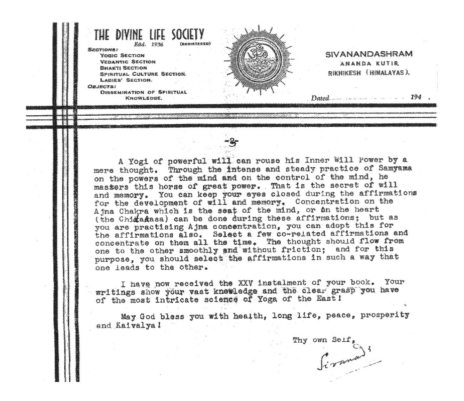

Figure 7.18. Letter from Swami Sivananda on samyama, April 1948.

Atma Vichara Meditation

Atma vichara means "inquiry into consciousness itself." I really love this meditation, and once Erich Schiffmann told me that it was one of his favorites too—in fact, he devotes a small section to it in his book *Yoga: The Spirit and Practice of Moving into Stillness.*[341] It is no wonder Erich loves this meditation—he has a firm grasp on the beautiful technique and continuously reminds his students to discriminate between what is real and what is unreal.

The ultimate practice of samyama is the discrimination of "Who am I?" All through our yogic path, we are told that we are not this body, we are not this mind. If this is the case, then who are we? *Aham Brahmasmi,* I am Brahman. We are the unchanging, everlasting Spirit. But how do we get to know our true Self? Swami Sivananda explained.

> Atma Vichar is negation of the unreal and assertion of the real; it is a process of sifting, of analyzing and picking out the wheat from the chaff. Whatever is subject to the working of the three Gunas is Prakriti. Whatever contains in it an element of these Gunas is Prakriti. Purusha is the Transcendental Being beyond the pale of the Gunas. Prakriti is the active principle; Purusha is the Static principle.
>
> But meditation is one continuous flow of a positive thought, like "I am Brahman," "Sat-Chit-Anandam Brahman," etc. Meditate on the Atman as Sat-Chit-ananda (Existence-Knowledge-Bliss Absolute); the ocean of light, bliss, all-pervading, Indwelling Presence. Samyama on the Atman, on these lines, will greatly elevate you.[342]

This meditation involves a process of negation known as *neti neti,* which means "not this, not this." *Prakriti* is all of the manifested Universe, which is subject to the effects of the three gunas. The gunas are the three potential qualities found in everything that is manifested. The three qualities are *sattva* (purity, light, harmony, and balance), *rajas* (activity and passion), and *tamas* (darkness and inertia). As an example, your asana practice can be perfectly harmonious and balanced (sattvic), or aggressive and potentially harmful (rajasic), or lazy and without any dedication (tamasic).

One's body and mind are prakriti, but the soul, the Atman, is not. So this meditation is to negate everything that is prakriti, which will eventually leave us with the Atman.

The essence of the Vedic Upanishads is that we are Brahman, *Tat Tvam Asi* (that Thou art), and this meditation is a process to guide us to the eternal Self by negating who we are not. Each time we ask the question "Who am I?" we answer with what we are not, until there is nothing left but the Self.

Swami Sivananda of Rishikesh explained to Hari that he could start the process with any *indriya,* or sense, by forming the appropriate question.

> If you rigorously enquire "Who is it that speaks? Who is seeing? Who is smelling? Who is hearing?" and so on—you will come to the conclusion that the gross and the subtle Indriyas are not the real speakers. It is the mind. If you ask the mind "Who is the real speaker?" you will come to the conclusion that even the mind is dependent on the Buddhi. That is the point up to which argumentation and intellection can go. If you persist in your enquiry, all thought will cease, and you will have immediate awareness of the Inner Pure Consciousness [that] alone lends light to the Buddhi, Mind, and the Indriyas.[343]

Who is this that hears the cars going by outside? The sounds will not last, therefore it is not I. Who is this that feels pain in the knee? This pain will not last, therefore it is not I. Who is this that is breathing? The breath will not last forever, therefore it is not I.

Subject after subject will rise into the mind, and each time it is negated. Only the permanent spirit within will remain.

Hari had a "chocolate" version, using this meditation when dealing with his temptation toward chocolate.

> I should at once utilize this moment, when a desire arises, and ask: "Who is it who wants a chocolate? Is it the body, Is it the Prana, Is it the mind, Is it the intellect, or is it the Self (Atma, Purusha)"?
>
> This kind of *vichara* [inquiry], if seriously pursued, can be of some temporary help, for it shows that the desire is not in *Me,* but in the pranamaya kosha, manomaya kosha, but *not* in *Me/* Atma)....
>
> But a practice I really do now, is to draw in the senses (pratyahara) and concentrate, or remember, that *I am above the mind.*[344]

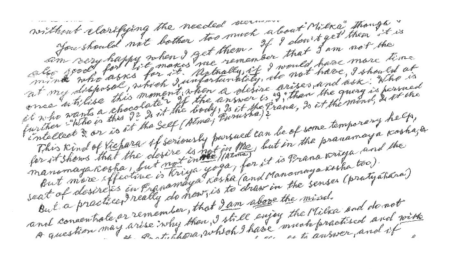

Figure 7.19. Letter to author from Hari, September 16, 1978.

Ramana Maharshi believed he had a more direct method to simply bypass all of this negation and be that "I," the true and pure Self. All else is an illusion, maya, so go right to the source. He wrote a book on this meditation method titled "Who Am I?" Hari helped translate the book into Latvian in 1933.

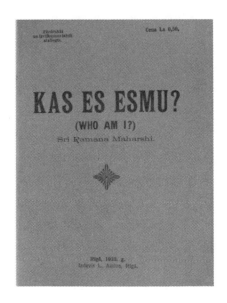

Figure 7.20. Sri Ramana Maharshi's book *Who Am I?* translated into Latvian by Hari and others at the Latvian Yoga Society. Photo of book cover: Dzintars Vilinis Korns.

Major A. W. Chadwick left the British army to become a disciple of Ramana Maharshi after he was inspired by Paul Brunton's book *In Search of Secret India*. In the ashram, he became known as Sadhu Arunachala.[345] Hari asked Mr. Chadwick to bring more clarification on how to practice this method of meditation. I share his response because it sheds so much light on the practice of this beautiful meditation.

Dear Mr. Dikman,

Personally I could see no point in taking someone as my guru if I did not at least endeavour to follow his advice. That I have been a poor example, I am quite willing to admit, but I did at least attempt Atma-Vichara and still continue. It has grown so natural to me that I should *now* find any other method difficult.

But I do consider a presumption on my part to attempt to make clear to others what He Himself [Sri Ramana Maharshi] never expounded more fully. Am I capable of succeeding where he failed? Did he fail? Or may it not be that there are certain things that cannot possibly be made more explicit, that belong to the realm of intuition rather than intellect? He has shown his method of approach in the little book "Who am I?," but is it possibly when we try to take these words of his too literally that we make a mistake.

You remember the description of his own awakening in "Self-Realization," when he lay on the floor and acted the death-scene? His was not just an intellectual discarding of objectives, "I am not the body," etc. He did not say to himself mentally, "Who am I?" alone, but it was a certain attitude of mind that he assumed. You yourself say that you have experienced no result from intellectual discrimination. Could you expect any? After all, such is only for beginners, it is only to turn the mind away from any and every possible object to which it must necessarily attach itself to live. For the mind is ranked by him with the senses, which without something to take hold of cease to exist.

Bhagavan said that it was almost impossible to make the mind subside completely, there would always be thoughts; so why not give it other and better employment, make it ask itself, "Who am I?" This was the whole secret of his method. And personally I have found that this in the end is the easiest.

When I sit to meditate I *turn* my mind inward to the source. Any thought that comes up I try to discard, trying at the same time to *see* or somehow catch hold of the thinker, the "I." Searching inwards toward the right side of the breast, but this latter is quite optional, because as Bhagavan said, "We cannot locate an experience."

Thoughts will constantly arise, but do not let them worry you, try and concentrate always on the thinker; if you cannot stop the thoughts, at least you can be the witness of them. Keep your mind turned always to the witness, and gradually the mind will become still. It requires constant practice and patience. But Bhagavan was never a stickler for sitting in any position at a fixed time for meditation, though most of us practiced it, we found it easier; he said, whatever we did, wherever we went we could keep up the enquiry, "Who is it who thinks he is doing this?" Watch the doer and not the deed. Though he did tell to Humphries [another disciple of Ramana Maharshi], if you remember, to practice for a short time every day at the same hour, and that the current then set up would continue subconsciously for the rest of the day.

Bhagavan found it almost impossible to explain all this so that our intelligence could understand. How can I hope to do better? I feel all I have said is very amateurish and that you will be disappointed. But one more thing I should like to add. You ask about my experiences. Now, experiences were definitely the one thing that Bhagavan did *not* encourage. They are, and must be, objective, and therefore in the realm of duality. What are they after all? Seeing a light, bearing a drawn-out note, a thrilling feeling? One is not the least better after them, in fact worse, as one is apt to go on enjoying such, thereby holding oneself back from further progress. He said that directly any such thing was experienced we must immediately try and undercut it with the usual formula, "To whom is such and such occurring?" Or as I said above by concentrating on the experiencer and not the experience, let *that* take care of itself, it will soon wither away like every other thing when one turns to the Self.

People do not always remember that the state to which Bhagavan had attained, and the only thing he was interested in teaching us, was the *Natural State,* the state behind waking, dreaming, and deep sleep, sometimes called in the Upanishads the fourth state, but this is really a misnomer, because it is not really a state, it is Ever-Being. So when we meditate we should not try to force the pace. We should just try to rest naturally in the Self. Let the world go on around, let thoughts come up, what does it matter? Cling on to the essential "I," the Now, pure Being in fact. Do not waste yourself in effort, for He often said: "Make an effort to be without effort." Enigmatic but the deepest truth.

There will *always* be difficulties, but these will grow less and less with practice. The ego is reluctant to die, and will do anything, go to any lengths, to hold on to its kingdom. But it is no use to worry. In fact, worrying is harmful, it is just another tie. Quietly try and turn the mind back when it tries to run away outwardly, this is all that we *can* do. Success will surely crown our efforts.

I hope that this will be of use to you. I am afraid it is very inadequate, but then you see I am not a jnani. Fraternally, yours, A. W. Chadwick[346]

Once you feel you have enough clarity, sit comfortably with an erect spine. Begin to observe your breathing. Notice how slowly it moves inward and outward. Notice any pauses at the top of the inhalation and the bottom of the exhalation. When settled and ready, begin the process of questioning all the events that arise during the meditation.

Ask, "Who am I?" If the answer is "I am a doctor" or "I am a teacher," etc., then ask: "Who is the 'I' behind the doctor (or teacher, etc.)?"

As experiences begin to arise ask about them, "To whom is this ache intruding on," then ask, "Who is the 'I' behind the ache?"

Ask, "To whom is (whatever is going on—sadness, discomfort, joy, etc.) occurring?" When the answer appears, ask, "Who is it that answers?"

If this answer is "I am," then keep taking yourself directly to the source of the answer. At first it will be your mind, thoughts from the ego-self answering the questions. Keep digging deeper beyond the thoughts to the source of the "I" thought. As each "I" thought arises, try to trace it back to its source.

"Who am I?" If the answer is "I am," then ask, "Who is it that is thinking about this 'I'?"

When the answer appears, ask, "Who is the I?" Trace the answer back to its source. The answer is beyond words, beyond thought. Remind yourself the "I" is not the physical, astral, or causal bodies. Not the *pancha koshas* or layers of your being. The "I" is Atman.[347]

Go through this process for each experience that arises for as long as feels comfortable. Over time, and with practice, the essence of your pure being will begin to reveal itself to you.

Consider these wonderful words of wisdom from T. K. Sundaresa Iyer:

Above all, it is a very necessary that the consciousness of our divinity should be so developed as to make us realize every moment, that we are not the body, but the Supreme, one Indivisible Being. "I and my father are one" will help us much in this respect. It is further important to bear in mind, that all the qualities of a divine nature that go to make a perfect man are not obtained by trying to develop each quality one by one. It should then take ages for us to perfect ourselves. The God in us is the repository of all that is good and beautiful, and only when we have lost or can lose our identity in Him do we begin to reflect outwardly the inner perfection. So the effort must be more toward the realization of the All Beautiful in us, that we might lose the craving for the beauties and pleasure that are but transitory.[348]

I like to follow this practice with the mudra for humility as described at the end of the chapter 5. The mudra is beneficial for the quelling of the ego, so our personalities may become a reflection of our soul within.

Paramhansa Yogananda on Meditation

I often say to my students that it is not so much the technique you are doing but rather the intention behind it. Paramhansa Yogananda had such deep, unwavering love for God that one cannot help but get caught up by it. Here in a letter to Hari, he discusses meditation. There are two wonderful points he makes. One is that the zeal you put into meditation is more important than the length of time. And the second is that God responds to love. His great words leave us with the wisdom we should take into every meditation we do.

> Forget time, forget everything but that you love God, you want Him only and your zeal must be such that when you sit to meditate you are determined to keep on knocking at the doors of eternity *until* you feel His blissful presence. It isn't always the length of time spent in meditation that is important, but rather the zeal, the ardor that one puts into his meditations. God responds to the love of the heart—he is more easily reached through love, whereas the devotee who seeks Him through dry reason may get there, but the route is longer. Devotion plus application of scientific techniques of meditations (as, for instance, Kriya yoga and the Om Technique) is the great highway to God-realization.[349]

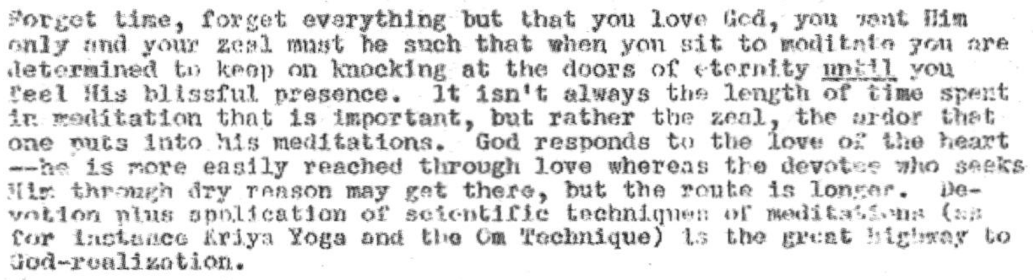

Forget time, forget everything but that you love God, you want Him only and your zeal must be such that when you sit to meditate you are determined to keep on knocking at the doors of eternity until you feel His blissful presence. It isn't always the length of time spent in meditation that is important, but rather the zeal, the ardor that one puts into his meditations. God responds to the love of the heart —he is more easily reached through love whereas the devotee who seeks Him through dry reason may get there, but the route is longer. Devotion plus application of scientific techniques of meditations (as, for instance Kriya Yoga and the Om Technique) is the great highway to God-realization.

Figure 7.21. Letter from Paramhansa Yogananda on meditation, September 13, 1949.

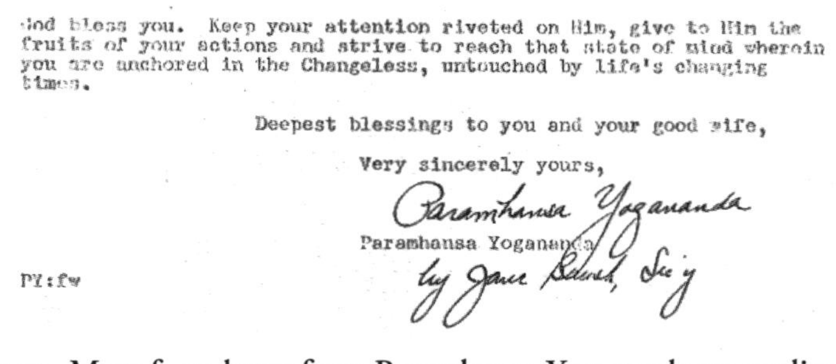

God bless you. Keep your attention riveted on Him, give to Him the fruits of your actions and strive to reach that state of mind wherein you are anchored in the Changeless, untouched by life's changing times.

Deepest blessings to you and your good wife,

Very sincerely yours,

Paramhansa Yogananda
Paramhansa Yogananda

PY:fw

by Jane Beloved, Sec'y

Figure 7.22. More from letter from Paramhansa Yogananda on meditation, 1949.

Chapter Eight

KUNDALINI AWAKENING
AND SAMADHI

MOST YOGA TEXTS WARN OF THE DANGERS OF AWAKENING the kundalini before one is ready, but it is impossible to comprehend what we should be cautious of when it is something that we have never experienced.

Swami Vishnu Tirth explained that the kundalini is a latent energy sleeping within a ganglion below the muladhara chakra, like a serpent coiled three and a half times. She cannot be experienced while resting in muladhara. Once awakened, she pierces the Brahma granthi and rises up to the svadhisthana chakra, which then becomes her resting place—*svadhisthana* means "her own place." Kundalini is the power through which one experiences the Lord, and she simply uncovers Him from the three gunas—*sattva*, "darkness, inertia," *rajas*, "activity, passion," and *tamas*, "truth, reality." Surrender to her and be simply a witness to her activities.[350]

The three gunas are the qualities of *prakriti*, "nature, matter"—all of the manifested universe. Everything that is manifested or part of our material existence is considered maya—that which appears to separate us from God. Whenever we feel separate from our Creator, our Source, this is the effect of maya. The more success we have in our yoga, our union with our Source, the less power maya has, and the more power is directed to awakening the kundalini energy.

Paramhansa Yogananda assured Hari that "Kundalini awakening is not a painful process requiring physical medication."[351]

So how do we awaken the goddess kundalini and what is a "kundalini experience"?

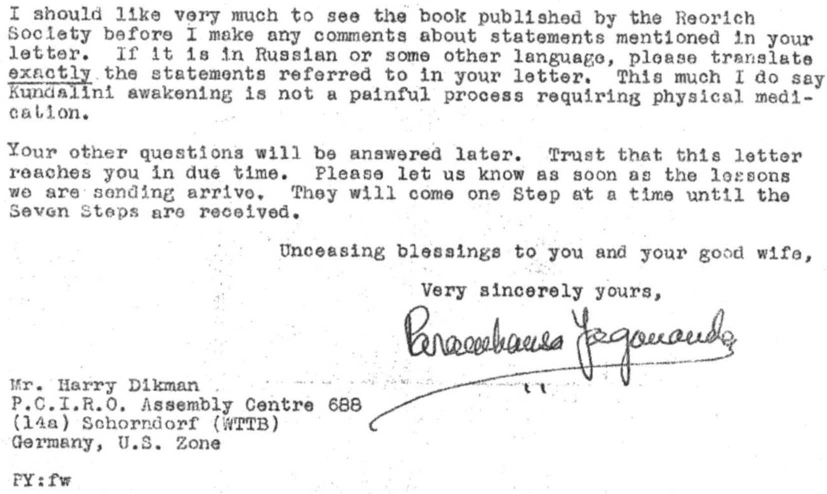

I should like very much to see the book published by the Reorich Society before I make any comments about statements mentioned in your letter. If it is in Russian or some other language, please translate exactly the statements referred to in your letter. This much I do say, Kundalini awakening is not a painful process requiring physical medication.

Your other questions will be answered later. Trust that this letter reaches you in due time. Please let us know as soon as the lessons we are sending arrive. They will come one Step at a time until the Seven Steps are received.

                    Unceasing blessings to you and your good wife,

                         Very sincerely yours,

Mr. Harry Dikman
P.C.I.R.O. Assembly Centre 688
(14a) Schorndorf (WTTB)
Germany, U.S. Zone

PY:fw

Figure 8.1. Letter from Paramhansa Yogananda stating kundalini awakening is not a painful process. September 22, 1947.

Hari and his friend Boris Sacharow were both in a DP camp in Germany in 1947–48. These men taught and practiced their yoga during these years in these camps. Life was not easy for them. This is reflected in a letter to Hari from Paramhansa Yogananda.

Am pleased to learn that the CARE package recently sent from the [SRF] Headquarters arrived in good condition and at a most opportune time. The Blessed Father works subtly, responding when we need Him most....

I am aware that conditions in Europe are extremely difficult to bear. Do not lose faith, but cling to the unseen hand of God, Who is aware of the difficulties you and many others are undergoing.

It is sad to learn about the suicidal deaths of the two aged persons who could no longer bear the troubles surrounding them. But death is no escape, for we carry impressions with us into the astral world. To take one's own life is to heap additional trouble upon the soul, for it must work out this action through the law of karma. The soul cannot return to earth for long until many attempts are made to enter it again.

So do not dwell on the fate of your friends, but rather look ahead, believing that a better life is in store for you, for all things are possible in God's sight.[352]

He means the soul of someone who has committed suicide will have to work through the karma that was caused by that suicide. The soul will incarnate a number of times, but it will die quickly (in infancy or in utero—in a miscarriage). Only after those many attempts will the soul be able to return to earth and live a life of normal length.[353]

Like Hari, Boris Sacharow was a keen student of yoga, and he got Paramhansa Yogananda's address from Hari to ask him some burning questions about kundalini. Both his letter to Yogananda and Yogananda's reply were among Hari's collection of letters. It is rare to actually read the question posed, as most of the letters are simply answers to Hari's questions. Boris asked, "Is it Muladhara or Ajna as a starting place in the Yoga Sadhana? Since there are two main paths, viz., Dhyana Yoga and Kundalini Yoga, the difference between the two being the arousing of the Kundalini Shakti in the latter and a mere meditative process in the first. The point is whether one is able by means of Dhyana alone to attain Samadhi and Mukti, or one is unable to do so without awakening the Shakti?"[354]

Paramhansa Yogananda answered.

One should use the Ajna Chakra as the place of preliminary concentration. Ajna means Christ Center, or Kutustha, which is located at the point between the two eyebrows. The eyes should be kept half open while the mind should be concentrated at this center (chakra)....

Man is in his present state of ignorance simply because his spiritual eye ("If therefore thine eye be single, thy whole body shall be full of light." Matt. 6:22) is not open. As soon as one consciously opens this eye, this eye of light, of intuition, one is able to see in every direction and through everything.[355]

When eyes are half-open and directed toward the ajna chakra, the meditator sees a light surrounded by flickering lights. This is considered the halo of the spiritual eye.

He also gave Hari a very encouraging piece of advice.

You must not think that you cannot reach higher states of realization, for this is not so. The more you meditate and earnestly seek God, the more you will realize this. Book learning cannot give this realization, but deep communion can produce these higher states of consciousness. Never cease to believe that you will find God, for without faith, little may be accomplished. Believe that He is with you, guiding your footsteps along whatever path He has set before you, and meditate long and deeply. Read less and meditate more, for then you will understand many things that books cannot impart to you.[356]

If I were in a postwar DP camp, these words of guidance would have been immeasurably valuable. Hari was full of respect for Paramhansa Yogananda, and his SRF lessons in kriya yoga. He encouraged me to take these SRF lessons at some point, because the instructions were so clear and the guidance so supported for sadhakas that they clearly would lead one to success in yoga. He was unable to teach me kriya yoga because he was never given the permission to do so in the United States, even though he was encouraged to teach portions of it in the DP camps. I have yet to take these lessons—if not in this lifetime, then perhaps in the next.

Over the years, Hari continued to study the awakening of the kundalini. Swami Narayanananda suggested to Hari a couple of ways to arouse the kundalini shakti.

Mother Shakti (Kundalini Shakti) can be worshipped in two ways.
　　1. Imagine a beautiful woman, who is All-powerful and full of all the Divine qualities, as if seated on a lotus of 4 petals (Muladhara).
　　2. Think of the Shakti, which is All-powerful, in a concentrated point in the centre of the 4-petalled lotus (Muladhara) and worship it.
　　In both cases, hold the vision in your mind, and whenever your mind wanders, return it to the vision.[357]

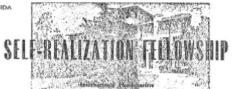

PARAMHANSA YOGANANDA
Founder

SELF-REALIZATION FELLOWSHIP

PUBLISHERS
East-West Magazine

September 22, 1947

Dear One:

Thank you for your most interesting letter written August sixth.
I am very happy to know that you have received and read Autobiography
of a Yogi, and that it has satisfied many questions in your mind and
soul. You may be interested to know that there are plans to have the
book printed in several different European languages as well as in
Bengali.

You must not think that you cannot reach higher states of realization,
for this is not so. The more you meditate and earnestly seek God the
more you will realize this. Book learning cannot give this realization,
but deep communion can produce these higher states of consciousness.
Never cease to believe that you will find God, for without faith little
may be accomplished. Believe that He is with you, guiding your footsteps along whatever path He has set before you, and meditate long and
deeply. Read less and meditate more for then you will understand many
things that books cannot impart to you.

Now about organizing a Self-Realization (Yogoda) group in Germany.
The secretary in charge of Center work will write to you shortly about
the instructions to be followed in conducting such a class, and I have
instructed her also to send you a new set of the Praecepts from which
you may teach the physical exercises and techniques. However, you must
not teach the Kriya Yoga without written permission from me, for this
is the promise which I gave to my Master. This condition is made
simply to avoid misunderstanding and incorrect teaching of this important technique. There must be a complete understanding of all the
previous teachings and the devotee must have followed them faithfully
in order to fully appreciate Kriya Yoga. It is a very sacred technique
of the highest order and must be given only to those who will faithfully
use it. If anyone is interested in knowing Kriya, have him study the
other techniques faithfully for a year at least, then write to me for
permission to give the Kriya Yoga.

You may teach the group from the Praecepts, and encourage any who are
able to enroll with the Fellowship and receive their own lessons. About
fees, I doubt if the people are able to contribute anything toward the
upkeep of the work. If so, let it be on a free will offering basis,

Figure 8.2. Letter from Paramhansa Yogananda on the higher states, September 22, 1947.

These seemed rather vague, and Hari was a man of detail, so he asked his
beloved teacher Swami Vishnu Tirth, who suggested that both hatha and raja
paths will arouse kundalini: "*Gheranda Samhita* is a treatise of Hatha yoga,
and 'thoughtless vacant mind' means simply Raja yoga. Kundalini is aroused
either way."[358]

Swami Vishnu Tirth continued to explain more about the conditions for awakening the kundalini.

Kundalini is a Tantric term, and Yoga Darshan appears to be an older work than the Tantras, and the word should not have been vague in Shri Patanjali's times. Awakening of Kundalini shakti is mentioned [in the sutras] as Pratyakchetnadhigam, sutra (1–29), which means literally an achievement of the experience of a distinct chetna (life) other than one's own through meditation of Ishwar (God) and japam (repetition) of His name, viz., Pranava (Om). Does it not imply that the distinct chetna must be divine, if so, what else can that be if not the same [as what] one experiences when Kundalini is aroused[?][359]

The "distinct" life is one of a sadhaka, a person who has completely dedicated his or her life to knowing God.

Further we have the term "kriya yoga," vide sutra (2-1), clearly indicating the kriyas (activities) following Pratyakchetnadhigam resulting from the sadhan of Tapas, Swadhyaya (repetition of Pranava) and Ishwar Pranidhan as defined in foregoing sutras.[360]

These are the practices of the niyamas, the second limb of Patanjali's ashtanga yoga—to be disciplined, to study the Spirit, and to surrender to the Divine.

When Kundalini is aroused, Kriyas are experienced, and hence the Kundalini is known as kriya Shakti. Thoughtlessness of mind comes automatically thereafter. Preliminary Dhyan also does, therefore, help to arouse Kundalini to some extent. All sorts of Sadhana awaken Kundalini, it is difficult to say which is more effective, because much depends on the aptitude of the sadhak. The easiest way of awakening Kundalini is through the direct contact of an adept.[361]

Like most of us dedicated to the path of yoga, Hari wanted to understand some of the experiences that occurred for him as a result of his practices. At one point, when Hari started experiencing a sort of "jerk" or jolt in his body while meditating (which I spoke of in chapters 4 and 6), he queried many of his gurus about it. Swami Shivananda Saraswati of Assam offered this explanation.

> It is clear to you that Yoga has to purify and cleanse your body and mind. You have got to transform yourself. You must have to be Divine. During the course of transforming yourself to divinity, many changes are wrought in the physical state also. Man comes to the world with unlimited possibilities. What is stored in him in the form of potential energy is laid at rest. Sadhana is the action which disturb[s] the energy at rest. Gradually by the force of Sadhana what remain[s] in potential form is transformed into kinetic form. The jerk you feel during Dhyana [meditation] is the result of this sort of effect on [the] body."[362]

In the same letter, Swami Shivananda Saraswati of Assam gave Hari specific instructions to pierce the Vishnu granthi to allow the kundalini to move beyond the anahata area. Although he suggested some physical techniques that would be helpful, he also mentioned that at Hari's stage of development, these were not going to be useful and that what he needed to do was purify his mind.

> As I can pursue the course of your progress in Dhyana, I feel that you are moving in the correct path. So far your sensation of some substance rising upward through your spine and the feeling of warmth in "Anahata" area are concerned, it is very much normal. It is the movement of Kundalini Sakti. This is the common experience of all beginners. It comes up to Anahata easily, but a great deal of Sadhana is necessary for its surpassing Anahata area and rising higher towards Sahasrar.
>
> Udghata Kriya should be performed first, for it opens Susumna, and so [is] very much helpful for pranayama. You want to devote more time and energy for Bhastrika pranayama in order to remove obstruction of Vishnu Granthi. At this stage of yours, devotion of more time and energy to this will not serve the purpose. The primary condition for it is to purify your mind through rigid observance of Yama and Niyama. You must have to cleanse yourself both in body and mind so that it becomes the true temple for divine

manifestation in you. Only at this stage Kundalini Shakti will move upwards and the obstruction of Vishnu Granthi will be removed. You proceed with your normal [program] of Sadhana, but utmost importance should be given in purifying and cleansing your body and mind. Any sort of impurity that still may disturb you must be purged to be completely stainless.[363]

Branch :
SHIVANANDA YOGASHRAM
471, Netaji Colony,
Calcutta-50

SHIVANANDA MATH
(UMACHAL YOGASHRAM)
Kamakhya, Gauhati-10
BHARAT (INDIA)

Dated.....5....10......1972

Dear Harry Dickman,

        I received your letters dated July 26 '72 and Sept, 1972 in time. Never I could answer to your letter in time and never you complained against my delay, and so I also do not apologize.

        I received your remittance of $3.50 in time. I received a letter from Mr. K. Grikupels and a remittance of $ 20 and I sent an answer to his letter.

        i) As I can pursue the course of your progress in Dhyana, I feel that you have been moving inthe correct path. So far your sensation of some substance rising upward through your spine and the feeling of warmth in 'Anahata' area are concerned, it is very much normal. It is the movement of Kundalini Sakti. This is the common experience of all beginners. It comes upto Anahata easily, but a great deal of Sadhana is necessary for its surpassing Anahata area and rising higher towards Sahasrar.

        ii) Udghata Kriya should be performed first for it opens Susumna ,and so very much helpful for pranayama. You want to devote more time and energy for Bhastika pranayama in order to remove obstruction of Vishnu Granthi. At this stage of yours, more devotion of a more time and energy to this will not serve the purpose. The primary condition for it is to purify your mind through rigid observance of Yama and Niyama. You must have to cleanse yourself both in body and mind so that it becomes the true temple for divine manifestation in you. Only at this stage Kundalini Shakti will move upward. and the obstruction of Vishnu Granthi will be removed. You proceed with your normal programe of Sadhana but utmost importance should be given in purifying and cleansing your body and mind. Any sort of impurity that still may disturb you must be purged to be completely stainless.

Figure 8.3. Letter from Swami Shivananda Saraswati of Assam on udghata kriya, May 10, 1972.

Yogindra Amar Nandy described *udghata kriya* as similar to bhastrika. Place your right hand in Vishnu mudra (see fig. 4.4) and close the left nostril with the ring and baby fingers of the right hand. Breathe rapidly in and out ten times through the right nostril. Inhale deeply and fill the lungs, then immediately shut the right nostril with the thumb and breathe out the left nostril slowly and fully. Now breathe rapidly in and out ten times through the left nostril. Continue the practice, alternating between the right and left nostrils, for up to ten minutes.[364]

When the sushumna is opened, the prana and apana can move into it and unite. Prana, the vital air, is broken down into five forms known as the pancha vayus: prana, apana, samana, udana, and vyana. All movement of the body is a result of these five vayus—moving the arms and legs, swallowing, digestion, assimilation and distribution of energy, and elimination of wastes. It is prana that brings life to the body, which is otherwise just a corpse, and each of the five constituents of prana plays a role.

Of these five vayus, prana is the incoming energy of the life force, and apana is the outgoing energy of letting go and elimination. When the sushumna is opened, these two forces are joined. Swami Vishnu Tirth explained how this feels so Hari could identify with it.

> Union of Prana and Apan, when they unite inside the spinal (Sushumna), their union leads to Samadhi and liberation from bodily bondage. But when they unite out (of Sushumna), death will ensue. Kumbhak long enough may help, but it is not an easy task and free from danger. Mental concentration is the easier method but needs long, deep concentration.... When you fix your mind on the mid-brow, Prana will tend to rise up the spine gradually. When prana enters sushumna, one feels divine intoxication and mind becomes stilled down to thought-lessness.[365]

Swami Vishnu Tirth told Hari that he was an advanced aspirant, and he suggested transference of energy from him to Hari.

> In my previous letter, I had advised you not to attempt Hatha yoga, as it is not necessary for an advanced aspirant, and instead to devote mostly to meditation. As a help from this side [of the world], you may imagine waves of Shakti coming to you from [India]. After some practice, I hope, you should actually experience the same in some form, not as light or electricity, as you say, but like some force. Five to ten minutes imaginative thinking for the purpose should be sufficient.

Your experience of feeling vibrations in the top of the head is in the right direction. The Shakti, while dormant, is seated at Muladhar, and when aroused, rises to swadhistha, as the name itself implies (swa—one's own, adhi—in relation to, sthan—place). Currents of Shakti rising from there, when feeble, may not be felt below sahasrara. But you say that you feel at times some sensation ascending up the spine. That is good. Sometimes it is felt as if ants are crawling up inside the spine. When the force is sufficiently stronger, it is strong enough to give jerks to the whole body, shaking it vigorously. They are the signs of an awakened kundalini. The intensity may vary from feeble to violent, according to one's personal, bodily, and mental aptitude. In most cases even highly advanced persons do not have any such experiences, except a peaceful silence.[366]

Hari described having these feelings in a letter to Swami Shivananda Saraswati of Assam: "I often feel as if a slight electric current or some kind of mild vibration passes from the place between the eyebrows to the place of Brahmarandhra."

The swami suggested that these vibrations of an awakened kundalini can be a focus of meditation, which can lead to *savikalpa samadhi* (a stage of samadhi in which the mind still retains material impressions between subject and object). Further, he described how one can focus on three specific chakras during meditation in order to raise the kundalini.

If you can advance further this state of your meditation, [it] will deepen more, and this electric current and vibration will be more intense. You will then be unconscious of your senses and mind. You will then feel a state of void—a kind of self-effacement or self lost in itself. This is the feeling of Sunya Brahma, as has been described in the Buddhist philosophy. When you will feel this kind of absorption or voidness, you will have nothing to do. Your conscious will automatically merge into God-Consciousness. As the river flows to [the] ocean and is lost there, so also you will lose yourself into God or Supreme Consciousness. This state has been named by Patanjali as the Savikalpa Samadhi.

I think you have read about the perplexed and restless state of [the] mind in Patanjali. Even at this perplexed state of the impure mind, Samadhi can be attained, but this kind of Samadhi is not desirable to us. The Frogs and Snakes can have this state of Samadhi. They remain underground in winter in a state of Samadhi and can go for long without any food, without the least effect to their body.

Hatha yoga is a process of developing mind with the help of body and nerves. Hence it includes Kundalini yoga. When one proceeds a little with the help of Kundalini yoga, the mind itself takes the charge of this Sadhana. But this Lay-Yoga, without purification of the mind, is of little value. It is just like the state of a toad or a snake, as I have already mentioned.

There are three points for meditation in which mind can be centralized. These three points are Manipur-Chakra or navel region, Anahata-Chakra or Heart region, Ajna Chakra or Bhrumadhya. We would advise a student of yoga to meditate first on the centre known as Manipur Chakra or the [navel] point. You have to sit straight in Padmasana or Siddhasana or Swastikasan, keeping the eyes fixed in [navel] point, and be absorbed in meditation. The object of meditation will be selected according to one's own choice. It may be the sky, the sun, the moon, or any idol of God, or [an] image of any Holy man as one pleases. The best time for meditation is morning, evening, mid-day, and mid-night. The minimum time to be covered in one sitting should be one hour.

If one continues this sadhana regularly for six months, one can hear the Anahata-dhwani [inner sounds, see "Meditation on Nad" in chapter 7], Susumna is opened, and the Kundalini becomes awakened. At this stage you will feel the rise of the Kundalini up to the Anahata Chakra and the sound of this Anahata-dhwani [will] be often heard; and with the help of this Anahata-dhwani, [the] mind can be concentrated. After this you have to select the place of Anahata Chakra for meditation. Lastly select the place of Ajna chakra or Bhrumadhya for meditation.[367]

It is worth noting here that the practice above focuses on moving the attention into the higher chakras, (from the manipura, which is the highest of the three lower chakras, which relate to the material existence and our walk on this earth), up into the anahata and ajna chakras, related to spiritual awakening. Paramhansa Yogananda explained to Hari that the chakras may have their petals either pointing down or pointing up. If we identify more with the body and mind, then the chakra petals point downward. If we identify more with the soul and the spiritual chakras above the navel, then the chakra petals are pointing upward. We must shift our identification from the body to the soul in order to attain samadhi.

> The word "star," as mentioned in the Christian Bible, is a better term to describe spinal centers than is the word "lotus," which is a term used by the Hindus. All the current in the body is travelling outward, because we are using the senses, but when we meditate, we withdraw the current through the spine toward God. When we are identified with the body, the current, or rays, of each center flow downward, and when we become identified with the soul, the current, rays, or petals of the lotus cells, travel upward toward the brain. This is what is meant by the statement that the chakras, or lotus petals, are turned downward or upward.[368]

He continued to clarify this for Hari in a following letter.

> They will remain in their upright position as long as you preserve that advanced state of consciousness. Through steadfast devotion to God and gurus and proper practice of Kriya Yoga, you will attain the highest reward—Self-realization.[369]

Brahmachari Animananda Dharmacharya, a disciple of Yogananda, described the aftereffect of this practice for Hari.

> First let me explain what "the after-effect of kriya" is. After-effect means the result. When the kriya is performed correctly with devotion for some time, breath automatically becomes slower and slower and ultimately ceases to function. At that time, the life force that is generally engaged to function various activities in the body turns inward and gradually accumulates in the spine. Instantly a tremendous sensation ensues in the spine, as if hundreds of [volts] of electrical current is flowing through it. The sensation begins from the coccyx and rushes toward the brain, where it becomes fixed in the Ajna chakra. The [lower chakras] becomes inactive as gone dead or

paralyzed. Some times the life force may not ascend so far. It may accumulate in the heart centre.

The tremendous flow of life force in the spine is the first symptom of the after-effect of kriya. Secondly the 27 thousand [billion] cells will be charged fully with [electricity]…. Thirdly the microscopic knowledge of the devotee becomes macroscopic, i.e., the perception of the sensory organs becomes very great….

What I have explained in the first [paragraph] may be achieved temporarily, but full control over the life force is what is known as self-control, i.e., When you can withdraw mind and life force at will by the force of kriya. Many [yogis] know what the after-effect of kriya is, but the difficulty is how to acquire it permanently. Here requires Guru Kripa.[370]

Guru kripa is "the grace of the guru." The grace of the guru can be bestowed upon a devotee at any moment, giving him or her all the power of self-control, but the devotee should deserve it first.

Boris Sacharow asked Paramhansa Yogananda about a possible alternate way of achieving Samadhi: "I wonder if I can attain Samadhi by making concentration on the pineal gland, which is supposed to tentatively represent the Sahasrara Padma, without awakening Kundalini in Muladhara?"[371]

Paramhansa Yogananda responded that this was impossible.

It is impossible to attain the state of Samadhi without awakening the Kundalini. The life energy passes through the coiled passage in the spine during Samadhi, travelling upward. All the life from the cells passes through the spine, for during Samadhi the life is withdrawn from the five senses into the spine and taken upward toward the Christ Center through the coiled passage. Samadhi is impossible to attain unless the life force goes through the coiled passage.

To believe that one can attain this state without the awakening of the Kundalini force is false. Such individuals have *imagined* themselves to be in that state of Samadhi, but this does not make it so.

Self-Realization Fellowship teaches the scientific *Kriya Yoga*, the practice of which brings about the state of Samadhi in a gradual manner, as the body becomes equipped for it.[372]

Samadhi is the goal, and as Paramhansa Yogananda said, without kundalini awakening there is no samadhi. Samadhi is a state of full knowledge. It is the eighth limb of yoga—a superconscious state in which one identifies with the ultimate Reality or God.

There are various stages of samadhi. *Samprajnata samadhi* is also known as *savikalpa samadhi* or *sabija samadhi*. It comes from successful concentration of the mind. This samadhi still has seeds of attachment pertaining to the material world (samskaras or patterns of behavior). It brings perfect knowledge of the gross and subtle elements of the object of meditation, but does not take one to the finer stages of samadhi. This samadhi includes:

> *Savitarka* samadhi—concentration on a gross object and its nature. Knowledge of the gross elements is acquired through inquiry and reasoning in relation to time and space, the name of the object, the form of the object, and the idea of the object in the mind.

> *Nirvitarka* samadhi—true knowledge of the object is acquired outside of time or space. The essence of the object alone remains without reasoning or argumentation.

> *Savichara* samadhi—the object is subtle. Knowledge of the subtle elements is acquired. Inquiry alternates between time, space, and object, but there is no thinking in words.

> *Nirvichara* samadhi—the subtle object has no connection with space or surroundings. There is no reflection, thinking or inquiry, only pure sattva.[373]

There are two other samadhis that are part of Samprajnata samadhi:

> *Sananda* samadhi—meditation on bliss. This is a joyful samadhi in which one moves beyond the five elements and rests in a sattvic mind, free of rajas and tamas. There is a real peace and intense joy in this samadhi.

> *Asmita* samadhi—concentration on the mind itself. Sattvic ego alone remains. The Self knows the Self. The yogi recognizes "I Am" as opposed to "I am the body." The sense of individuality shifts into pure awareness.[374]

Swami Sivananda explained these to Hari.

Regards the query on Savichara Samadhi, it is all a matter for direct personal experience. When one reaches that stage of development the Meditator is able to perceive many things that are not ordinarily visible to the gross eye. Samadhi is a state wherein one gets direct perception of Brahman Itself; then what to say of Tanmatras [the qualities of the elements (earth, air, fire, etc.)]? The difference between Sananda Samadhi and Asmita Samadhi is that in the former one meditates on the mind as pure Sattwa perfectly devoid of Rajas and Tamas and in the latter as Pure Consciousness or "self-awareness". In Sananda the emphasis of the dhyana is on the joy or ananda of the pure sattwic mind and in the Asmita the emphasis is upon pure experience.[375]

The final stage of samadhi is *Asamprajnata samadhi,* also known as *nirvikalpa samadhi* or *nirbija samadhi.* It is samadhi without any seeds of attachment to this material world—no samskaras or thought. It is a state in which we stop thinking and are still conscious. There is complete stillness of the mind. It is the highest superconscious state; the mind and the ego-sense are completely annihilated, and one is freed from the cycle of karma and reincarnation. This is the Absolute state, the goal of yoga, leading to final liberation.[376]

The different kinds of planes in Samadhi, the mental states of Bliss, Vichara, etc., are denoted by the Savitarka, Nirvitarka, Savichara, Nirvichara, Sananda, Asampragnata Samadhi, etc. These experiences can be clearly understood when the aspirant reaches the advanced stages through purification and regular meditation and introspection. All can have a general idea from books, but real truths can be grasped and understood when the aspirant who is well established in Dhyana.

Figure 8.4. Letter from Swami Sivananda explaining samadhi, October 25, 1946.

The different kinds of planes in Samadhi, the mental states of Bliss, Vichara, etc., are denoted by the Savitarka, Nirvitarka, Savichara, Nirvichara, Sananda, Asampragnata Samadhi, etc. These experiences can be clearly understood when the aspirant reaches the advanced stages through purification and regular meditation and introspection. All can have a general idea from books, but real truths can be grasped and understood when the aspirant who is well established in Dhyana.[377]

Through these various stages of samadhi we evolve. This means we are tasting delicious moments of samadhi all through our journey of yoga, as we purify our mind and body. Each stage should not be discounted as "not enough," for each is a step leading to deeper and deeper awareness of the Self.

Hari said when one comes out of a sound sleep, one awakens with a memory of ignorance: "I knew nothing," whereas one who comes out of a state of samadhi has memory of knowledge: "I existed only there." Outwardly, there appears to be no difference, but the inner experience is nowhere near the same.[378]

Chapter Nine

DELICIOUS STORIES

Jesus As a Yogi

When I first became a yoga teacher in the 1970s, the idea of Jesus being a yogi was rather unknown in the West. Hari told me that many Eastern yogis believe that Jesus was in India during his lost years. This was not discussed freely with others.

It was not difficult for me to understand why this information would be kept quiet. I was raised as a Christian in the United Church of Canada and was taught that Jesus was "the way, the truth, and the life." If I did not embrace the teachings of Jesus, I was never going to get to know the heavenly father. I was also taught that I was fortunate to have the opportunity to be a Christian.

When I became a yoga teacher, I found many people from the Christian community feared the teachings of yoga. Concerns were expressed that meditation would open up my mind to the devil. The occult was dangerous. Mantra repetition was saying God's name in vain. I needed to be born again through Jesus, and no other way would work. I needed to be baptized as an adult, fully submersed in water. I needed to be saved.

Once a couple who attended my yoga classes had to stop coming—the parents of their babysitter were going to ban their daughter from babysitting for them if they attended yoga classes. The couple did not want to lose their babysitter, so they quit coming to my classes.

After living in the ashram and embracing the teachings of yoga, I was confused. The yogis I had encountered accepted Christians and those from all walks of faith. They believed one could be Christian and practice yoga, because yoga is a way of life that fits nicely with any religion—or none at all.

I decided that I needed to study Christianity more thoroughly in order to feel peaceful about what I was teaching. I really hadn't paid much attention as a youth in Sunday school, so at this time in my life, I had more knowledge of yoga philosophy than of Christianity. It was perfect timing, because I was unemployed. I enrolled in numerous Bible study classes in an attempt to make some sense of all the contradictory information.

Over several months, I studied at the Baptist, Alliance, Lutheran, United, and Mormon Churches. Each group was studying a different book from the Bible with their own favorite translation. I learned so much about Jesus and the people of the Bible. I loved the teachings of Jesus and the stories of people's burning love for God. It was heartwarming and reassuring. As a result, I knew that my path of yoga was just another pathway. We all had the same goals, just different methods and terminology to define them. Swami Sivananda said, "The paths are many, but the Truth is One." All the worries and contradictions I felt were replaced with an umbrella of peace.

Many years have passed since then, and attitudes have changed. People's minds have opened up to accept yoga more readily. Knowledge often replaces fear, and as more and more people came to understand yoga, the threat of the unknown diminished. Today many churches hold yoga classes in their basements. Medical professionals refer patients to yoga as an aid to help them heal. Colleges and universities run yoga classes for health and welfare. In 1984 I presented at the International Yoga Teachers Congress in Barcelona, Spain. The theme was integrating yoga. My presentation was followed by a Catholic priest, Father Paul Brossard, from Switzerland, who had done his doctoral thesis on yoga and the Christian mystics. He shared how he had integrated yoga into his spiritual path.

The United Church of Canada changed, too, expanding to embrace diversity in religious and spiritual paths. I ended up working for a United

Church Continuing Education Centre and taught yoga in this Christian environment for more than twenty years. I still continue to teach yoga to Christians. One of my greatest resources is the book *Christ, the Yogi: A Hindu Reflection on the Gospel of John*, written by Ravi Ravindra.

So we come back to the secret of Christ the yogi. Hari had queried his Indian teachers about Christ, and some of the most interesting information he received came from the Sri Gorakhnath Temple in Gorakhpur, India. A letter from Mahant Dig Vijai Nath, dated April 20, 1963, included an article regarding the time Jesus spent in India.

Indo-Christian Legend by Surath Kumar Sarkar

It is indeed very strange that we hear nothing about Jesus Christ from his thirteenth year till his thirtieth year. The Bible is unfortunately silent. One therefore naturally asks, where he was these 17 years and how he spent this time.

It is interesting to note that some rare Hindu and Buddhist Shastras record the interesting belief that he was in India and spent those 17 years in this country. This is corroborated in *Natha-Namabali*—a very old manuscript, dearly and zealously preserved by a section of Natha-Yogis. In this book it is also said that after his resurrection he came to India again and did a good deal for the welfare of the Yogis.

Long before the birth of Christ, there was a class of saints in Palestine, who were almost like the Hindu Yogis. They were called *Essenes*. Arthur Lillie writes in his "India in Primitive Christianity" that "Jesus was an *Essene* and the *Essenes* like the Indian Yogis sought to obtain Divine Union and the Gifts of the Spirit by solitary reverie in retired spots." ... Essene is the foreign pronunciation of the Indian name *Eeshani*. *Eeshani* is *Shiva*. *Eeshani* (or Essene) is the worshipper of Eeshana or Shiva.

John the Baptist : -

In their modes of worship the Essenes and the Yogis of the Natha community were very much alike. John the Baptist was an Essene. He, along with the other great Yogis of the Natha community, is held in high esteem in certain sections of the community. Even in the remotest parts of Bengal where no missionary has ever set foot, John the Baptist is still the subject of many folk songs. John baptized

> Long before the birth of Christ, there was a class of
> saints in Palestine, who were almost like the Hindu Yogis. They
> were called Essenes. Arthur Lillie writes in his "India in
> Primitive Christianity" that "Jesus was an Essene and the
> Essenes like the Indian Yogis sought to obtain Divine Union and
> the Gifts of the Spirit by solitary reverie in retired spots."
> (Pg. 200). Essene is the foreign pronunciation of the Indian
> name Eeshani. Eeshana is Shiva. Eeshani (or Essene) is the
> worshipper of Eeshana or Shiva.
>
>   John the Baptist : -
>
>   In their modes of worship the Essenes and the Yogis of
> the Natha community were very much alike. John the Baptist
> was an Essene. He, along with other great Yogis of the Natha
> community, is held in high esteem in certain sections of the
> community. Even in the remotest parts of Bengal where no missionary
> has ever set foot, John the Baptist is still the subject of many
> folk songs. John baptised Jesus. Ernest Renan, the famous author,
> has written,-" The Essenes resembled the Gurus (spiritual masters)
> of Brahmanism".

Figure 9.1. Letter from Mahant Dig Vijai Nath on the Indo-Christian legend of Christ, April 20, 1963.

Jesus. Ernest Renan, the famous author, has written,— "The Essenes resembled the *Gurus* (spiritual masters) of Brahmanism."

Jesus was initiated into the Indian yoga form of religion. To gain more knowledge of the subject, he came to India. This is related in a very old manuscript preserved in a temple at Marbur—a very inaccessible region of Tibet. A copy of the manuscript can also be found at Himis Temple situated on the Frontier of India and Tibet. Some years back a Russian tourist named Dr. Notovitch slipped from a hill near Himis and was severely wounded. The kind Lamas took him to Himis Temple. Here he happened to learn from the Lamas that a very important book on Jesus Christ was in their possession. He borrowed the book from them and translated it into English. On the basis of this translation he later wrote a book called the "Unknown Life of Jesus" in America. The American Government thought that there were passages in that book ... [that were] uncharitable attacks on the Christian community. The book was therefore banned.

The Translation : -

The original book at Marbur is written in Pali; whereas the book of Himis Temple is the Tibetan translation. From its pages we learn that Jesus came to India at the age of thirteen. Swami Abhedananda of the Ramakrishna Vedanta Society has himself seen the book and translated a portion of it. Swami Abhedananda and the Tibetan Lamas are of opinion that the book was written some three or four years after the Crucifixion. There are 14 chapters and 244 Shlokas in this book. Jesus has been called Eesha. Philologists tell us how Jesus of Palestine came to be Eesha in India. The Hebrew name "Jeshua" is of Greek "Issoas," and in India it is "Esshai" or "eesha."

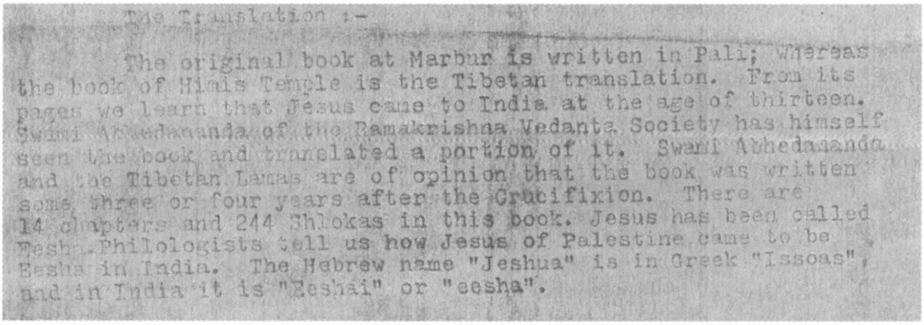

Figure 9.2. More from letter from Mahant Dig Vijai Nath on the Indo-Christian legend of Christ, April 20, 1963.

A summary of the translation is as follows: -

"Eesha attained his thirteenth year. Admiring his knowledge and learning, most of the rich folks and the *Kulinas* of the country became eager to give their daughters in marriage to him, but Eesha had no mind to marry. At the talk of marriage he left his father's home. He became desirous of attaining perfection by acquiring all the merits which the Former Buddha had attained. He started for Sindh with some merchants and at the age of 14 he arrived at the land of the Aryans. The Jains were very much attracted by his sober figure and requested him to live with them. He did not accede to these requests and did not wish for anybody's favour. Afterwards he arrived at *Jagannatha-Dhama* (Puri), and became a disciple of Brahmanas and learnt the Vedas and Shastras. Then for six years he travelled in the holy places such as Rajagriha, Benares, etc., and came to Kapilavastu. With the Buddhist monks he read the Buddhist Scriptures for 6 years. From there he travelled in Nepal and the

Himalayas, and returned to Persia. He was now 29. On attaining his
30ᵗʰ year he returned to his own land, and began to preach his message of peace and good will to his oppressed relatives."

Son of God : -

Jesus was well acquainted with the teachings of the Vedas and
from these he got the justification for calling himself the Son of God.
Is it not proclaimed in the Vedas that all men and all gods are the
Sons of God, -*Amritasya Putrah?*

Nath-Namavali : -

The Nath-Yogis possess a very old manuscript, called *Natha Na-
mavali*. In this manuscript is found the following :- "Jesus came to India at the age of 14, and after long 16 years' prayer was enabled to see
Shiva, the Great God. After that he went to his native land and began
to speak about God among his countrymen. But many of his contry-
men [*sic*] were of materialistic temperament and they could not bear
this light of knowledge. They conspired against Ishai-Nath [Jesus]
and tortured him by driving nails unto his hands and feet. Ishai-Nath,
who saw God, went into *Samadhi* by means of *yoga*. He did it for the
welfare of the three worlds. The brutes thought him to be dead and
put him in the grave. When Ishai-Nath was crucified, one of his Gurus, the great Chetan Nath, was in deep meditation in the vicinity of
the lower regions of the Himalayas. Through meditation he came to
know of the tortures practiced upon Ishai-Nath and making his body
lighter than air, in 3 days he crossed to the land of the Israelites. Here
in a forest he assumed his real form. It was a rough day, and there was
thunder and rain because the gods were very angry, and the world
shook. He cared not for these, and raised the body of Ishai-Nath from
his grave and broke his *Samadhi*.

After that both of them returned to the holy land of the Aryas
[*sic*] and established a *Math* in the lower regions of the Himalayas. At
the end of the three years of meditation and wrship [*sic*] here, the all-
merciful Sankara kindly saw him again and gave out that Ishai Nath
should explain to the world all the mysteries of the Creation. Accord-
ingly Ishai Nath placed the trident of Sankara, which was the emblem
of Sankara's Knowledge, Power and Force, on the *Yonipitha* of Sankara (the Goddess Durga) and introduced the *Puja* called the *Yoni-
lingam Shiva Puja*. Then holy men of all parts came to show respect to

him. He left his mortal body through yoga at the age of 49 in the *Math* established by him.

The manuscript "Nath-Namavali," though very rare, is neither unavailable nor a myth. I myself have seen a copy recently, and the late Vijay Krishna Goswamy also had the opportunity to read a copy of the same. The book may be found among the Sannyasis of the Natha Yogi Community. It contains 17 more biographies of great men of the Natha community over and above the biography of Jesus Christ here described.[379]

Today there are many books and articles about Christ as a Yogi. It is a fascinating link between East and West, leaving us with much to ponder and meditate on. Since yoga was here long before Christ, it does not seem unfathomable for Christ to have learned this ancient practice that guides us to know God within. When we study the masters of all the pathways, we cannot help but notice how they were all teaching the same thing—how to know God within.

There are many parallel teachings from the yoga masters and Jesus. I mentioned near the beginning of chapter 6 the similarity of Om in the *Mandukya Upanishad* and the Word in John 1:1 of the Bible.[380] Another example that stands out for me is found in the *Bhagavad Gita*.

In John 14:6–20, there is a conversation between Jesus and his disciples:

I am the way and the truth and the life. No one comes to the Father but by me. If you had known me, you would have known my Father also;

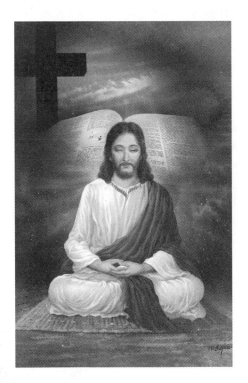

Figure 9.3. Jesus beyond Crucifixion, painted by Vyankatesh Sapar for author.

henceforth you know him and have seen him." Philip said to him, "Lord, show us the Father and we shall be satisfied." Jesus said to him, "Have I been with you so long, and yet you do not know me, Philip? He who has seen me has seen the Father. How can you say, 'Show us the Father'? Do you not believe that I am in the Father, and that the Father is in me? The words that I say to you I do not speak on my own authority, but the Father who dwells in me does his works. Believe me that I am in the Father and the Father in me; or else believe me for the sake of the works themselves....

Even the Spirit of truth, whom the world cannot receive, because it neither sees him nor knows him; you know him, for he dwells with you and will be in you. I will not leave you desolate; I will come to you. Yet a little while, and the world will see me no more, but you will see me; because I live, you will live also. In that day you know that I am in my Father, and you in me, and I in you.[381]

These verses speak to me of the God, the Father, within. This God is within us all. Krishna, a widely worshipped god in Hinduism, is said to have been God in human form, on this earth to help the people. In chapter 9 of the Bhagavad Gita, a text from around 500 BCE, Krishna speaks to Arjuna (the son of the Pandava family, who fights for righteousness), assisting Arjuna as he struggles with the battle of life's challenges. What he says is similar to what Christ says.

I will tell thee a supreme mystery, because thy soul has faith. It is vision and wisdom and when known thou shalt be free from sin. It is the supreme wisdom and the purification supreme. Seen in a wonder of vision, it is a path of righteousness very easy to follow, leading to the highest End. But those who have no faith in this Truth, come not unto me; they return to the cycles of life in death....

But the fools of this world know not me when they see me in my own human body. They know not my Spirit supreme, the infinite God of this all....

But there are some great souls who know me: their refuge is my own divine nature. They love me with a oneness of love: they know that I am the source of all....

I am the Father of this universe, and even the Source of the Father. I am the Mother of this Universe, and the Creator of all. I am the highest to be known, the Path of purification, the holy OM, the Three Vedas. I am the Way, and the Master who watches in silence; thy friend and thy shelter and thy abode of peace. I am the beginning and the middle and the end of all things: their seed of Eternity, their Treasure supreme....

I am the same to all beings, and my love is ever the same; but those who worship me with devotion, they are in me and I am in them.[382]

Thais Thomas shared another story of Jesus with Hari. It contains some information that he learned from his teacher Yogeshwar Muni, also known as Charles Berner.

Muniji does not think Jesus had a Divine body because [a divine body] cannot be physically destroyed or deformed. Also, when blood and water ran from his side—does not show that the water element had been destroyed. Lately there have been articles in Indian periodicals and newspapers about the recent publication of the Jesus in Kashmir story. According to the compounding of all the research on the subject, Jesus was not completely dead when taken down from the cross. (P. Pilate was against killing him in the first place.) The tomb, actually a room, was the recovery room in which Jesus, with the help of Joseph of Arimathea, regained strength and fled Palestine. According to the story, they went back to India, where as a young man, Jesus had spent many years. Mary died on the way in a place in Pakistan, which is to this day called by her name. Jesus lived in Kashmir until his nineties and had a family of which there is a Srinagar family claiming lineage. The scriptures left in a monastery of Leh and first discovered by some German missionaries tell of Jesus' earlier experiences in India, where apparently he upset brahmanical order and religion by preaching to sudras and calling for equality of mankind. He is known to have resided in Orissa, Benares, and other places.[383]

I am one who finds peace in the Oneness of All and the acceptance of all spiritual paths. All devotions, all prayers, all mantras find their way to the same Source—the One within.

Spiritual Beginnings

Hari asked Swami Shivananda Saraswati of Assam, whom he corresponded with from 1959 to 1976, about his spiritual beginning and what it was like to leave his family for spiritual callings. The swami shared freely about his childhood.

You have expressed your desire to know about my past and those old days of my early and initial stage of the spiritual begining [*sic*]. To begin with I may say that it was at the age of nearing eight that I felt the urge for spiritual begining. A novice as I was then and without guidance, I would at occasions sit in a lonely place in an attempt for Dhyana. You know of course that our Hindu religion [Vedanta] follows Advaitabada. And I am sure you know where lies the difference of this Advaitabada [non-duality] of ours and the Western theory of Ekeshwarabad [one ultimate principle]. In Advaitabada there are indeed many modes for the worship [of] Gods. How this procedure of DVAITABADA [duality] can fall in accord with the ADVAITABADA within the same framework of our religious boundary is something that may pose to many of the Western philosophy as a peculiar point of [query]; but that sounds nothing strange to us. In our society there is a class who professionally or in some cases as a gainful pastime preach, rather explain the stories of PURAN, etc. in all family circles of the village by rotation once a week or so and they are known as Puran-Bakta, the word Bakta meaning one who talks or explains. Through the medium of religious songs and stories they unfolded the philosophical mysteries, logical technicalities, the spiritual problems, etc., to all who assembled there in a very lucid way which always pierced through the busy and apparently negative mind and touch[ed] the very core of the inner mind. Even the boys and girls who accompanied the elders to such circles got very much impressed when they found the morals of our religions after the removal of the screen of mystery and technicality. Such preachers helped to build up the moral and religious backbone and served the purpose of mass religious education to a large extent.

When such Baktas spoke in a touching language about the stories of Dhruba, Prolhad, etc., for their urge to meet the God, I would feel an inspiration and a twist in my little heart to fall in line with them for such attainment. Apart from the time which was strictly fixed for my studies by my guardians, I would make out opportunities to be lonely and sit for Dhyana and Japa. I would any time that I could, make out in this way which I could have otherwise spent in games with my friends. And all this I did when I was about to touch the fringe of eight only. Yes, games and other recreation were no charm to me. Among the Gods I heard in such circles, I took Krishna as my idol. I felt thoroughly moved when I heard the Bakta narrating the heroic acts of the early days of Lord Krishna, His love for the comman [sic] man, His sacrifices. I thought it over in my latter days, and I can speak judiciously that it was the expert hands of those most charming and revered Baktas who moulded my mind through their most piercing language and made my heart full of Krishna, the Hero and my Lord. There are boys in every society some of whom love their fathers, and there are some who love their mothers more. Equally you will find that some amongst us prefer to offer their love to God as father while the others do the same liking the God as mother, which is always a matter of individual choice or taste with them. The Bakta would explain five modes of Upasana [worship] of Lord Krisna. They were Shanta Bhava [an attitude of peace], Dashya Bhava (the surrender of the self as a servant to a master), Sakhya Bhava (the friend-like feelings of equity and of love), Batshalya Bhava (loving the God with the filial feelings of a mother for her son), and the Madhur Bhava [the attitude of lover]. The Shanta and Madhur Bhavas were then difficult for me to understand. But I could very well feel myself drawn to Sakhya Bhava of the three which appealed to me. Yes, I selected the Lord Krishna as my friend, my Hero, and started to feel for Him as a true friend for a friend.

One can concentrate better, as I guess, in the early days. I can quote from my heart some of the lengthly poems at this late age which I liked in those days. I would in those early days concentrate in Japa and Dhyana. I could feel the presence of my Lord, my Friend in my tender [heart] and would become full of joy. Occassionally at nights I would have some special feelings in my heart. I felt as I had been lost in an all pervading darkness which was beyond description. After some time, from this darkness came out a luminous circle making the darkness to give way gradually. The circle would ultimately form into the shape of my Lord—my beloved. The bright white sparkling light would turn into charming bluish colour of my Lord. Again it would fade away and darkness engulfed. I would at this stage come out of sleep and look at the clock to find that it was about 3 A.M. or so. From those days ... up to the twelfth year I would frequently dream such dreams. A long gap [between the dreams] would pain me. It even happened in occasions more than once that I kept a knife in my bed at night and uttered words of warning in my childish tone that should He not come and meet me at night in dream, I would make an end of my body with that knife. Strange as it was, I felt the presence of my Lord on those nights. The truth remains in such events that there was no lack of honesty of purpose and no duality of mind. Such things, boyish as it may seem at this length of time, I can very well satisfy myself after a careful analysis that there was no mockery, no self-hypocrisy in it and that the feelings were indeed genuine....

The two third of the Indian population is vegetarian. In the Eastern India, the States of Bengal, Assam, Orissa are nonvegetarian save a small fraction. The family I belonged to was nonvegetarian, and I made an exception in them. I heard my mother saying in latter days that every attempt was made to convert me to their custom, but that was not successful even though I was [a] very tiny boy. I would vomit spontaneously if fish or meat was mixed up in my food. My elders left me in utter dissappointment [sic]. I myself never knew what prompted me in those days of early childhood to react in such a manner. My friends would catch fish with nets and rods and such things indeed pained me. I never stayed with them during such games. There are some fishes of the variety of Kai, Magoor, etc., who live days together when kept in small pots in homes for progressive consumption of the children and sick members of the house who need it for their protein value. Our house was no exception. But I could never stand the sight of my sisters, mother or aunties cutting them while they were still living and struggling for life in vain. I felt a kind of pain and discomfort that words cannot express. Sometimes my elders laughed at me. At length I found my mother to feel syspathetic [sic], and it was through her decree that they granted some concession for me that is they would not cut living fish during my presence in the house. They would do it when I was away at school. Yes, I was partly successful that such things were brought to a minimum in latter days.

India was under the clutch of the Muslims for long 700 years. These rulers were staunch opponent to education to the women. It was a credit and custom with them to carry away the handsome Hindu girls from their homes to serve their purpose. The Hindus decided to marry their daughters as early as eight years of age as a protective measure. As a result of this forced child-marriage and abolition of women education, our women remained very back-ward. There were a few girls who could exchange letters with their husbands who were staying at distant places. Now these girls of the village naturally needed the help of some third person who could do the letter-writing job for them. Some elderly who might serve the purpose, were not likened by them. I became a hero to them because my reputation in those days as a first boy of the class was taken to be a splendid success and won their praise always. When invited to do the letter-writing job for them, I would in return make them to promise that they would not torture the living fishes. They might kill them with one blow and then make pieces, instead of mak-ing pieces of the living one still struggling on point of knives. Some readily agreed but the others would not give way so soon. Yes, al-most all of them took pity on me and at length came to terms. It was a gain to me as I considered it.

Another interesting and humurous [*sic*] side of this letter writing career of mine may be given here. As you know, I would write these letters on dictation from these married girls. It so happened at times that they would dictate "you accept my __" [not giving the final word of the sentence]. In such cases I would try to convince them that ... there must be some word to be placed in the gap. Now the girls blashed [blushed] and insisted that it would remain so. It hurt my knowledge and authority in grammer [*sic*] and I would fight to convince my point very hard. Often a quarrel ensued. The girls ulti-mately made a compromise, saying that they would fill in the [space on] their own. The theory of such reaction of the girls [was] that they wanted to convey "kisses" to the husbands which they could not do through my medium. In our country it is blamable even for the husband & wife to kiss in open which is contrary to yours. Our parents even stop kissing their boys and girls when they reach the age of ten or so. Hence these married girls on the one hand could not check their feelings to offer their kisses to their husbands at the same time get baffled to send it through the pens of a letter-writer about the age of 9 or ten. During my visits in European Tea Estates in Assam I have seen frequently the husband & wife kiss in open, mothers kiss the boys, sisters kiss the brothers. It raised a question in my mind as to which of the system is better, yours or that of ours. There is in fact nothing wrong in a kiss, which is an expression of the feelings affection and love. In our country it is thought that kisses at a certain age raise the latent feelings of passion, and as such it has been kept with the bounds of husband-wife relation. The elderly express their feelings of love and affection to the youngers by touching them on their heads with the hands by way of blessing, and the youngers express it by touching the feet of the elders.

It was probably due to Dhyana [meditation] practice that I could [complete] my [school] lessons in a very short time and this would give a better margin [of time] for me to devote in devotion. Now this trend of my mind and the way I spent for devotion became known to my friends and relatives far and near, and they called me Gurudeva jokingly. I would pray to God that, born in a Rishi Family, as was ours, I might be worthy of it and might come in the care of guidance of one who was really the greatest of the Sages of the time.

I was aged 11 only when I read the book JNANI-GURU and I came to find out that the author of the book was no less a Sage than the Great Swami Nigamananda Paramhansa. I wrote to him immediately for my admission in his Ashram. He wrote to me in return to obtain the consent of parents. I could not speak it face to face and hence I wrote to my father about my desire but nothing to mother. On the first day father spoke nothing. The following night I heard there was weeping sound from the room next to my own, where my parents stayed. It was none else than my mother who was weeping and father was heard to have been consoling. He said that it was a custom in our family to spare one boy of the house in each generation for Sannyas Life, of course from him who had more than one son. [No] one ever thought of me because I was the only son of my parents. Yet my father spoke in emphatic terms to mother that the tradition begged of her this gift—gift of her boy. Further talks were choked with emotion and did not reach my ears. Enough all that I heard then. Yes, the kind consent came to me after a couple of days and I wrote to my Gurudev. He then wrote to me that I was a mere boy and that he advised me to stay 6 months more. That I should see him when he would visit Dacca at that time. That I did and it gave me a new turn in life.

I hope to give you some details of my early Asram life in my next letter.[384]

Ashram Life

Hari was curious about life in an ashram, as many people are. It is quite different than living in the "world," as time is always made for sadhana in an ashram. In fact, that is all that daily life is about: sadhana—be it karma yoga, devoting time to support the ashram or others in need, bhakti yoga devotions, raja yoga time for meditation, or hatha yoga time for asana. How yoga sadhana is done varies from ashram to ashram, but in all, the days are filled with sadhana. Swami Shivananda Saraswati's beautiful story came in his reply.

I like the Umachal Ashram best. The natural beauty of the place is incomparable. The river Brahmaputra flows by the side of the hill on which the Ashram is situated. The entire surrounding of the hill from 400 feet to 1000 feet is in our possession. At the peak of this hill, the space near about five or six hundred feet is quite plain [i.e., flat]. It is just like a field for playing foot ball. So this peak is quite nice for the purpose of walking.

Here the river Brahmaputra is about two miles in breadth. Many ships and boats with various coloured sails are constantly passing in. Gauhati, the second city of Assam is situated in the plain by the eastern side of this hill. The moving vehicles and the pedestrians of the city seem to be very small and tiny liliputian figures.

One will never be able to turn one's eyes back from the superb beauty of the surrounding place, which has been created by the hills and rocks, river, city, and the verdant plains all around here. The whole thing appears as a land of dream.

About thirty years back when we first situated this Ashram, the land was full of jungles and ferocious wild animals. Tigers, snakes, and deers were our constant companions. There were dens for three tigers within the area of our Ashram. Two of three were the Royal Bengal tigers and one was a leopard. We had a somewhat intimacy with the Royal Bengal Tigers. Sometimes it happened that I had to sit for meditation on a stone which is spread like a throne. When my meditation was over, it grew dark, and I found one of my tiger friends lying comfortably beside me just like a pet cat.

Sometimes again it happened that I was to come down from the peak while my friend the tiger was to climb up by the same path. We were then in a position at face to face with each other. My tiger friend then used to move aside and waited for my passing. I then passed by his side without the least fear.

But I had never any friendly term with the leopard. As the Englishman never believed us and thought us to be anarchists in the disguise of monks, so the leopard also never believed us.

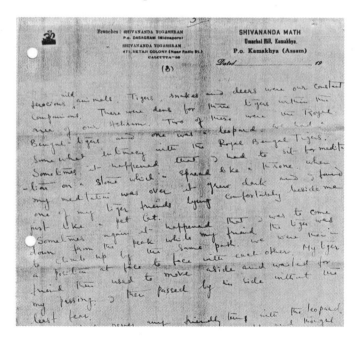

Figure 9.4. Letter from Swami Shivananda Saraswati of Assam on ashram life, October 14, 1961, p. 3.

When I came across [the leopard] at day time he used to frown at me and moved into the bush, and if we met at night it never gave me way. But our Royal Bengal tiger friends were not so unmannerly in their behavior. They gave us way whenever we met at day or at night. But the leopard cared little for good behavior. He used to get angry if we lighted the torch upon his face, and begin to growl in fury. If in spite of that we lighted the torch in his face, he became ready to fall upon us. His anger alleviated only when we stopped lighting the torch. These tigers living in our Ashram with us were called Matul (maternal uncle) by us. The two Royal Bengal Tigers were called as "Bara Matul" (elder uncle) while the leopard was taken to be the Chhota Matul (younger).

Our Bara Matul sometimes went out in search of prey in the surrounding villages, near about the Kamakhya Temple, and if could kill a cow, carried it over to our Ashram. We could not but be surprised to see how they could carry so easily such a big animal from so far. When they could do it, they gave a loud roar which made the whole hill tremble! We could easily guess from such a roar that they had a good prey that day. When they could get such a good prey, they used to stay near about it, and it took seven or eight days for them to finish the entire dead animal. They used to be there near their prey from four P.M. in the evening to 7 A.M. in the morning and went away to sleep only for a few hours in the midday. I used to go at evening to see their feast. When they saw me they stopped eating and stood silent. I sometimes said to them in joke "Oh Matal how you are behaving like a non-Hindu while you are staying in a Hindu Ashram! A Hindu never kills a cow but you are committing this sin."

But I had never seen them to kill any deer or any animal within the area of our Ashram. They killed it outside the area. One day I had a chance to see their process of having a prey of monkeys. The monkeys took shelter on the branches high up a tree. The tiger stood under it and gave a loud roar. Many of the monkeys fell down on the ground just as the ripe fruits fall down when the tree is violently shaked.

This flock of wild deers used to roam about the whole day in our Ashram, just like pet deers. Sometimes one or two of them stepped on the verandha of my room and used to stare at my writing table in wonder. I have the picture of their beautiful eyes even now in my mind. When sometimes I used to give them rice, banana or pulses to eat, other deers of the flock came and struggled to take share from them.

There were wild elephants in other hills by the side of our hill but they never came to our hill.

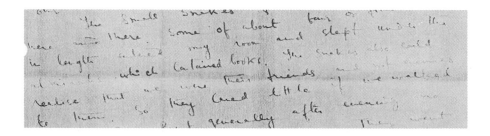

Figure 9.5. Letter from Swami Shivananda Saraswati of Assam on ashram life, October 14, 1961, p. 6.

The small snakes often used to roam about here and there. Some of about four or five cubit in length [four cubits is about six feet] entered my room and slept under the [set of shelves] which contained books. The snakes also could realize that we were their friends and not enemies to them, so they cared little if we walked about them. But generally after evening no snake could be seen in our room. They went out in the evening. Sometimes it had happened that while I had to walk in the dark, I trampled down on them. The snake being hurt had clung round my leg. I had no other way than but to stand with the leg up. It was natural for them to bite after being so [severely] hurt. But it did not bite me. Slowly it unclung its clasp and moved away silently. We have spent ten years here having such a friendly relation with the wild animals.

Their silent love charmed me like anything. It seemed to me that these wild animals even knew that man is the last creation of God and that they are to be respected at all costs. If man could be non-violent, these animals could live happily and man also would not have been treated with so much malice by them.

No body except a few brave came to our Ashram at this time. We like best such seclusion. Once a French lady appeared in this inaccessible forest abode of ours with a Bengal boy.... She was in "garik sari." She had a very calm and quiet appearance, just like a good Indian woman. The "garik sari" suited her well in her healthy beautiful body. I told her to take sit and then asked, "Mother, on what purpose have you come here in this forest region full of wild animals?" She did not know English well. She answered in broken English, "I have read some books on Tantra by Arthur Avalon (Woodroffe). I want to learn the process of Tantra ... from a higher tantric sadhak. Generally the tantriks practice their Tantra in places inaccessible to others.

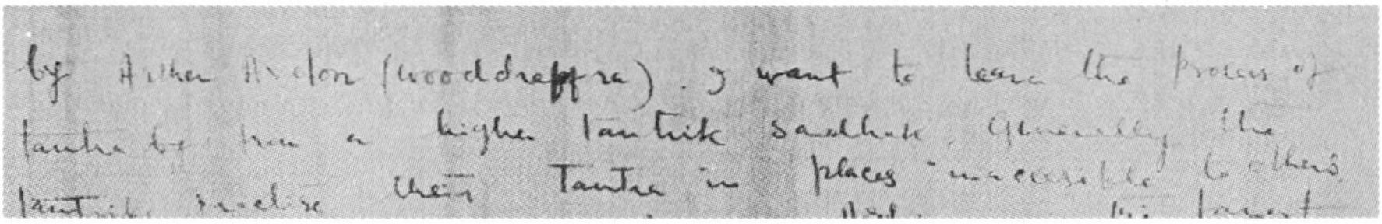
by Arthur Avalon (Woodraffe). I want to learn the process of
tantra by from a higher tantrik sadhak. Generally the
tantriks practise their Tantra in places inaccessible to others.

Figure 9.6. Letter from Swami Shivananda Saraswati of Assam on ashram life, October 14, 1961, p. 7.

I have heard that there is an Ashram in this forest region so I have come to find it out. Will you please satisfy my desire?" I replied then, "Oh mother, we are not the tantriks but we are vaidiks, we have some theoretical knowledge regarding Tantra, but no practical knowledge. Kamakhya was at a time the centre for Tantrik practices, but now there is not a single person here who can be called a real Tantrik. Of course, there are still some real good Tantriks in India, but I do not know their whereabouts. The person from whom Arthur Avalon learned, he has become very old now, and I have heard he is now in Burma."

In the course of our conversation this French lady related that she belonged to a rich family and had no want of money. She had no intention to get married. If she could find a good Tantrik Preceptor, she would like to stay with him in his hermitage and will spend her life for tantrik sadhana. At last I told her, "Mother, do not dare to travel all alone like this. In your country there is no difficulty for women to travel alone. Nobody would dare to insult a woman there. But our India is a land of both the civilized and uncivilized nations. There are many animals—men here who would not miss a chance to insult a woman if she is alone, nor even hesitate to outrage her modesty. So I advise you to go first to the Pondicherry Ashram of Sri Aurobindo. The organizer of the Ashram herself is a French lady. I think you would be able to get information of a good Tantrik Preceptor from there." As she appealed to me to allow her to stay for a few days in our Ashram, I did so. She also walked fearlessly in this region of wild animals. Her fearless spirit charmed me, and I thought if this lady could get good guidance, she would be a real "Sadhika."

We spent thus ten years here quite peacefully, and then the Second World War started. We lost the calm and tranquil life for ever. There were camps on all sides of our Ashram, and the Japanese began bombing in these camps. As a consequence of bombing on or near our military camps, glass panes of the windows of our Ashram house were shattered to pieces. All the other members of the Ashram moved to other places for safety. I was alone left here. The tigers left the hermitage, being frightened at the roaring sound of the bombs and anti-air craft guns.

The soldiers, coming to know about the deers in the forest nearby, began to kill the innocent animals cruelly. A great misfortune came over the quiet life of our Ashram.

The English soldiers began to retreat successfully, but a good number of English soldiers were crushed down by Japanese bomb. The law and order of this zone broke down. Three years thus passed. In the mean time, the war took a different turn. A huge regiment of American soldiers with arms and ammunitions and bombing planes were sent to India to help the English. The retreating English soldiers again proceeded to Assam victoriously. New camps for the incoming soldiers were tented again in the surrounding areas of our Ashram hill.

The American soldiers used to come to our Ashram just at 4 P.M. They spoke highly about the natural beauty here. Some educated soldiers amongst them used to enter in our library room and asked permission to take out some English books from the [bookshelf] to read.

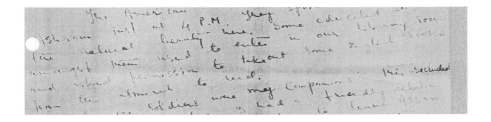

Figure 9.7. Letter from Swami Shivananda Saraswati of Assam, on ashram life, October 14, 1961, p. 10.

These American soldiers were my companions in this secluded hill. Those with whom I had a friendly relation, when they got a transfer order to leave Assam, they came to bid me good bye. At the time of this parting, I felt like parting with some near and dear ones!

Here I stop relating my story of our Ashram. Yours —Swami Shivananda Saraswati.[385]

About a Guru

Hari inquired to know more about the guru of Brahmachari Punyabrata of the Shivananda Yogashram. I believe the guru he was referring to was Swami Shivananda Saraswati of Assam, the author of the above story and the head of the ashram where the Brahmachari lived. The letter is not dated, but the author stated that he was replying to Hari's letter of October 15, 1959.

You have desired to know about His Holiness our revered Gurudev. I am giving you in brief the little bit I have been able to know about him so far. From the very childhood he was very akin to religious aptitudes. While he was a boy of only six–seven years, from that very tender age he used to absorb in meditation under the tree-shade or inside the temples. Parents of His Holiness also were very religious-minded, and they did never stand in the way of his religious practices. At the age of twelve, he cut off his connection with his family and adopted the life of a monk and joined an Ashram of a Sannyasin, Swami Nigamananda Saraswati by name, who was a "Jnana-panthi". There he studied the different Hindu Shastras. After that he practised sadhanas (meditation, etc.) for ten years in the loneliness of the mountains, where he realized his own Self. Once we dive [deep] in Samadhi or Self-realisation, we do not require any further Sadhanas. As those who have come out of the Universities after obtaining degrees do not need going through school-college books, similar is the case of the Self-realised Sannyasin.

Still we find, our Swamiji sleeps very little at night and spends the last part of night in deep meditation. We do not see him doing anything spiritual at day time, when either he remains engaged in various kinds of humanitarian work or writes books and essays on religious subjects.

To say about his virtues, we can quote a verse of the Upanishads:

"Naham Mahye Suvedeh, No Na Vedeh Veda Cha
Yo Nastadveda Tadveda No Na Vedeh Veda Cha"

- Kenopanishad 2/2

I.e., I do not think that I know the Brahma well; I do not think that I know not him at all.

Similarly, this verse is applicable in case of our Gurudev. We do not claim that we have understood him; we also cannot say that we have not understood him at all.

All the virtues of the "sthita prajna" (wise) as described in Shree-mad Bhagabat Gita Canto 2, are found in his nature. He is always serene, steady, and calm. In his character we see the combination of Supreme Knowledge, divine love, and indefatigable worker. We never see him to be angry, despite reasons for anger. When we do anything wrong, we are reproached, but that reproach is mixed with such tenderness and sweetness that touch the very core of our heart. Now we understand, after coming in his touch, how much magnanimous—how much godly a man could be. His instructions arouse in us great thirst for wisdom and a strong desire for sadhana. He particularly insists on us to practice meditation in the morning, evening, and in the third part of the night.

The letter is going to be a lengthy one. No more to-day. Hope you are well. With love and best wishes, yours—Brahmachari Punyabrata.[386]

Astral Beings for the Good of All

Swami Shivananda Saraswati of Assam was quite the storyteller in many of his letters to Hari. The following is a story about miracles performed by astral beings in India. I have edited it slightly so the sentences flow more smoothly.

> What I narrated in my previous letter in respect to an incident experienced by my Gurudeva is a common experience with many Sadhaks or pious souls all over the world. Let me tell you another incident of a Sadhak. He went to a remote village. He came to know that many persons in difficulty came to the temple of that village in order to get rid of their difficulties. In a dream they would receive instructions and guidance to avoid a danger that might befall of them. The Sadhak was curious, because his path was the path of Jnanamarga [path to enlightenment through wisdom] and he had never any faith in such supernatural happenings. However, he wanted to make an experiment.

> (v) What I narrated in my previous letter in   P.T.O.
> respect of an incident experienced by my Gurudeva, is a common expe-
> rience with many Sadhaks or pious souls all over the world. Let me
> tell you another incident of a sadhak. He went to a remote village.
> He came to know that many persons in difficulty came to the
> temple of that village   in order to get rid of their difficulties.

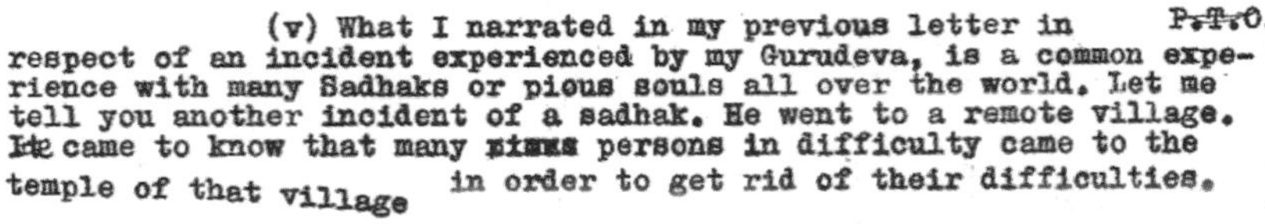

Figure 9.8. Letter from Swami Shivananda Saraswati of Assam regarding astral beings, May 10, 1972.

> He went to the temple at night and decided to spend the night in meditation there. Deep in the night he fell into a trance, and he happened to meet someone not in his gross physical body but in the subtle, or astral, body, the Sukshma. In his trance he had a talk with him. The astral being told the Sadhak that he was the priest of the temple and that he had a deep attraction for the presiding deity of the temple. He also had deep affection for the people of the place, so he could not leave this place.

> He explained to the Sadhak that in this astral body, his vision was not obstructed by any material fetters, so he could see what was coming to the people. When some danger or misfortune approached

them, he cautioned them in their dreams and advised them as to how they were to avoid the danger.

The Sadhak requested the priest to leave the temple and to go to the higher region where he could be free. The being expressed his attachment for the deity in reply, to which the Sadhak proposed that he would destroy the deity inside the temple so that this being might be free from his attachment for the deity. The astral being importuned him not to do so. At this stage the Sadhak lost his trance and came back to his worldly consciousness.

To speak the truth, the world is beset with these kind and high spirits, always eager to help the pious ones or the Sadhaks. My Gurudev was helped by such a spirit. These spirits can create a house or a light or anything they like to construct to meet the need or requirement for helping the pious ones. When the real Sadhak offers food to his deity, as in when prasad is offered in the temple, it is this sort of spirit who accepts it. The devotee thinks that his offering is accepted by God the Master. But actually it is the action of the kindly spirits who may be considered as the angels or Debdut described in the Bible or the Koran. Like our Government, there is also a spiritual Government. Officers of this Government do the needful things that will help a Sadhak in his higher mental evolution and self-realization.[387]

The Lady and Lord Krishna

Swami Shivananda Saraswati of Assam explained to Hari that any story he hears from his Guru he never doubts as truth. He then went on to tell a story of a woman and her miracle. Once again, I have only edited this slightly for easier reading, but the content is not changed.

We never question the reality of a story from Gurudev. When a child hears a story from his elder, he never doubts the reality of the story. In India this kind of miracle often happens, so we never become astonished to hear it. I have also my personal experience about it. So I will also tell a story to you.

When I was 25 years old, I was in my tour in Himalayas. I met a pious Lady devotee there. The object of Dhyana for this Lady was that she was the Divine mother and Lord Krishna was her son. The boy Krishna used to come to her in a physical body. I and a young boy met this pious Lady. The young boy had a camera. He took a photo of the Lady. When the photo was washed [exposed], we were astonished to see that the boy Krishna, with a heavenly smile, is [at] her back-side, embracing her neck. The camera never tells a lie. So we should not nourish any kind of doubt about this miracle. If you are interested, I can tell you more stories like this.

As the pious Lady always thinks the boy Krishna is always with her, so you will always think you are not the body, not the soul, not the intellect nor the ego—you are the Self. You are one with the Supreme Divinity. This kind of thinking or Dhyana will be helpful for your union with the Infinite or Supreme Divinity—this is real Yoga.[388]

Ambubachi

Swami Shivananda Saraswati told Hari about a special day, June 25. Ambubachi is a yearly gathering in Guwahati, Assam, in the Kamakhya Devi temple during monsoon season. It is considered a Tantric fertility festival to celebrate the menses of Mother Earth, after which she can conceive.

I am writing to you on a significant day—today—i.e. "Ambubachi Day"—which means [living] on simply water—i.e., liquids only, and it has an inner significance according to the Hindu Scripture. The religious people observe it in strict ardour—i.e., living on unboiled plain milk and fruit juice and avoid all cooked edibles—for three successive days. Besides, none shall dig the earth, which means—giving peace and rest to Mother Earth, which is an imperative.

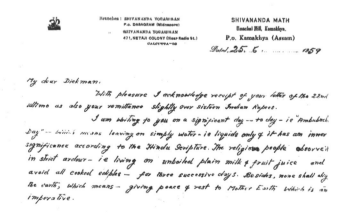

Figure 9.9. Letter from Swami Shivananda Saraswati of Assam regarding the Ambubachi Day festivities, June 25, 1959.

Regarding the theory of Creation, the Hindu Idealists have some peculiar ideas and this observance point at on these. Namely—this Earth is [a] living personality and not at all an insensible mass. There are millions and millions of living organism[s] and microbes inside our body-world, they live in families, are subjects to the laws of birth and death, they freely move inside our bodies. Their personality also freely move within our greater personality.

The organs like liver and spleen, etc., inside our body are as large as the Himalay[a]s to them, the great arteries seem to be oceans and small arteries are like large rivers to these minute creatures. To them, of course, our body appears to be certainly inert, since they cannot comprehend that their vast living place has a great consciousness, a large personality. Similarly—we also fail to comprehend that the Earth has a consciousness, a personality, a life, and we wrongly estimate her to be a mere mass of earth only. But really she is not insensate; she is throbbing with life. Thus the Hindu Idealists maintain that the eternal manifestation of life from the earth could not be possible if the Earth herself is insensate.

These three days of Ambubachi remains fixed for the menstruation period of Mother Earth, after which she is designed to conceive, just like a human mother. Directly hereafter, the rains start, and the cultivator jubilantly goes out to his field to till and sow. Father vital force, father's semen. With the showering rains—the down-pour of life falls upon the Mother Earth, and she does receive it, which results in numerous and varied "life" upon her.

Not only the Earth, but also the sun, the moon, the stars are all living things, vibrating with consciousness. Would you take such ideas of the Hindus as mere unbalanced mooning [dreaming]—or you are prone to believe them?[389]

Swara Yoga

Swami Shivananda Saraswati of Assam elucidated in great depth the mystery of swara yoga (or svara yoga). The source is a tantric text known as *Swarodaya Yoga*, which goes into great detail about the tattvas (or *tattwas*, as it appears in Swami Shivananda Saraswati's letters—the elements earth, water, fire, air, and ether) and how they are represented within the flow of prana in ida and pingala nadis. There is a natural shift of energy between the flow of prana in the ida and the pingala nadis approximately every hour. You can tell which is flowing by checking which nostril is more open—the left nostril for ida and the right for pingala. Within this hour, each element has a period of dominance. According to the tantric text, and as we know, prana is the life force, the energy behind all movement, and therefore this flow between the nadis has great impact on the success of our daily actions. Swami Shivananda Saraswati explained this in several letters. (These letters have been edited for flow, and some of the terminology has been made consistent.)

The aim of Swarodaya Yoga is to reveal the science of breathing. By controlling the breathing system, one can fulfil one's cherished desires. Irregular breathing foretells to one 15 days ahead that he would be attacked by some serious disease. One can take preventive measure with the help of this Swarodaya Yoga and can easily resist the disease. At the time of a journey either by boat, rail, or by aeroplane, we can, with the thorough knowledge of the Swarodaya Yoga, prophesy whether our journey will be pleasant or beset with danger.... We can also know by Swarodaya Yoga the monthly and annual readings of our individual fortunes and also the fortune of the States as a whole. With thorough mastering of this Swarodaya Yoga, married couples can give birth to accomplished children up to their own liking. One can get oneself prepared for death one year ahead of time, if one is adept in this Swarodaya Yoga. There are probably errors in astrological readings, but the indications of Swarodaya Yoga are free from errors and mistakes. This Swarodaya Yoga is a wonderful and very useful chapter of the Yoga Science.[390]

We can also increase our span of life if we follow swarodaya yoga. So to know the science of breathing is a boon to human society. Yogins have noticed that there is a rule or process of breathing.

The Lighted fortnight (sukla paksha [the period of the waxing moon]) begins after a moonless day (New Moon day or Amavasya). At the time of sun-rising on the first 3 days of sukla paksha, breathing commences in ida nadi, or the left nose. This breathing will [continue for] ... one hour, and then breathing in pingala will begin, and it will [continue] for an hour. In this way breathing alters from ida to pingala, from pingala to ida, throughout the day and night until full moon-day (Purnima). After full moon-day, it is the reverse.

Then the dark fortnight (Krishna paksha [the period of the waning moon]) begins. From the first day of Krishna paksha, at the time of sun-rising, pingala commences instead of ida.

Everyone should notice whether [his or her] breathing system is acting this way or not. If your breathing system does not follow this rule, then you will understand there is something wrong in your body system. Disease germs are increasing, so you should be careful. If the growth of disease germs [in your body is] slow and weak, then altering of breathing will continue from ida to pingala and pingala to ida, though irregularly. But when disease germs are stronger, then altering of breathing of ida and pingala will be stopped, and one-nose breathing will continue. You will notice that you are breathing [only] by ida or pingala for hours; it is not changing. If this one-nose breathing continues for seven days or more without any stop, you will be attacked with dangerous disease without delay. At this stage you will have to change your breathing by force. If your breathing is in ida, change it into pingala. If it is in pingala, change it into ida. By this way you will be able to prevent your dangerous disease. It is needless to say that it will be very difficult for you to alter breathing at the time of disease if you have not practiced it when you were in perfect health.[391]

Learning to change the flow of breath in the nostrils is not difficult. Hari taught me one way. If you wish to open the right nostril, lie on your left side and put the fingers of your right hand in your left armpit and the thumb pressing on the visible space between the shoulder and the breast (the pectoralis major). Lie on the left side for at least one minute, and the right nostril should open. If you wish to open the left nostril, lie on the right side, with your left fingers in the right armpit, with the thumb as above, and stay for at least one minute.

There is also a method to open both nostrils or the sushumna. Stand or sit and put your right fingers in the left armpit and the left fingers in the right armpit. Thumbs are visibly pressing into the space between the shoulder and the breast. Hold for at least one minute. This is called *padadhirasana*, or breath balancing pose. Swami Shivananda Saraswati offered Hari another way to change the flow in the nostrils.

In this way when a holy spiritual man sits for meditation, sushumna then naturally flows. When sushumna does not flow naturally, then

Indian yogins use a pair of wooden sticks. Size [here he means the shape] of the sticks is like this [a Y shape].

When these two sticks are fitted underneath the two armpits, sushumna begins to flow. Those who do not wish to use sticks should meditate fixing his eye-vision on the navel region. After a few weeks of meditation, sushumna will naturally flow at the time of the meditation. With the help of this process, when sushumna begins to flow naturally, remove your glance from navel region to forehead region between the eyebrows. If health is perfect and mind is pure, then sushumna becomes active after a few days meditation. Time of meditation should be kept fixed [that is, an established time every day]. If the body is not free from all kinds of disease, then it is difficult to keep the sushumna flow.

Once he had explained how to change the flow in the nostrils, the swami continued, espousing the benefits of swarodaya yoga for digestion and stomach ailments.

When you suffer from headache or pain in the stomach or pain in your heart, please change your breathing, and your pain will subside slowly. In your attack of fever, you will notice that ida or pingala is continually breathing [that is, one nostril is continually open; it is not changing every hour]—if you can change it, the strength of disease will decrease,... and the disease will subside soon....

There is also a special rule which acts freely [naturally, of its own accord].... Digestion glands can secrete the necessary secretions for digestion when pingala is active. This is why when a healthy person sits down to take his meal, activity of ida stops, and pingala flows. But if any disorder [disrupts] pingala when you take your meal, all kinds of stomach disease, such as indigestion, acidity, gas, ulcer, etc., will gradually develop.... If ida flows when you take your meal, change it just after taking your meal, so that pingala may flow at least half an hour continually after the meal. If you can control your breathing system in this way, you will be saved from painful stomach diseases.

The pingala nadi is activating, and the ida nadi is more passive. Hari explained that when pingala nadi is flowing, it is a good time to be active, such as eating, walking, running, and doing asana. When ida nadi is flowing, it is the best time for passive activities—meditation, pranayama, and spiritual study. If I was unable to sleep at night, he suggested that I lie on my right side with my left hand in my right armpit and block my right nostril with the right thumb. This would cause me to breathe only through the left nostril while opening the ida nadi, which is beneficial for insomnia. Equally, if I was feeling sleepy mid-afternoon, during one of our philosophical discussions, I should do the opposite—lie on my left side with my right hand in the left armpit and my left thumb blocking my left nostril. Then the pingala nadi would open, and I would feel more energetic again. Swami Shivananda Saraswati of Assam affirmed the effect of swara yoga during meditation.

> If you do your Japa-Dhyana [meditation using the japa mala] when ida is active, you will have your partial concentration, but if you do it when pingala is active, your mind will not be concentrated. You will have your full concentration in Japa and Dhyana when sushumna is active.... When a spiritually advanced person sits down for meditation, sushumna will flow then naturally. Without the help of sushumna, it will not be possible for a sadhak to enjoy deep concentration or samadhi. When a sadhak wishes to raise kundalini, the flowing of sushumna is necessary at that time. So control of sushumna is essential for self-realization or God-realization.

Followers of Swarodaya yoga feel its impact in all aspects of life. The swami explains how to pay attention to the flow in ida and pingala during any worldly work or business.

> When you go anywhere for any business, please notice your breathing. If ida is flowing when you depart,... your first step should be with the left leg. If pingala flows, your first step should be with the right leg. If you follow this rule, your aim of journey [that is, your goal] will be fulfilled; no inconvenience, no danger, not any kind of obstruction will come in your way....
>
> If you start ... when sushumna is in full flowing, you will have a fatal accident. Your life will be endangered. You may die a painful death. Breathing clearly by both nostrils is called full sushumna. When one nostril is clear breathing, and ... the other nostril is a

bit less clear, breathing is called half-sushumna. Or a few seconds of breathing in ida and a few seconds of breathing in pingala—this rapid change of breathing is also called half-sushumna. So half-sushumna and full sushumna is very bad for worldly affairs. This is why swarodaya yoga has advised all not to do any worldly work when half-sushumna is active—All these injunctions of swarodaya yoga are like gospel Truth. We have tested it, so one should not doubt about it.[392]

In other words, when the sushumna is open, it is not a time to be conducting business—it is clearly a time for spiritual activities. The ancient text describes in great detail how to achieve success in all activities, including the ability to identify the tattvas (elements) within the breath. When the ida nadi is flowing for one hour, each of the tattvas has a presence during that hour. When the flow switches to the pingala nadi, the presence of the tattvas cycle through that hour. So not only does a swara yogi need to know which nadi is flowing, it is also necessary to know which tattva is present at any given time. Knowing which tattva is present in ida or pingala nadi for both the man and the woman at the time of conception can determine the sex of the child. The ability to identify each tattva is important if one wishes to attain mastery over the body using swarodaya yoga.

Swara Yoga As Related to Tattwa Sadhana

Now I will begin the discourse on pancha Tattwa [the five tattvas]. Everything in this creation is made of Supreme energy or prakriti. This Supreme energy manifests herself in five ways—this is why the creation is called pancha Tattwa.... In the lower stage, we see the creative energy is divided into five parts—prithivi [earth, also known as "kshiti"], apa [water], teja [fire, also known as "agni"], vayu [air], and vyoma [ether, also known as "akasha"]. In the macrocosm, we find the combination of these five elements in a refined form. In [the microcosm], there is also the combination and activity of these five elements, which are comparatively gross.

In our body—the bones, flesh, skin, arteries, and hair—these gross things are a product of prithivi Tattwa. Both internal and external secretions of all the glands—such as semen, saliva, digestive juice, etc., blood, bone marrow, and urine—these liquid things have come out of apa Tattwa. Appetite, thirst, sleep, exhaustion, and lethargy—these are from teja Tattwa. Retention, ejection, motion, contraction, and expansion—these five are from vayu Tattwa. Love, shame, hatred, fear, and confusion emanate from vyoma Tattwa.

The yogins have precisely calculated the time of arising, duration, and predominance of any particular Tattwa over the human body. The prithivi Tattwa [earth element] supervises our body as we inhabit the lowest stratum of the physical world, i.e., the earth, and it holds on the longest time. The vayu [air] and vyoma [ether] Tattwas hold supreme over the bodies of the inhabitants of higher worlds or Deva-Loka; for this reason, they can freely move about from one corner to other in a moment like air or lightning. Their body is also made of lightning or air. Their hearts are also illumined with the radiance, knowledge, purity, and Bliss.

The five Tattwas appear in our body one after another. First we should know the rules and regulations of our breathing. In every hour, it is changed from one nostril to the other. Sushumna flows for a few seconds when the air is changed from one nostril to the other. Breathing through the right or left nostril for approximately one hour. In every one hour, prithivi Tattwa lasts for ... 20 minutes, apa Tattwa ... 16 minutes, teja Tattwa ... 12 minutes, vayu Tattwa ... 8 minutes, and lastly vyoma Tattwa holds for ... 4 minutes only.

METHODS OF ASCERTAINING THE TATTWAS

There are eight various methods of ascertaining the different Tattwas arising at different times in our body when breath flows through either channel. Only four, which appear easier, are mentioned here.

1. If we breathe out on a mirror, the shape of the vapour left upon it indicates the different Tattwas—a four-cornered [shape] indicates prithivi Tattwa, a semicircular one is the apa Tattwa, a triangular one signifies teja Tattwa, a circular one vayu Tattwa, and if it is dotted all over the glass signifies vyoma Tattwa.

2. When breath blows through middle of the nostril, then prithivi is active in your body. If breathing through the lower side [of the nostril], it is Apa Tattwa; blowing by the upper edge denotes

Teja Tattwa; by the sides, Vayu Tattwa; and fully through the nose shows the activity of Vyoma Tattwa.

3. It appears that shutting our eyes—we only see darkness; but in fact, if one closely looks through the darkness, different colours will appear at different times. Thus the yellow colour indicates the activity of prithvi Tattwa. White indicates Apa Tattwa; Red, Teja Tattwa; black or blue colour in cloudy form will indicate the rise of Vayu Tattwa; and shades of different colours indicates Vyoma Tattwa.[393]

4. A mouthful of water, if sprayed out against the rays of the sun will spread over in dewy particles showing the colour of the rainbow in it. The colour of the Tattwa prevailing at that time will be reflected in the sprayed background....

People who are guided by these indications of the Tattwas and swarajnana [knowledge of swara yoga] while starting to go out or performing any auspicious job will always succeed in enterprises whatever they will undertake.[394]

Swarodaya Yoga is a simple process which will help one to be master of the breathing system. At will, if I can control ida and pingala, it will be easy for me to stir up Sushumna. And Sushumna always helps the Sadhak to realize his Supreme self.

The chief aim of Tattwa Sadhana is to protect us. Hatha Yoga can save us from disease but cannot save us from accident or accidental death. In our normal breathing, when Vayu or Teja Tattwa is active, we should not go out anywhere; if we start, we will meet an accident, but this accident will not be serious or fatal. But in Vyoma Tattwa, Sushumna is active; if we go anywhere in Vyoma Tattwa or in full sushumna, we will meet fatal accident or death.

Higher types of Indian Sadhaks do not like to spend time [studying] this kind of Sadhana, because they do not care about an untimely death. They do not like to stay longer in this lower world. If God wishes to keep him alive longer, he may do it. It is good to spit out [release] the body and start for higher world. This nonattachment for this lower world is a peculiar mentalism of Indian Sadhaks. You may call it foolish orientalism or anything else you like, but it is a fact. I also sometimes wish to be free from the bondage of the material existence.[395]

Prana is the life force, and the more we can learn the subtleties of the breath, the more we are able to attune ourselves with it. The science of swara yoga is clearly outlined in the Shiva Swarodaya Yoga scriptures.

The Seven Lokas—Life after Death

We all struggle with death and the loss of those we love. When Ramana Maharshi died in April 1950, Hari wrote to Swami Sivananda of Rishikesh regarding his loss. Swami Sivananda had visited Ramana Maharshi and received darshan from him.

> Regarding Bhagawan Ramana's passing away. The body of even a Jnani is controlled by the Prarabdha Karma which made it! And, he is unattached to the body. Karma takes its course; the Jnani who has attained Cosmic Consciousness stands aside as a witness of its decay and death, even as we stand at the bedside of a dying man.

Swami Sivananda went on to add:

> It is not wise to expect to halt the work of nature! This body, which is composed of five elements, is bound to decay. We should not use Yoga-methods to its preservation beyond its natural course. We should, on the contrary, let it takes its allotted course, dissociating our real Self from the body. Better give up reading at night and utilize the time in divine contemplation.[396]

As we all are, Hari was very interested in life after death, even more so after his wife, Isabella, died. He had experiences that made him believe there was so much more than meets the eye. He asked his good friend Swami Shivananda Saraswati of Assam about life after death. The Swami wrote him about the seven lokas (worlds) and the stages after death. The seven lokas can be related to the seven chakras.

The first three chakras (muladhara, svadhisthana, and manipura) relate to the first three lokas *(bhur, bhuvah,* and *swar)*. These are the foundation for our existence on earth, in this material world. Our basic needs of food, clothing, and shelter must be met. We have a sense of belonging, reproduce, and have the willpower to succeed. The heart chakra (anahata) relates to *mahar* loka and is a center of choice. It is where we choose to dwell in these three lower worlds or move upward into the more spiritual chakras. The choice depends on the development of our consciousness—if we believe that we are merely a body and mind, we will remain attached to the lower worlds. If we begin to understand that we and everyone else are spiritual beings, then we will be attracted to the higher worlds. The higher chakras (vishuddhi, ajna, and sahasrara) are connected to the spirit world and relate to the *janah*, *tapah*, and *satya* lokas.

Swami Shivananda Saraswati of Assam explained to Hari how each loka relates to a stage of consciousness—waking, dreaming, deep sleep, and so forth. I have edited the following only slightly so the sentences run together more smoothly.

We daily enjoy the three stages of life: the waking, dreaming, and deep-sleeping stage. In this material world, our waking stage is prominent, where we enjoy the waking stage for at least 18 hours. After death, the dreaming stage will be prominent. We will enjoy more than 18 hours in the dreaming stage. If there is good dream, then we enjoy happiness. If there is bad dream, we suffer. This suffering and happiness may be called heaven and hell.

So just after death, the soul gets a body. It is the body of a vapour-like white cloud. In winter, dew-drops or snow come down from the clouds, but we don't see the winter cloud. In this same way, we cannot see the body of the departed soul. They roam in the sky. As long as they are in the dreamy stage, they are separate from others and only enjoying their dream. When they awake from dream, their memory of the worldly life is awakened, and they go to their beloved and try to talk with them. But alas! It is not possible. Again the dreamy stage comes, and they forget the memory of the relatives. In dreams also, they talk with their relatives, but it is their own dreamy mental function.

Generally, the human soul lives in this way for 100 years, enjoying this dreamy stage and sometimes the waking stage. The remaining time is spent in the sleeping stage, and then, again, he is promoted to another higher region where sleeping is prominent—18 hours of sleep and 6 hours in either the dreaming or waking stages.

In this way, two hundred years is passed, and then the departed soul takes his re-birth again. Over this long period, we cannot remember the events of our previous birth. High-minded souls do not come back into this lower world again—they cross this dreamy land.

In our Indian terms, this dreamy land is called Bhubarlok [*sic;* bhu-var loka]. They also cross the sleeping land, which is called Swarlok and move into the higher worlds. Only the people who have been enlightened and who have no attraction for this mortal world can enter into these higher worlds, which are free from all sufferings and are the abode of eternal bliss. Crossing the three higher worlds, called Mahah, Janah, and Tapah, the enlightened soul will be united with Supreme Divinity, or God. This is Deva-janpadh for the pure-minded devotees.

Some Indian Yogis, at night, leave this material body and can go to the dream land and sleep land, i.e., Swarloka and Bhuvarloka, to meet the departed soul. Bhuvarlok and swarlok are not separate worlds. As a big circle covers a small circle within, so Bhuvarlok covers Bhulok, the material world. Swarlok covers Bhuvarlok and Bhulok. More in next letter.[397]

And in the next letter, Swami Shivananda of Assam continued his explanation of life after death and addressed how Hari's departed wife, Isabella, might visit him every day.

I am satisfied to know from your letter that you are really much more interested in the subject of "Life after Death." Your experience in the dream is a vivid and correct one. It is even possible to remember all the facts in the awakened stage. It becomes possible only in deep meditation and sound concentration.

You have mentioned in your letter that while you were sleeping in Riga, you were seen at Tuckum. It is, of course, a rare case. It sometimes happens that while you were asleep, your intense desire from the awakened stage to appear in Tuckum became more intense or super conscious, and the desire manifested in that place. But your body remained unconscious in the sleeping condition in Riga. Conversely, the persons in Tuckum, having intense desire to see you there, saw you at Tuckum. It is coincidence of thought. I, however, cannot understand clearly what really happened to you.

I have already told you lot of things about the "Life after Death." I have already told you that the departed soul normally enjoys dreams most of the hours and awakens for one or half-an-hour only in every 24 hours. It is, of course, presumed that the departed soul comes to their beloved or near-and-dear one, or to touch this materialistic world almost every day in the first year (after death). You can, however, see the departed soul of your wife only in that plane while you are in the dream-stage and the departed soul is in awakened stage. It is possible to remember the happenings of the dream in the awakened stage too.

In my last letter I have told you about the departed souls of Adhah-tri-loka, which is related to the affairs of the lower world, and we shall have to come back again in the earth. But if you wish to hear about the souls of the Udhah-tri-loka (the higher world), I will discuss in my next letter.[398]

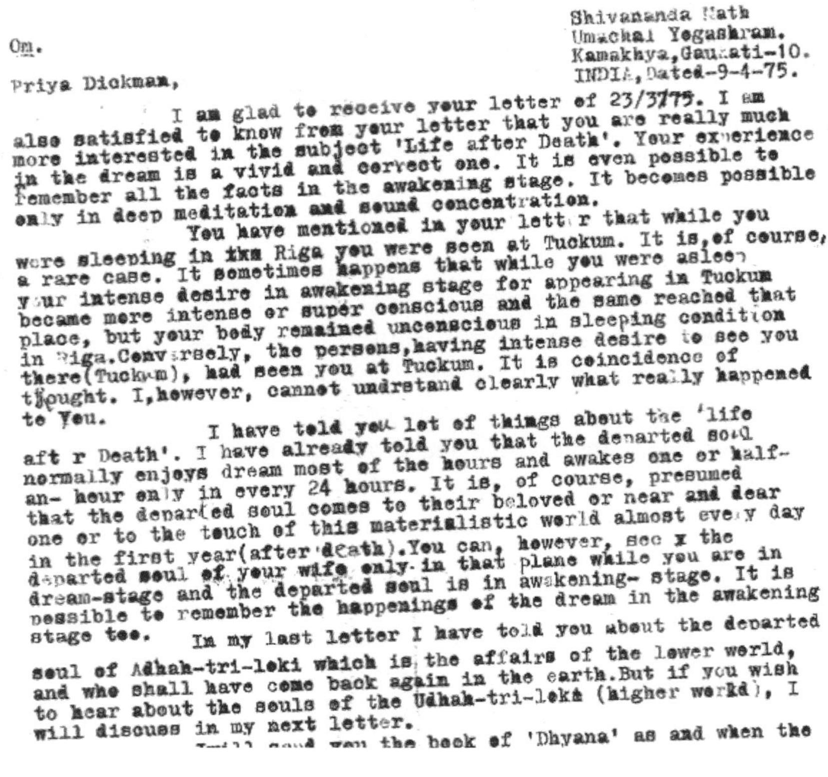

Om.

Priya Dickman,

Shivananda Nath
Umachal Yogashram,
Kamakhya,Gauhati-10.
INDIA,Dated-9-4-75.

I am glad to receive your letter of 23/3/75. I am also satisfied to know from your letter that you are really much more interested in the subject 'Life after Death'. Your experience in the dream is a vivid and correct one. It is even possible to remember all the facts in the awakening stage. It becomes possible only in deep meditation and sound concentration.

You have mentioned in your letter that while you were sleeping in the Riga you were seen at Tuckum. It is, of course, a rare case. It sometimes happens that while you were asleep your intense desire in awakening stage for appearing in Tuckum became more intense or super conscious and the same reached that place, but your body remained unconscious in sleeping condition in Riga.Conversely, the persons,having intense desire to see you there(Tuckum), had seen you at Tuckum. It is coincidence of thought. I,however, cannot undrstand clearly what really happened to You.

I have told you lot of things about the 'life after Death'. I have already told you that the departed soul normally enjoys dream most of the hours and awakes one or half-an- hour only in every 24 hours. It is, of course, presumed that the departed soul comes to their beloved or near and dear one or to the touch of this materialistic world almost every day in the first year(after death).You can, however, see the the departed soul of your wife only in that plane while you are in dream-stage and the departed soul is in awakening- stage. It is possible to remember the happenings of the dream in the awakening stage too. In my last letter I have told you about the departed soul of Adhah-tri-loki which is the affairs of the lower world, and who shall have come back again in the earth.But if you wish to hear about the souls of the Udhah-tri-loka (higher world), I will discuss in my next letter.

I will send you the book of 'Dhyana' as and when the

Figure 9.10. Letter from Swami Shivananda Saraswati of Assam on life after death. April 9, 1975.

Swami Shivananda Saraswati continued sharing with Hari about life and death, although it took almost a year; his letters were mailed to Rutherford, New Jersey, but by that time, Hari had moved to San Rafael, California, and so the Swami's letters were returned. They caught up with each other in April of 1976.

                    This vast universe is divided into seven divisions
Man's body and mind have the same corresponding divisions. 'Bhu',
'Bhuva' 'Swas' are the three stages at the primary level. So long our
mind remains attached to those levels, we suffer from sorrow. When we
succeed in liberating our mind from the bondage of these three stages
we become free from suffering. As we go on elevating ourselves – we
gradually transcend lower planes of creation. As we go on transcending the lower planes of creation, our brain unfolds itself towards

Figure 9.11. Letter from Swami Shivananda Saraswati of Assam on life after death, April 16, 1976.

This vast universe is divided into seven divisions. Man's body and mind have the same corresponding divisions. "Bhu," "Bhuva" "Swas" are the three stages at the primary level. So long as our mind remains attached to those levels, we suffer from sorrow. When we succeed in liberating our mind from the bondage of these three stages, we become free from suffering. As we go on elevating ourselves—we gradually transcend the lower planes of creation. As we go on transcending the lower planes of creation, our brain unfolds itself toward the Eternal, and as a result, the mind casts off all evil and selfish longings, and it embalms itself in pure, serene, and exalted aspirations that gradually elevate him beyond the three lower stages.

    When the mind surpasses the lower three stages and enters the 4th higher stage he enters the domain of "Maharlok," which is Antariksha or the middle stage. He may come down to the lower stages (Bhu, Bhuvah, Swah lokas) or go up from this Mahah stage (to Jana, Tapah, and Satyam). It depends on the tendency of his mind. The mind may maintain equilibrium between the lower and higher stages, or the spiritual urge may become more potent to inspire him to rise above. It is also possible that he may lose the stage through pre-domination of lower urges on his mind. But once mind can surpass the stage of Maharlok and he enters into Janalok—the world of Divine Bliss—where love remains free from passion, and works become free from self-interest. Once this stage is attained, he gradually ascends toward the Tapalok, the world of pure knowledge.

He may enjoy these worlds of Bliss and pure knowledge as long as he wishes; then he enters into Satyalok, where he becomes one with God consciousness, the region of Supreme Truth, Supreme reality, where there is unification of pure Bliss, pure knowledge. This stage is called chidananda.

This earth is a very tiny place, where one may suffer during his short stay. This also happens when he violates the law of nature. One who knows how to live according to the Divine Law does not suffer at all. To such a man, the world appears to be a blissful place. Again I repeat—the first stage—we get Bhu, Bhuva, Swa—these three lokas. Maharlok stands in between the lower stages and the higher stages ... Janalok, Tapalok, and Satyalok. When the mind surpasses Maharlok and enters Janalok, he enters the world of bliss; after surpassing Janalok, he enters the stage of Tapalok, or the world of pure knowledge. In Satyalok, both Bliss and knowledge become one. This contains the whole creation.

Even after death, the mind continues to have its finer body, which is transparent. Clashes continue in the gross plane. There is no clash in the finer plane. In the finer plane, the ego survives in the subtlest way so long as it does not merge itself with the Supreme Being or God. Just as a river merges into the sea and loses its identity, so the ego is dissolved as soon as one merges with the universal soul and loses individuality. At this stage, he is tranquilized into a perfectly tranquil and serene Being. All actions cease to exist at this stage.[399]

Further discussion on the lokas came from an interesting letter from Sri Satyakam explaining how the eight-pointed star represents the lokas. Again, I have edited minimally for clarity.

In my opinion, the meaning of the eight-petaled star is to unite ourselves with the seven worlds, praying sublime happiness for all. Ourselves + Bhu + Bhuva + Swa + Maha + Jana + Tapa + Satya (sapta lokas or seven worlds) = 8 (eight). The star is the symbol of promotion and permanent knowledge and the swastika is the symbol of happiness and peace. Let us promote our knowledge to the seven worlds, praying peace for all. Acharyadeva said "Bhu, Bhuva, and Swa—these three worlds are [worldly] worlds. Here is the chain of life, death, desire, and cravings, which is always revolving. Only by yoga can we cut off this chain of life and death. Maha, Jana, Tapa, and Satya—these four worlds are dhyanaloka—worlds of meditation. Persons of these worlds live on meditation and not on food, and they pass their whole time in meditation. It is needless to say that those who can cut the chain of worldliness by yoga get here to this place.

The swastika denotes Om or Brahma. Also it is its integral meaning. In this sense "Om Swasti" means "Brahma is peaceful." Who is this peaceful (Swastika) person? The answer is "He is Om" or Brahma. In this sense swastika denotes Om or Brahma.

Figure 9.12. A closeup of the letterhead from Sri Satyakam showing the Om plus the eight-pointed star with the swastika in the middle, undated.

EPILOGUE

HARI KNEW HE WAS DYING. He didn't tell me, though. He had been sick for four days with a "nauseated tummy," and although I kept asking him if I should call a doctor, he implored me not to. "Wait until tomorrow," he kept saying. I remember him telling me how much he regretted calling the doctor when his wife was dying. She was all hooked up to tubes at the end, and he just wanted her to be able to release from her body naturally. He told me he wanted to go naturally and not like she had.

The afternoon before he died, he brought me a bag of cookies and his half-empty bag of M&M's. It was not like Hari to go without his chocolate. Chocolate and yoga were his mainstays! I told him the he couldn't give me his M&M's, but he insisted he didn't need them anymore. I, naively, didn't get it.

That evening he called me to his room. He asked me about Canada and how cold it was. We chatted for a while, and then he looked at me lovingly and said, "You are so good." He would often say this to me for the littlest thing I did for him, be it mending his books or studying hard at the yoga subjects we were covering. I replied back, "That is because I love you." And I did, so deeply—so very deeply. He took my hand and said, "How can I help but love you when you are so good." Then we hugged, and I went to my room.

The next morning Hari did not get up at his usual time. At noon I knocked on his door, and there was no answer. I asked one of the men renting at the house to please check in on him, and he found Hari had passed away. Hari had the peaceful, natural parting he wanted. It was February 11, 1979, and he was eighty-four.

During the month we had together, we shared so many happy times. We would ask and answer questions, practice our sadhana together, and never work too hard. We shared our meditations, and he loved to watch me do my asana practice. I absolutely loved cooking for him, doing his laundry, mending his books, and shopping for his groceries. The little hugs he would give me always meant so much.

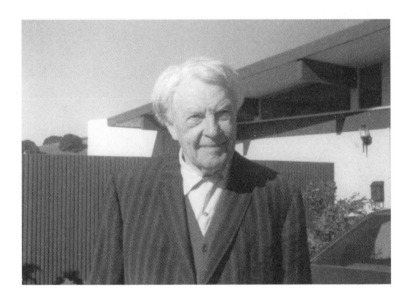

Figure E.1. Dr. Hari Dickman, January 1979, in San Rafael, California. Photo by author.

Katherine returned from India, and soon letters poured in from yogis in all corners of the world as news spread of Hari's passing. One letter came to me from my mother. She likely had no idea how important that letter would be to me, even to this day.

I have tried so many times to tell you how badly I feel about Hari; he has been someone so special to you, & even if we didn't know him, he was important to all of us because of your love for him.

I feel very much that he felt he did not need to live any longer, because he had given you what you needed, & he needed to pass on. He has taught many people, but I feel you were his special one, & he can be sure you will not waste what he has given you.[400]

Katherine permitted me to stay on at the house for a couple of months. I feverishly typed notes from the letters where we had left off. He had been so specific about what he wanted me to know, and we hadn't gotten through it all yet.

Eventually it was time for me to go. My sister and I were leaving to walk the Pacific Crest Trail from Mexico to Canada. The first leg, which would take four months, was to take us to the Oregon border. I clearly remember one day on the trail being completely overwhelmed by Hari's presence. It felt like he was hiking the trail with me, and it was the closest I have ever felt to God.

At some point I began to put M&M's on my altar. If I forgot, I carried a picture that I drew of M&M's. They became prasad, sacred food for the gods.

A few years ago, as I was preparing to drive to Penticton to lead a yoga teacher-training session, I was lamenting the fact that I had been so young when I studied with Hari. Had I been older, I would have been more mature, a better student, and I would have gotten more out of it. As I pondered this, I turned on the radio to the CBC, and there was a man being interviewed. He played a cello, or some beautiful instrument like that, and he was telling a story of how he had studied music with a great master, but had never the opportunity to play in a symphony with him. And then he realized that every time he plays, he plays with him.

And then I realized that Hari has never stopped teaching me. Hari is always teaching me.

Guru Om Guru Om
Sadguru Datta Hari Om
He is OM, The Word. He is the true teacher. He is Hari.[401]

APPENDIX I

Yogis Who Corresponded with Hari Dickman

Those marked with an asterisk* are referred to or have been quoted in this book.

KAIVALYADHAMA INSTITUTE OF SCIENTIFIC RESEARCH

*Swami Kuvalayananda 1930–1958
Balkrishna, undated (refers to *Yoga Mimamsa* Vol. 10, No. 1. Vol. 7, No. 1 is referred to as "at the press" in Feb. 1958 letter)

ARUNACHALA ASHRAMA OF BHAGAVAN SRI RAMANA MAHARSHI

Sri Ramana Maharshi—Hari states that they communicated with each other via cassette recording; no letters exist. There is evidence of letters before the Second World War, from 1929–1940 (see Niranjanananda letter, 1951, requesting copies of these letters for their records)
*T. K. Sundaresa Iyer (cousin to Krishnamurthy), 1931, from Tiruvanna-malai, Madras, India

*Niranjanananda Swamiji, 1933–1951, from Tiruvannamalai, Sri Ramana
 Ashrama, S. India
*Major A. W. Chadwick (a.k.a. Sadhu Arunachala), 1951, from Tiruvanna-
 malai, "At Puri"
*Arunachala Bhakta Bhagawat, 1976, from Arunachala Ashrama, 342 East
 6th St, New York

Sri Aurobindo Ashram

Swami Shuddhananda Bharati, 1938 and 1946, from Pondicherry,
 S. India, Also in 1954, 1965, 1968, and 1977, sent from Yoga Samaj,
 Adyar, Madras–20, India. By 1977, also known as Kaviyogi Marashi
 Shuddhananda Bharati
T. R. Sundararajan for Anbu Nilayam Book Publisher for books,
 Sept. 5, 1946

Kriya Yoga

Bupendranath Sanayal, 1956, disciple of Lahiri Mahasaya
Jnanendra Nath Mukherji, 1948–1951, Calcutta (gave Paramhansa Y
 ogananda permission to translate the Pranab Gita commentary into
 English—as noted in letter April 3, 1951)

Paramhansa Yogananda Lineage

Yogoda Sat-Sanga Society/Self-Realization Fellowship
*Paramhansa Yogananda, 1934, as Swami Yogananda, 3880 San Rafael
 Ave., Los Angeles, CA
*Paramhansa Yogananda 1939–1952
*Faye Wright, Confidential Secretary to P. Yogananda, 1936–1952, from
 Mt. Washington Estates, Los, Angeles
Sister Gyanamata, March 1948, from Hermitage, Encinitas, CA
Viola Como, SRF Center Department, 1951, from 3880 San Rafael Ave.,
 Los Angeles, CA
*Dr. Minott W. Lewis, 1952–1954, from Golden World Colony, SRF,
 Encinitas, CA
Sister Sri Daya Mata, 1953–1966, 3880 San Rafael Ave., Los Angeles, CA
Sister Radharani for Rajasi Janakananda, 1953, from 3880 San Rafael Ave.,
 Los Angeles, CA

Swami Premananda, 1953–1965, from SRF, 4748 Western Ave., Washington 16, DC

*Rajasi Janakananda, 1954, from 3880 San Rafael Ave., Los Angeles, CA

*Brother Bhaktananda 1967 from 3880 San Rafael Ave., Los Angeles, CA

"Mother Center," for Mother Dayamata, 1976, 3880 San Rafael Ave., Los Angeles, CA

YOGODA SAT-SANGA AND SHYAMACHARAN MISSION, RANCHI, MIDNAPUR, PURI AND DAKINESHWAR.

Swami Satyananda Giri (Dharmacharya), 1937–1971, sometimes from Ranchi, Bihar, India in the 1930s, then from Sevayatam, Jhargram, Midnapur, West Bengal, India

Swami Satchidananda Giri, 1955–1979, (1955–1958, from Ranchi, Bihar, India, then May 16 & June 7, 1958, from Woodfield, Simla 5, Punjab, India, then Feb. 11, 1962–Jan. 27, 1963, Dakineshwar, PO Ariadaha, 24—Parganas, W. Bengal, India, then back to Sevayatam, Jhargram, Midnapur, West Bengal, 1979)

*Niranjanananda Giri, May 1975–Oct. 1976, Sevayatam, Jhargram, Midnapur, West Bengal

*Brahmachari Animananda (Dharmacharya), 1952–1954, Ranchi, Bihar, India

*Swami Sevananda, 1937–1946, Karar Ashram, Puri, India

Swami Kripananda, 1958, from Ranchi

Chandra Ghose for Brahmachari Sreeprakash, 1951, Dakineshwar, PO Ariadaha, 24—Parganas, W. Bengal, India

Joseph Chandra Battacharya, 1969–1977, from 166 Belilios Road, Howrah-1, West Bengal

B. C. Nandi 1947 from Glenloch Rd, London NW

M. P. Thyagarajan BA, 1951–1961, Kanaka Vilas, 14 Warren Road, Mylapore, Madras 4, India. Also a Siddha Yogi and disciple of Guru Saravanbava when he was sixteen years old (Oct. 29, 1951 letter)

*Swami Kriyananda, 1978, from Ananda, Nevada City, California, and undated, 220 16th Ave, San Francisco

Swami Hariharananda Giri, 1974–1975 or 1978, Karar Ashram, Puri India

Swami Premananda Giri, 1975–1976, Karar Ashram

Swami Shuddhananda Giri, 1976–1979, from Sevayatam, Jhargram, Midnapur, West Bengal, India

DIVINE LIFE SOCIETY OF RISHIKESH

*Swami Sivananda Saraswati of Rishikesh, 1946–1962

*Swami Thapovanam, 1949–1950, (founder Thapovana Kutee, Uttarkashi UP India)

*Swami Satchidananda, 1953–1974, (founder of Integral Yoga Institute and Yogaville)

*Swami Venkatesananda, 1971–1978, (founder Chiltern Yoga Trust)

*Swami Shivapremananda, 1975–1978, (founder Centro de Yoga Sivananda-Vedanta, Santiago, Chile)

*Swami Vishnudevananda, 1951–1978, (founder International Sivananda Yoga Vedanta Society, Montreal)

Swami Chidananda, 1958–1970

Swami Sasmathananda, 1951

Gauri Prasad, 1955

Swami Jyotir Mayananda, 1974, (founder International Yoga Society and Yoga Research Foundation, Miami Florida)

BIHAR SCHOOL OF YOGA, MONGHYR, BIHAR, INDIA

Swami Chaitanyananda, 1968

Swami Yogeshwaranand, 1970

Swami Shantananda, 1976

Swami Yogananda, 1976

Swami Agnimritranand, 1978

Swami Haripremananda, 1978

SHIVANANDA MATH, UMACHAL HILL, KAMAKHYA, ASSAM

*Swami Shivananda Saraswati of Assam, 1959–1976, Disciple of Swami Nigamananda Paramhansa of Assam.

Swami Bignananda for Swami Shivananda Saraswati of Assam, 1959

*Brahmachari Punyabrata, undated, likely 1959

YOGA NIKETAN TRUST

Brahmachari Vyas Deva, 1960–1961, Rishikesh, India (he later became known as Swami Yogeshwaranand)

*Swami Yogeshwaranand Saraswati, 1962–1967, Swargashram, Dehradun, UP India

Swami Omanand Saraswati, Rajyogacharya, 1972, Gurukul, Hoshangabad,
  Madhya Pradesh, India
Des Raj Trehan, 1967–1973, Rishikesh, India

Kapil Math of Swami Hariharananda Aranya, Madhupur, Bihar, India and Kapilaram, Kurseong, Darjeeling, Bengal, India

Satya Prakash Brahmachari, 1960
Swami Dharmamigha Aranya, 1938–1979
*Sri Satyakam, 1957–1964, from Amritayan Yogapeeth, Jadarpur, Calcutta
  32, India
Adinath Chatterjee, 1976–1978, from Calcutta, follower of Swami
  Dharmamigha Aranya

Siddha Yoga

*Swami Vishnu Tirth, 1957–1968, from Narayan Kutir Sanyas Ashram,
  Dewas MP India and from Rishikesh, District Dehradun, UP India
*Chandra Singh Yadav answering for Swami Vishnu Tirth, Oct. 1957, from
  Snehlataganj, Indore, India
Swami Shivom Tirth, 1978, 1979
Swami Shankaracharya, 1978
*Tarachand Garg, 1957–1959, from Indore, MP, India and from University
  of Minnesota, Minneapolis 14
M. P. Thyagarajan, 1951–1961, Kanaka Vilas, 14 Warren Road, Mylapore,
  Madras 4, India. Also with Self Realization Fellowship, Madras Branch
  (Oct. 31, 1955 letter)
Srimat Brahmananda Abadhut, 1958, from Sri Siddhayogashram,
  Chhotigaibi, Varanasi
Shri Balaram Brahmacharya, 1958, from Sri Siddhayogashram, Chhoti-
  gaibi, Varanasi
Swami NarayanAntha, 1978, from Sri Siddhayogashram, Chhotigaibi,
  Varanasi

Natha Yoga

A. K. Banerjea, 1964, Gorakhnath Temple, Gorakhpur, UP, India
*Dig Vijay Nath, 1961–1963, Gorakhnath Temple, Gorakhpur, UP, India
Nilakanth Madhao-Rao Ghiri, 1964, from Shri Dnyaneshwar Sansthan
Shreenavas G. Supekar, 1961–1966, Deccan College, Poona, India

Narendra Kumar, 1976, from Goraknath Mandir
Devendra Vigyani, 1960–1962, disciple of Sri Yogendranath Vigyani
R. D. Sant, 1962

VED-SANSTHAN, NEW DELHI, INDIA

Vidyanand Vedeh, founder, 1969–1973

SAI BABA SAMAJ, MYLAPORE, INDIA

Signature unreadable, 1947

JAIN PHILOSOPHY, SRIMAD RAJCHANDRA MISSION

Bhogilal G. Sheth, 1961–1964, Bombay, India
Sukhlal M. Mehta, 1961, for Bogilal G. Sheth

ICYER (INTERNATIONAL CENTER FOR YOGA EDUCATION AND RESEARCH)
AND ANANDA ASHRAMS

*Dr. Swami Gitananda Giri, 1976

SRI YOGENDRA INSTITUTE

Devendra Vigyani, 1960–1962, from Vigyan Press, Rishikesh

OTHERS:

* Sri Shyam Sundar Goswami, Goswami Yoga Institute, Sweden
*Thais Thomas, 1978–1979, from Madurai, S. India. Student of Swami
    Rajarshi Muni, Life Mission, Gujarat
VG Patwardan, undated, from Guru Mandir, Shri Ballappa Math, Solapur,
    Bharat
Hanuman Swami, undated, Shanti Ashram, Kotamgaon, Nasik
Seth Mukundas, 1953–1964, from Alinagar, Gorakhpur, UP, India
*Balshastri Phadke, a.k.a. Shri Shrikrishna Shridhar Phadake, 1965, Gayatri
    Mandir, Nasik, Maharashtra
*Swami Narayanananda, 1951–1960, Jagratiniketan, Rishikesh
P. S. Bhatnagar, 1968, Vishwayatan Yogashram, New Delhi, India

*Vijayendra Pratap, 1969–1971, Yoga Research Society, Philadelphia

Niranjan Dhang, 1970–1971

*Yogindra Amar Nandy, 1972, Yoga Cure Centre, Dtt. Hooghly, West Bengal, India

Swami Nirmalananda, 1974, Viswa Shanti Nikethana, B.R.PO. Chamarajanagar, Karnataka

Karai Siddarji, 1962, c/o Sri S. Ambrijammal, 96 Mowbrays Road, Madras 18, India

Selvarajan Yesudian, 1956, from Zurich—refers to Vivekananda

*Madhavananda, 1969, Bombay

Swami Shankaracharya, 1978, Vishwa Bharati Sanskrit Yoga Parishad, New Delhi

Peter Birnbaum, 1960, studied with Swami Kesavananda

Andrew Berwizky, 1976, Binghamton, NY

Victoria Lacas, 1973, Connecticut

Unknown from Gangotri, 1952

*Dr. Henry A. Carns, 1962, College of Divine Metaphysics, Indianapolis

APPENDIX II

Addresses of Letters Written to Hari Dickman

It is difficult to know how often Hari and his family had to move while living in the DP camps. The addresses below were on the letters to Hari. With help from others in Latvia, it seems Hari was moved at least three times, if not more. I have been told that the administration transferred people from one camp to another without giving any reasons for the change. At other times, labor camps were closed or "reformatted." In an email, Dzintars Vilnis Korns in Lativa, who was trying to help me sort out where Hari stayed, said, "We can think in one way or another way, but cannot say exactly. It will stay a secret for us, I think."

Liela iela No. 20., Tukum, Latvia; 1933
Zigfr. Meierovica iela 20, Tukum, Latvia; 1936
M. Minsterejas iela No. 5 Dz. 2, Riga, Latjija (Latvia) Europe; 1939
224/D Camp, 224 D.P. Assembly Center, 800 Central Unit, B.A.O.R. (Via Gt. Britain); Jan. 31, 1946

(14) Bad Mergentheim (WTTB), UNRRA Team 69, Germany, US Zone; Aug.–Sept. 1946

UNNRA Assembly Center 650, Bad Mergentheim (WTTB), Kr. Mergentheim, Germany, US Zone; May 1947

IRO Assembly Centre 688, (1a) Shorndorf/WTTB, Germany, US Zone; Sept. 1947

Gutleut Kaserne, 8710 Labor Service Company (Lativan), Frankfort a/M Germany, US Zone; Dec. 1948

(17a) Karlsruhe Baden, D.P. Camp (Latvian), Forstne, Kaserne, Germany, US Zone; Feb. 1949

7318th Labor Service Sq, APO 57, US Army, c/o Postmaster, NYC, NY; Sept. 1949

(17a) Karlsruhe Baden, D.P. Camp (Latvian), Forstne, Kaserne, Germany, US Zone; April 1950

Artillerie—Kaserne, Bi—4-100, Schwab, Gmund, Germany, US Zone; Jan. 1951

(22b) Bruchmiihlbach, Pfalz, Postfach 100, Germany, French Zone; March 1951

Schwabenhof, Block 11-57, Heilbronn/A.N., Germany, US Zone; Oct. 1951

7132 Labor Service Company, c/o 11th Labor Supv. Center, APO 227, US Army, c/o Postmaster, New York; Dec. 1951*

c/o K. Eichvalds, 5225- 14th Ave, Brooklyn 19, NY; March 5, 1952

826 President Street, Brooklyn 15, NY, Feb. 3, 1954

290 Lincoln Place, Brooklyn 38, New York, USA; June 1954, and 1969

20, Hackett Place, Rutherford, New Jersey, 07070; Feb. 1975

5 Mount Tioga Court, San Rafael, California, 94903; May 1976 until Hari's death, Feb. 1979

* Hari was in New York February 5, 1952, according to a letter from Paramhansa Yogananda, in which his prayers expressed his thanks for Hari's safe arrival, having crossed the seas, but no address was given. (Hari might have been living at the 14th Avenue address in Brooklyn.)

GLOSSARY

abhyantar kumbhaka	A breath retention held after an inhalation. It is also known as antara kumbhaka.
abhyasa (abhyas) krama	A habitual or customary order of practice. Often related to the order one practices asanas or mudras or their entire yoga practice.
abhyast asan	Your accustomed or usual way of sitting for meditation or pranayama.
adham pranayama	Breathing into the lower lungs (see vibhaga pranayama).
adharma	Sin. Unrighteousness or immorality.
adhikari	One with authority. A qualified person.
adhi mudra	A hand mudra with the thumb tucked into the palm of the hand and fingers wrapped around the thumb like a fist.
adhyam pranayama	Breathing into the upper lungs (see vibhaga pranayama).
advaitabada	Non-duality, as in Vedanta philosophy, in which God and Self are one, not separate.
agni	The fire element.

agnisara	A kriya, or cleansing technique, in which one pumps the abdomen in and out while holding uddiyana bandha and abhyantar kumbhaka.
Aham Brahmasmi	One of the four mahavakyas, meaning "I am Brahman." From the Brihadaranyaka Upanishad of Yajur Veda. See "Atma Vichara Meditation" in chapter 7.
ahamkara	The ego.
ahimsa	Non-violence. One of the yamas.
ajapa gayatri mantra	An unconscious and involuntary repetition of the mantra "hamsa" or "so hum," which is the sound (meaning "I am That") created with every breath. Represents the cosmic force flowing in an out. An involuntary form of devotion.
ajapa japa (ajapajap)	The repetition of the sacred word Om mentally with every breath.
ajna chakra	The third eye, or brow chakra.
akasha	Ether, the element for the throat chakra. Also space. Ether is finer than air.
Ambubachi	A tantric fertility festival to celebrate the menses of Mother Earth.
amrita	Celestial nectar of immortality, also known as soma nectar or ambrosia.
amritpan khechari	An alternative to khechari mudra, in which the tongue is rolled back into the soft palate in the roof of the mouth.
anahata chakra	The heart chakra.
anahata-dhwani	Inner sounds that one hears, as described in "Meditation on Nad" in chapter 7.
ananda	Pure joy or bliss, unaffected by emotions—an aspect of Brahman.
antara (anthara) kumbhaka	Internal breath retention.
antaranga yoga	Yoga of the inner limbs, referring to the inner limbs of Patanjali's Yoga Sutras: dharana, dhyana, samadhi, and sometimes pratyahara.
anuloma viloma	Alternate nostril breathing. Literally means "with the grain, against the grain."
anusandhana	Investigation or inquiry into the truth. For example, chakra anusandhana is to investigate or gain an inner knowledge of the chakras.
apana vayu	The outgoing breath. A form of prana.

aparigraha	Non-possessiveness. One of the yamas.
aprakasha bindu	The respiratory center of the lower brain. It is divided into two segments, one for inspiration and one for expiration.
arohan	The ascending psychic pathway in kriyas.
asana	Posture or position.
asamprajnata samadhi	A final stage of samadhi, without any seeds of attachment to the material world. No samskaras or thoughts remain. Same as nirvikalpa or nirbija samadhi.
ashram (asram)	A monastery retreat where gurus and their disciples live immersed in the practices of yoga.
ashtanga	Eight limbs, generally referring to Patanjali's eight-limbed path of raja yoga.
ashvini (ashwini) mudra	A mudra in which one contracts the anal sphincter to assist in awakening the kundalini.
asmita samadhi	Concentration on the mind itself. Sattvic ego alone remains.
asteya	Non-stealing. One of the yamas.
Atharva Veda	One of the four vedas (Rik, Yajur, Atharva, and Sama Vedas). The oldest yogic texts known.
atma gyana	Knowledge of God within.
atman (atma)	The individual soul or the Self.
atmic jyotis	The light of the atman that appear during meditation.
avastha	A state of consciousness, such as waking, dreaming, deep sleep.
avidya	Spiritual ignorance.
awarohan	The descending psychic pathways in kriyas.
Ayam Atma Brahma	One of the four mahavakyas, meaning "The Self is Brahman." From the Mandukya Upanishad of Atharva Veda. See "Upanishad Mantra Meditation" in chapter 7.
ayurveda	An ancient science of Indian medicine—the science of life.
bahiranga yoga	Yoga of the outer limbs, referring to the outer limbs of Patanjali's Yoga Sutras: yama, niyama, asana, pranayama, and sometimes pratyahara.
bahya kumbhaka	External breath retention. One holds the breath out after exhalation.
bahyantar	To regulate pranayama according to place, time, and number during the inflowing and outflowing breath.
bahyantarakshepi	The stopping of the breath during inhalation and exhalation.
bandha	A lock, generally a technique to lock the flow of prana.

bandha traya (bandha treya and bandhatraya)	When all three major bandhas are applied—jalandhara, mula, and uddiyana.
basti	One of the shat karmas. A yogic enema for cleaning the lower intestines and colon.
Bhagavad Gita	The gospel of Hinduism. The Song of God. An excerpt from the Mahabharata.
bhakta	Devotee.
bhakti yoga	The path of love and devotion.
Bhanumati	The author's spiritual name, meaning "the Light that shines on everything," according to Swami Vishnudevananda.
bhastrika	Bellows breath. A pranayama technique to awaken kundalini and break through the granthis.
bhavana (bhav, bhava)	Concentrated thought related to love toward God.
bhramari (brahmari)	Bee breath. A pranayama in which one creates a nasal humming sound during inhalation or exhalation. Bhramari is the sound of a female bee on exhalation, and bhramara is the sound of a male bee on inhalation.
bhrumadhya drishti	To direct your gaze toward the third eye, with eyes open or closed.
bija mantra	Bija means "seed." A seed sound. Often a single-syllable mantra, but not always.
bindu	A point or dot, like the dot in the Om symbol. Bindu is a psychic center above the ajna chakra and below the sahasrara.
Brahma	The creator. One of the gods of the Hindu holy trinity.
brahmacharya	Celibacy, or control of the sexual energy. One of the yamas.
brahmamuhurta	The last several hours before sunrise, beginning approximately at four in the morning. The best time for sadhana.
Brahman	God, the Absolute Reality. Pure consciousness.
brahmarandhra	The place at the crown of the head where there is a soft spot in infants. The top of the sushumna. The soul is said to leave the body through this spot at the time of death.
Brahma Tejas	The aura of Brahman, Source itself.
buddhi (budhi)	The discriminating aspect of the mind. Intellect.
chakra	Centers of psychic energy in the body.
chandra nadi	The lunar or left nadi.
chatur	Four.

chin mudra	A hand mudra with the tip of the index finger touching the tip of the thumb, palms facing downward.
chinmaya mudra	A hand mudra with the tip of the index finger touching the tip of the thumb, and the remaining fingers curled into the palm of the hand.
crore	An Indian unit of measurement. One crore is ten million or one hundred lakhs.
dakshina	Right, as in the right side.
danda	A staff or stick.
darshan (darsana)	The blessing or purification felt in the presence of a holy one. Truths seen in a higher state of consciousness. Direct perception of God.
desh	A place.
desh paridrishti	A place where you focus your attention during pranayama, such as a drishti.
Deva (Devata)	A god.
Devi	A goddess.
dharana	Concentration.
dhyana	Meditation.
dirga pranayama	The complete or three-part breath. Also known as mahat yoga pranayama.
dirgh	Long. A term related to pranayama in how long you can make the breath pranayama.
drishti	Gaze. Seeing. The place in which you focus your eyes and attention.
Durga	A Hindu goddess. Wife of Siva. She fiercely protects her children.
dvaitabada	Duality, as in a religion based on duality (where God is separate from the Self).
Ganesha	The son of Siva and Parvati. Ganesha has an elephant's head and is the remover of obstacles on your spiritual path.
Gayatri mantra	From the Rik (Rig) Veda, one of the most sacred and powerful mantras.
Gheranda Samhita	One of three classic texts on hatha yoga, as taught by Gheranda. The other two classic texts are Hatha Yoga Pradipika and Siva Samhita.
goad	A tool used to train elephants. Often it is in one of the hands of a god or goddess. This represents our elephant mind or ego ... to goad our mind along towards God consciousness. If the goad can train the largest of land animals, it surely can train our mind!

granthi	A psychic knot. There are three granthis—Brahma granthi at the muladhara chakra; Vishnu granthi at the anahata chakra; Rudra granthi at the ajna chakra.
guhya (guha) chakra	Mystical or hidden chakra said to be somewhere in the middle of the brain. Sometimes called the Brahma chakra.
guna	A quality or attribute of prakriti, "nature, matter." Prakriti consists of three gunas—sattva (purity and light), rajas (activity and passion) and tamas (darkness and inertia).
guru	A spiritual teacher. A guide to the Spirit.
guru inspiration	To be inspired by the grace of one's guru.
gurubhai	Brother or sister under the same guru.
guru kripa (guru-kripa)	Grace or blessing of the guru.
hamsa (ham sa)	A swan. Hamsa or so ham is a sacred mantra always on our breath, meaning "I am That."
Hari	An incarnation of Vishnu. A being who destroys the evil deed of those who take refuge in him.
hatha yoga	A system of yoga developed by Svatmarama, focusing on physical practices to cultivate strength and control over the physical body, including asanas, pranayama, kriyas, and mudras.
Hatha Yoga Pradipika	The yoga of light. An ancient text describing the pathway of Hatha Yoga written by Svatmarama around the 1500s.
hridaya	The heart area.
ida nadi	The psychic nerve related to the left nostril and a major nadi on the left side of the body; lunar, cooling, feminine energy.
Indra	A vedic deity; king of the gods.
indriya	Organ. There are karma indriyas (organs of action: hands, feet, mouth, genitals, and anus) and jnana indriyas (organs of knowledge: sight, sound, taste, touch, and smell).
Ishta Devata	Your chosen ideal form of God to focus your meditations and mantras in order to develop those divine qualities within you.
ishvara pranidhana	Surrender to the Divine. One of the niyamas.
jada samadhi	An artificial or inert samadhi.
jal neti	Cleaning the nasal and sinus passages with water (jal), generally using a neti pot.
jalandhara banda	Throat lock.
janu	Knee.

janu sirsasana	Head to knee pose.
japa (jap)	The practice of repeating a mantra or God's name. Usually used with mala beads or a rosary.
jaya	Halleluja! Victory, triumph.
jihva	Tongue.
jihva bandha	Tongue lock.
jiva atman	The individual soul.
jnanamarga	The path to enlightenment through wisdom and knowledge.
jnana yoga	The path of wisdom or knowledge. There is only God—all else is maya, illusion.
jnanins	Those devoted to the path of jnana yoga.
jyoti (yoti) mudra	When eyes are half-open and directed toward the ajna chakra. A light surrounded by flickering lights appears to the meditator. This is considered the halo of the spiritual eye.
Jyotsna	The name of Swami Brahmananda's first publication of his commentary on the Hatha Yoga Pradipika.
kaal (kal)	Time.
kaal (kal) paridrishti	A term related to the time during pranayama—counting the seconds or minutes during the process.
kaki mudra	Pursing one's lips like a crowbreak. Kaki means a "a female crow."
Kali	A fierce Hindu goddess who removes the ego. A wife of Siva.
kamalasan (kamal asan)	Another name for lotus pose.
kamandalu	A holy vessel, such as a copper bowl to hold water.
kanishth	Short. A term related to pranayama in how short you make the breath for pranayama.
kanth	Throat.
kapalabhati	Shining skull. A cleansing technique and pranayama.
karana sharira	The seed or "causal" body. It carries the seeds of your learnings from one life into the next.
karma	The law of action and reaction or cause and effect.
karma yoga	The path of self-less action.
kevela kumbhaka	An unintended breath retention.
khechari mudra	A mudra in which the tongue rolls back and up into the throat to capture the soma nectar (see amritpan khechari mudra).

kleshas	The obstacles to enlightenment (ignorance, egoism, attachment, aversion, and the desire to cling to life).
koshas	A sheath covering the spirit.
krama	Order or sequence of your practice.
Krishna paksha	The period of the waning moon.
kriya yoga	A system of yoga revived by Mahavatar Babaji, Lahiri Mahasaya, and Paramhansa Yogananda. Certain actions recharge the body, including pranayama and meditation techniques to accelerate one's spiritual grown and reach the goal of union with the Infinite.
kriyas	Cleansing or purification exercises drawn from hatha yoga.
kumbhaka (kumbhak)	Breath retention.
kundalini	Spiritual or psychic energy said to be coiled like a serpent at the base of the spine, waiting to be awakened.
kundalini yoga	The system of yoga to awaken and raise the kundalini energy.
kutustha	The Christ Center, or the ajna chakra.
Lakshmi	A Hindu goddess who is a bountiful provider. Wife of Vishnu.
lalana chakra	An esoteric chakra above the soft palate at the back of the throat, and just below the ears, near the glottis. Also known as talu chakra.
laya yoga	A system of yoga whereby the mind is absolved into the Self. It is devoted to cultivating and raising kundalini through awareness of the chakras.
likhita japa	Writing a mantra continuously.
linga sharira	The astral body. Also sukshma sharira.
lingam	A symbol representing Shiva.
loka	A world or vast space.
madhyam (madhya)	Medium, middle.
madhyam pranayama	Breathing into the middle area of the lungs.
Mahabharata	The famous Hindu epic from the fifth century BCE or earlier. Possibly the world's longest poem, with 110,000 couplets. The Bhagavad Gita is a portion of this poem.
maharaj	Great king. A name of respect for a yoga master.
maharshi	A great seer or sage.
mahatma	A title given to those who have advanced mentally and spiritually. It means "great soul."

mahat yoga mudra	Same as Brahma mudra. Gesture of grand integration.
mahat yoga pranayama	The complete breath, or three-part breath. Also known as dirga breath.
Mahavakya (mahavakya)	Literally, "a great sentence." These are four declarations of Vedantic Truth from the Upanishads. These are: Prajnanam Brahma (Consciousness of Brahman) from the Aitareya Upanishad of Rik Veda (see "Upanishad Mantra Meditation" in chapter 7); Aham Brahmasmi (I am Bramhan) from the Brihadaranyak Upanishad of Yajur Veda (see "Atma Vichara Meditation" in chapter 7); Tat Tvam Asi (That thou art) from the Chandogya Upanishad of Sama Veda (see "Atma Vichara Meditation"); Ayam Atma Brahma (This Self is Brahman) from the Mandukya Upanishad of Atharva Veda (see "Upanishad Mantra Meditation").
mahayogi	Great yogi.
mahavratam	A great vow or a great duty. Our life's purpose.
mala	A string of beads used for meditation. The yoga mala has 108 beads plus a meru.
manas	The recording faculty of the mind that takes in information through the senses.
manasika japa	Repeating a mantra mentally, in silence. The lips do not move.
manipura chakra	The solar plexus chakra.
matra	A unit used to count, as in pranayama, to measure how long a breath should be.
maya	Illusion. In the Vedanta philosophy, maya is mind and matter.
mayurasana	Peacock pose, in which the elbows push into the stomach area while balancing on them.
meru	The main starting bead on a mala.
moksha	Liberation from karma and reincarnation. Same as mukti.
mudra	A physical posture to awaken the kundalini, or a hand gesture to connect external actions with spiritual goals.
mukhi	Face, mouth, or gate.
mukti	Liberation from karma and reincarnation. Same as moksha.
mula bandha (mulabandha)	Root lock near muladhara chakra.
muladhara chakra (muladhar chakra)	The root chakra at the base of the spine.

murccha (murcha, murchha)	A pranayama that leads to a loss of awareness.
nabhi	Navel.
nada (nad)	Sound. Nada yoga is the yoga of the inner sound.
nadi	An astral nerve through which the prana flows.
nadi shodhana (nadi sadhana)	A pranayama technique to cleanse the nadis, similar to alternate nostril breathing.
nari	Nadi. Some yogis, such as Swami Yogeshwaranand, spelled nadi as "nari" in letters to Hari.
nasagra (nasikagra) drishti	Gazing at the tip of the nose.
natha yoga	Natha means "Lord," "protector," or "ruler." A system of yoga founded by Matsyendranath and Gorakshanath, designed so one can achieve liberation during this life and avoid the cycle of reincarnation. Svatmarama, author of the Hatha Yoga Pradipika, is said to be a disciple of Gorakshanath; therefore, natha yoga is similar to hatha yoga.
nauli	One of the shat karmas, or cleansing kriyas. A deep exhalation is followed by the abdomen drawn back and up toward the spine, then the rectus abdominis are dropped forward.
neti	A technique to clean the nasal and sinus passages. One of the kriyas.
nirgarbh	Without. To perform pranayama without adding the mantra Om with each count.
nirodha	Restraint.
nirvichara samadhi	A stage of samadhi in which there is no thinking or inquiry, just pure sattva.
nirvikalpa samadhi	A stage of samadhi without seeds of attachment to the material world. Without thought. Same as asamprajnata samadhi and nirbija samadhi.
nirvitarka samadhi	A stage of samadhi in which one acquires true knowledge of an object.
niyamas	Ethical observances of virtues to develop in yoga.
obhyas	Repeated effort to concentrate the mind on one thought.
ojas	A potent spiritual force that gives us vigor, vitality, and bodily strength.
Om (aum)	The sacred word for God. Sometimes spelled Aum.

Omkara	The Word of God.
padadhirasana	Breath balancing pose.
padahastasana	A standing forward bend pose in which feet and hands meet.
padatal	Foot.
padmasana	The lotus pose.
pancha	Five, as pancha koshas is "five koshas," or pancha vayus is "five vayus."
panchikarana	The doctrine of quintuplication in which, through meditation, one discards each of the five elements of matter (earth, water, fire, air, ether) until one comes to the source (Self).
papa purusha	A sinful or evil person.
Param Atman	The Supreme Spirit.
paramhansa	A name bestowed upon a sannyasi who has reached the highest level of spiritual development.
Parvati	A Hindu goddess. Wife of Siva, mother of Ganesha. Parvati is credited with writing down the scriptural knowledge Siva acquired during meditation.
Patanjali	Author of the yoga sutras.
paschimottanasana	A seated forward bend pose.
pavana (pawana)	Relates to the movement of wind or air.
pingala nadi	The psychic nerve related to the right nostril and a major nadi on the right side of the body; solar, warming, masculine energy.
plavini	A pranayama that reduces the effect of gravity on the body by swallowing air. Plavini means "to float."
pradipta	Inflamed or burning.
Prajnanam Brahma (Pragnanam Brahma)	One of the four mahavakyas, meaning "Consciousness of Brahman." From the Aitareya Upanishad of Rik Veda (see "Upanishad Mantra Meditation" in chapter 7).
prakriti	Nature. Manifested matter, always in combination with Purusha, "spirit."
prana	The life force or vital air (vayu) that brings life and all movement to the body.
prana shuddhi	The process of making the prana pure and untainted.
pranatasana	A name for child's pose. Prana flow is restricted in the legs as they are folded under the body, effectively moving the prana freely up the spine in fetal position.

prana vayus	Prana is broken down into five vayus: prana (heart region; inward moving such as breathing in or taking in food), apana (abdominal region; outward moving such as exhalation or excretion), samana (navel region; balancing force between prana and apana; relates to assimilation and digestion), udana (throat area; upward moving, related to growth physically, mentally and spiritually), vyana (distribution and circulation throughout the body).
pranava mantra	The sacred mantra Om, the primordial sound.
Pranayama	Control of prana. It enables the body to make use of prana.
prarabdha karma	Karma bearing fruit in this lifetime.
prasad	A spiritual offering of food.
pratyahara	Withdrawal of the senses at will, so if one wishes to concentrate or meditate, the senses are not a distraction.
prithivi	Earth element.
puja	A sacred Hindu ceremony to concentrate the mind on God and intensify devotion.
puraka (purak)	Inhalation.
purnam	Fullness.
Purusha	The Supreme Being.
pushpaputa mudra	A mudra for emotional balance. Gesture of offering a handful of flowers to the Divine.
raja yoga	The eight-limbed system of yoga developed by Patanjali to understand and control the mind in order to understand the true Self.
rajas	Activity. Passion. One of the three gunas.
rechaka (rechak)	Exhalation.
Rik (Rig) Veda	One of the four vedas (Rik, Yajur, Atharva, and Sama Vedas). The oldest yogic texts known.
rishi	A saint or seer.
Rudra	A name for Siva.
saanjali mudra	A mudra for humility. Gesture of offering one's own self. Saanjali means hallowed hands joined together as in prayer position.
sabda brahman	The mystical inner sound. The Omkara (Om), the Word of God.
sadguru	True guru (God) within.
sadhaka (sadhak)	A spiritual aspirant or seeker who practices sadhana.

sadhana	Spiritual practices or disciplines.
sadhus	One who practices sadhana—an ascetic.
sagarbh	To perform pranayama with the mantra Om with each count. E.g., Om one, Om two, Om three, and so on. This method of counting should equal about one second per count.
sahasrara chakra	The crown chakra.
sahita kumbhaka	Any intentional breath retention.
samana vayu	One of the five vital airs, or prana vayus. Samana vayu controls the digestive process in the body. It is a balancing force midway between prana and apana.
Sama Veda	One of the four vedas (Rik, Yajur, Atharva, and Sama Vedas). The oldest yogic texts known.
samadhi	The superconscious state in which one perceives or experiences the identity of the soul or spirit with the Infinite.
samprajnata samadhi	Same as savikalpa samadhi and sabija samadhi.
samskaras	Patterns of behavior. Can be subtle impressions from past lives carried forward through the karana sharira or seed body.
samyama	The practice of dharana, dhyana, and samadhi fused into one process. The yogi understands fully the truth of anything concentrated upon.
sananda samadhi	Meditation on bliss. A place of real peace and joy when one moves beyond the five elements and rests in sattva, without any rajas or tamas.
sanchalana	Moving to and fro, as in pawana sanchalana—a movement of breath consciousness.
sankalpa	Intention. One sets an intention before yoga practices.
sankhyā	Number. A term related to pranayama—the number of pranayama rounds you practice.
sankhyā paridrishti	Looking from the point of number, as in reducing the number of breaths taken in a minute.
sannyasi	A renunciate of attachments to worldly desires and ambitions. A monk or Swami.
santosha	Contentment. One of the niyamas.
sapta	Seven.
Sarasvati (Saraswati)	The Hindu goddess of creativity and fertility. Wife of Brahma.

sarvangasana	The shoulderstand pose.
satsang	Fellowship or gathering together to share in truth.
sattva (sattwa)	Truth. Reality. Purity. Harmony. One of the three gunas.
satya	Truthfulness. One of the yamas.
saucha	Purity and cleanliness. One of the niyamas.
savichara samadhi	A stage of samadhi in which knowledge of the subtle elements is acquired.
savikalpa samadhi	A stage of samadhi in which the mind still retains material impressions between subject and object.
savitarka samadhi	A stage of samadhi in which knowledge of the gross elements is acquired.
shakti	The creative power of the Universe. Feminine energy. A name for kundalini.
shakti-chalana (shaktichalani)	To churn or manipulate the shakti.
shaktipat diksha (deeksha)	The transferring of spiritual energy from one person to another.
shambhavi mudra	A mudra where the eyes are directed upward toward the space between the eyebrows.
shara-ripu (shat-ripu)	The six passions or negative tendencies: desire (kama), anger (krodha), greed (lobha), delusion (moha), egotistic tendencies (madha) and jealousy (matsarya).
sharira (sarira)	A body. A human being is considered to have three bodies; physical (sthula sharira), astral (sukshma or linga sharira), and causal (karana sharira).
shastras	Sacred books.
shunyaka (sunyaka, shunya)	Void, emptiness.
shwasa (shvasa)	Breath.
siddhasana (siddhasan)	Adepts or perfect pose.
siddhis	Powers that come when one attains perfection.
sirsasana (sirshasana)	Headstand pose.
sit karma	A cleansing exercise for the nasal passages in which water is put in the mouth and pushed out through the nasal passages.
sitali	A cooling pranayama in which the breath is drawn in through the tongue, which is rolled like a tube.
sitkari	A cooling pranayama in which the breath is drawn in through the mouth with the tip of the tongue placed behind the top front teeth.

Siva (Shiva)	The destroyer or remover. One of the gods of the Hindu holy trinity.
Siva Samhita	One of three classical texts on hatha yoga written by an unknown author. The other two classical texts are the Hatha Yoga Pradipika and the Gheranda Samhita.
soham (so ham)	A sacred mantra meaning "I am That." See hamsa.
soma chakra	The chakra between the third eye and crown chakras. This chakra is said to drip the soma nectar known as ambrosia or amrita.
stambh	Stop. Become stiff.
sthitaprajna	One who is established in wisdom.
sthula sharira	The physical body.
sukha purvak pranayama (sukh purvak)	Easy, comfortable pranayama. Alternate nostril breathing impling exertion without struggle.
sukshma	Subtle. A term related to pranayama—how subtle and slow you make the breath.
sukshma sharira	The astral body. Also called the linga sharira.
surya (soorya)	Sun.
surya (soorya) bheda (bhedi, bedha or bhedana) pranayama	A type of pranayama to pierce the sun nadi—breath inhaled through the right nostril.
surya prana mudra	A name for the mudra for psychic balance. Gesture of receiving the solar energy. Also known as trimurti mudra.
sushumna	The central nadi or energy channel within the spinal cord, through which the kundalini energy travels from the muladhara chakra to the sahasrara. It is said to open when there is balance between the ida and pingala nadis. Also known as Brahma's canal.
sutra neti	Cleaning the nasal passages with a cotton thread (sutra) drawn through the nose and out the mouth.
svadhisthana (swadhisthana) chakra	The sacral or pelvic chakra.
svadhyaya (swadhyaya)	Study of the self, the spirit, including the reading of scriptures. One of the niyamas.
swami	A name bestowed to one who takes vows of sannyasa. It means "he who is one with his 'Self' (swa)."
swastikasan	A seated meditation pose.
tadasana	Mountain pose. An upright standing pose of aligned posture.
tamas	Darkness. Inertia. One of the three gunas.

tanmatras	The qualities or essence (seed) of the elements; earth, water, fire, air, and ether.
Tantra or Tantrik yoga	A path of spiritual discipline in which kundalini shakti is the main deity worshipped through rites and rituals. There are three schools of Tantra: Kaula (external practices), Mishra (a mix of internal and external practices) and Samaya (internal practices). Kaula may be left-handed or right-handed. Left-handed means rituals may involve meat, fish, intoxicants, mudras, and sexual contact.
tapas	Self-discipline. One of the niyamas.
tattva (tattwa)	An element or substance. The essence or truth of it. There are five tattvas: vyoma tattva (or byoma, the ether element, also known as akasha), apa (or apas, water), prithivi (earth, also known as kshitri), teja (or tejas, fire, also known as agni), and vayu (or bayu, air).
Tat Tvam Asi	One of the mahavakyas, meaning "That Thou Art," from the Chandogya Upanishad of the Sama Veda. See "Atma Vichara Meditation" in chapter 7.
tratak	A kriya or cleansing technique for the eyes and third eye. Generally it is candle gazing, but one can gaze at the tip of the nose, the third eye, the Om symbol, or a mandala.
trikute	The third eye.
trimurti mudra	A mudra for psychic balance. There are three forms, like the triangle shape in this mudra—Brahma, Vishnu, Siva as the holy trinity; or the physical, astral, and causal bodies that we are. Also known as surya prana mudra.
udar	Stomach.
uddiyana bandha	One of the bandhas to draw the kundalini energy upward. A diaphragmatic lock.
udghata kriya	A general term for yoga practices to open the sushumna for the awakening kundalini lying dormant at the muladhara chakra.
ujjayi pranayama	A breathing technique with sound created by a slight closing of the glottis.
upamsu japa	Whispering or humming a mantra.
Upanishads	The sacred scriptures drawn from the Vedas. Upanishad means "to sit at the feet of the master," which symbolizes the student listening to the guru who shares these spiritual truths.
upasana	Worship.

uttam	Long.
uttanasana	A standing forward-bend pose.
vachika japa	Verbally repeating a mantra. Same as vaikhari japa.
vaikhari japa	Verbally repeating a mantra. Same as vachika japa.
vairagya	Dispassion or renunciation.
vajrasana	The thunderbolt pose. Kneeling and sitting on heels, with the spine very straight, so the kundalini can move up through the sushumna.
vajroli mudra (bajroli mudra)	A technique to control sexual urges.
vamana	To vomit or eject. It also means left, as in doing vamana nauli to the left side.
vasana aka basana	Subtle desire. Latent tendencies of our nature.
vayus	Vital airs or forms of prana.
Vedas	The oldest known scriptures on yoga, considered the original scriptures of ancient India.
vibhaga pranayama	Sectional breathing into the lower, middle, and upper lungs.
vichara	Deep inquiry or systematic thought. Intended to follow sadhana in order to gain knowledge that otherwise cannot be acquired.
vidya	Knowledge, science.
vijnana nadi	The carotid sinus—the nadi of nerve consciousness.
viparitakarani mudra (viparita karani mudra)	A mudra described in the Hatha Yoga Pradipika, similar to a half-shoulderstand.
virasan (virasana)	Hero pose.
Vishnu	The preserver. One of the gods of the Hindu holy trinity.
Vishnu mudra	A hand mudra used for closing the nostrils in pranayama.
vishuddhi (vishuddha) chakra	The throat chakra.
vritti (writti)	A wave or flow of movement. Can be the movement of the breath or the movement of thought, for example.
vyahriti	A statement or words, such as the sapta vyahritis, the seven great utterances.
vyoma chakra	A space where the nasal passage, pharynx, and trachea (or ida, pingala, and sushumna) meet. The space is closed by khechari mudra.

Yajur Veda	One of the four vedas (Rik, Yajur, Atharva, and Sama Vedas). The oldest yogic texts known.
yamas	Ethical restrictions or abstentions to establish self-control.
yantras	A mystical diagram said to hold occult powers.
yoga	To yoke, to join. Union with the Divine.
Yoga Mimamsa	A scientific journal of yoga initiated in 1924 by Swami Kuvalayananda and published at Kaivalyadhama.
yoga nidra	Yoga sleep. A state of pratyahara or sense withdrawal. One hour of yoga nidra is equal to four hours of regular sleep.
yoga sutras	The most famous aphorisms of Hinduism, written by Patanjali.
yogins	Those who practice yoga.
yogiraj	A title for yoga masters.
yogoda	One that bestows unity and harmony. Yogoda is formed from two Sanskrit words—yoga, which means "unity" and "harmony," and da, which means "one that bestows."

ENDNOTES

1 Harry Dickman was born Harijs Dīkmanis. Dīkmanis became westernized to Dickman and sometimes Dikman. Harijs became Harry and sometimes Hari (a name for Vishnu) to many of his yoga acquaintances. In his letters, he was called Harry or Hari Dickman, Harry or Hari Dikman.

2 Dr. Phil. Solveiga Krumina-Konkova, leading researcher, Institute of Philosophy and Sociology, University of Latvia, pers. comm. November 6, 2012.

3 Dr. Hari Dickman, San Rafael, CA. *Letter to Marion Kneẓacek*, September 16, 1978.

4 Dr. Hari Dickman, San Rafael, CA. *Letter to Marion Kneẓacek*, October 1, 1978.

5 Paramhansa Yogananda, Los Angeles, CA, *Letter to Dear Mr. Harry Dikman*, December 6, 1946.

6 *Skylight Journal of Yoga* 1, no. 2 (spring/summer 1974). Provided by SKY Foundation, Philadelphia.

7 See Nicolai Bachman, *The Language of Yoga* (Sounds True, 2004) 3.

8 The minutes of the Latvian Society of Parapsychology (earlier name for the Latvian Yoga Society) state the Harijs Dikmanis was born on July 5, 1895, in Tukums, Latvia (see LVVA, fund 2135, entry 1, case no. 1, pp. 41, 73). Solveiga Krumina-Konkova, author of "A Glimpse Into the History of Yoga Movement in Latvia," checked the report to Riga prefecture, dated April 25, 1939, which says "Chairman of the Board Harry Dikmanis was born in Tukums on July 5th 1895," and this report was signed by Hari. Hari told me he was born on July 4 and that his birthday was always celebrated in the United States with fireworks and parties for Independence Day. He states July 4, 1895, as his date of birth on a cassette recording made January 11, 1979.

9   Notes taken by author during studies with Hari Dickman, 1979, General p. 1

10 *Skylight Journal of Yoga* 1, no. 2 (spring/summer 1974). Provided by SKY Foundation, Philadelphia.

11 Shri Shrikrishna Shridhar Balshastri Phadke, Nasik City, Maharashtra State, Bharat, India, *Letter to Mr. Dickman*, February 5, 1965.

12 Arunachala Bhakta Bhagawal, Arunachala Ashrama, Bhagavan Sri Ramana Maharshi Centre, Bridgetown, Nova Scotia, Canada, *Letter to Dr. Harry Dickman*, December 10, 1976.

13 Dr. Henry A. Carns, President, College of Divine Metaphysics, Indianapolis, *Letter to Dr. Harry Dickman*, January 31, 1962.

14 Minutes of the Society "The Center of Yoga Sciences in Latvia" No. 1, April 25, 1935// LVVA, fund 2135, entry 1., case no. 3, p. 13., as shared by Solveiga Krumina-Konkova in her paper "A Glimpse Into the History of Yoga Movement in Latvia," 13.

15 Dr. Hari Dickman, San Rafael, CA, *Letter to Marion Knezacek*, July 12, 1977.

16 Dzintar Vilnis Korns, Latvia, *Email to Marion McConnell*, July 8, 2013.

17 Dr. Hari Dickman, San Rafael, CA, *Cassette recording of Dr. Hari Dickman*, January 11, 1979.

18 Dr. Hari Dickman, San Rafael, CA, *Letter to Marion Knezacek*, December 28, 1977.

19 Dr. Hari Dickman, San Rafael, CA, *Letter to Marion Knezacek*, July 23, 1977.

20 Swami Yogananda Los Angeles, CA, *Letter to Harry Dikman*, October 17, 1934.

21 See N. Ananthanarayanan, *From Man to God Man: the Inspiring Life-Story of Swami Sivananda* (Indian Publishing Trading Corp., 1970) 168.

22 See http://en.wikipedia.org/wiki/Displaced_persons_camp.

23 Paramhansa Yogananda, Los Angeles, CA, *Letter to Mr. Harry Dikman*, January 31, 1946.

24 Paramhansa Yogananda, Los Angeles, CA, *Letter to Harry Dikman*, May 8, 1947.

25 Paramhansa Yogananda, Los Angeles, CA, *Letter to Harry Dikman*, August 3, 1946. Also letter dated December 1, 1948.

26 Paramhansa Yogananda, Los Angeles, CA, *Letter to Harry Dikman*, April 20, 1946.

27 Paramhansa Yogananda, Los Angeles, CA, *Letter to Harry Dikman*, August 3, 1946.

28 Paramhansa Yogananda, Los Angeles, CA, *Letter to Harry Dikman*, December 6, 1946.

29 See http://en.wikipedia.org/wiki/Displaced_persons_camp.

30 Paramhansa Yogananda, Los Angeles, CA, *Letter to Mr. Harry Dikman*, December 1, 1948.

31 Faye Wright, Self-Realization Fellowship, Los Angeles, CA, *Letter to Mr. Harry Dikman*, July 11, 1947.

32 Paramhansa Yogananda, *Letter to Mr. Harry Dikman*, September 22, 1947.

33 Paramhansa Yogananda, Los Angeles, CA, *Letter to Harry Dickman*, February 5, 1952.

34 Paramhansa Yogananda, Los Angeles, CA, *Letter to Harry Dickman*, March 5, 1952.

35 Swami Sivananda, Rishikesh, *Letter of Reference for Harry Dickman*, February 18, 1954.

36 Yogiraj Sri Harry Dickman, *Yoga Chakravarty, Sri Swami Sivananda* (Rishikesh, India: Yoga-Vedanta Forest University, 1958), back cover.

37 Dickman, *Yoga Chakravarty Sri Swami Sivananda*, 11–12.

38 Dickman, *Yoga Chakravarty Sri Swami Sivananda*, 15–16.

39 Dickman, *Yoga Chakravarty Sri Swami Sivananda*, 18–19.

40 Dickman, *Yoga Chakravarty Sri Swami Sivananda*, 26.

41 Swami Shivapremananda, Belgium, *Letter to Revered Hari Maharaj*, December 10, 1976.

42 Swami Shivapremananda, Montevideo, Uruguay, *Letter to Revered Hari Maharaj*, February 6, 1976.

43 Swami Sivananda, Rishikesh, India, *Letter of Reference for YogiRaj Harry Dickman*, February 18, 1954.

44   Swami Venkatesananda, *The USA and Canada Revisited, 1971,* Swami Venkatesananda reports #25, Venkatesalibrary; record drawn from author's memorial notes, p. 9.

45   Swami Venkatesananda, *The USA and Canada Revisited, 1971,* Swami Venkatesananda reports #25, Venkatesalibrary; record drawn from author's memorial notes, p. 11.

46   Swami Sivananda, Rishikesh, *Copy of Letter of Reference for Harry Dickman,* addressed to Dr. Sri Robert Ernst Dickhoff, February 29, 1952.

47   Swami Sivananda, Rishikesh, *Letter of Reference for Harry Dickman,* February 28, 1954.

48   See N. Ananthanarayanan, *From Man to God-Man: The Inspiring Life-Story of Swami Sivananda,* (n.p.: Indian Publishing Trading Corp., 1970), 167–69.

49   Dr. Hari Dickman, San Rafael, CA, *Letter to Marion Kneẓacek,* December 28, 1977.

50   Dr. Phil. Solveiga Krumina-Konkova, leading researcher, Institute of Philosophy and Sociology, University of Latvia, "A Glimpse into the History of Yoga Movement in Latvia" (July 2014), 16–17, n. 90.

51   "Maharshi's Foreign Bhaktas," *Sunday Times* (city unknown), August 13, 1933.

52   A Tamil text that Hari had, discussing the disciples of Sri Bhagavan Ramana Maharshi, title and publisher unknown; this page was copied from the book by the author during her studies with Hari, to remember how Hari was appreciated by his teachers.

53   Niranjanananda Swamy Sarvadhikari, *Letter to Sri Harry Dickman,* June 8, 1951, Tiruvannamalai.

54   Swami Niranjanananda, Sevayatan-Ashram, Satsangha Mission, West Bengal, India, *Letter to Dear Dr. Dickman,* May 16, 1975.

55   Mahant Dig Vijai Nath, Gorakhnath Temple, Gorakhpur, India, *Letter to Dear brother,* August 30, 1961.

56   Brahmachari Animananda (Dharmacharya), Yogoda Sat-Sanga Society of India, Self-Realization Fellowship, Ranchi, India, *Letter to Dr. Harry Dikman.* Dec 9, 1952.

57   The author of this statement is unknown, but the statement is copied widely.

58   Swami Shivananda Saraswati of Assam, *Letter to Hari ... date unknown ... only pages 3–5 found ... no other info.*

59   *Yoga Mimamsa* 3 (April 1928), Kaivalyadhama Institute for Scientific Research, Lonavla, Bombay, India (founded by Swami Kuvalayananda), 138.

60   *Yoga Mimamsa* 3 (April 1928), 138–39.

61   Srimat Kuvalayananda, *Yoga Mimamsa Vol. III,* Vijaya Press, 1928. Poona, p. 138.

62   *Yoga Mimamsa* 3 (April 1928), 140.

63   *Yoga Mimamsa* 3 (April 1928), 141–42.

64   *Yoga Mimamsa* 3 (April 1928), 142–43.

65   *Yoga Mimamsa* 3 (April 1928), 144.

66   Swami Kuvalayananda, Bombay, India, *Letter to Harry Dikman,* September 11, 1930.

67   Swami Kuvalayananda, Bombay, India, *Letter to Harry Dikman,* November 2, 1933.

68   Swami Vishnudevananda, *Commentary on The Hatha Yoga Pradipika* (New York: Om Lotus Publishing: 1997) 106.

69   Swami Vishnudevananda, *Commentary on The Hatha Yoga Pradipika,* 105.

70   Swami Vishnudevananda, *Commentary on The Hatha Yoga Pradipika,* 106.

71   Swami Shivananda Saraswati of Assam, L268, Netaji Colony, Calcutta 36, Bharat, India. *Letter to My Dear Harri Dickman,* April 16, 1959.

72   T.K. Sundaresa Iyer, Tiruvannamali, India, *Letter to Hari Dickman,* September 18, 1931.

73   Paramhansa Yogananda, Los Angeles, CA, *Letter to Mr. Harry Dikman,* June 2, 1946.

74   Paramhansa Yogananda, Los Angeles, CA, *Letter to Mr. Harry Dickman,* June 26, 1946.

75   Paramhansa Yogananda, Los Angeles, CA, *Letter to Mr. Harry Dickman,* December 6, 1946.

76   Sri Swami Sivananda Saraswati, *Practical Lessons in Yoga,* 5th ed. (Rishikesh, India: Divine Life Society, 1971), Tehri-Garhwal, 79.

77   Sri Swami Sivananda, *Hatha Yoga (Illustrated)* (Rishikesh, India: Divine Life Society, 1939) 4, 10, 13, 46, 63, 79, and 81.

78   Notes taken by author during studies with Hari Dickman, 1979, Asanas p. 3–4.

79   Dr. Hari Dickman, San Rafael, CA, *Letter to Marion Kneẕacek,* July 23, 1977.

80   See Phil Liney, "Discussion on Pranayama—'Why Exhale Bottom-to-Top?,' " *International Light Magazine,* International Yoga Teachers' Association, Australia (July–September 2011), 28–29, http://icyer.com/documents/phil_pranayama.pdf.

81   Srimat Kuvalayananda, "Ujjayi Pranayama Explained," *Yoga-Mimansa* 4, no. 1 (July 1930) 68–69.

82   Unknown Author, for Manager at Yoga-Mimamsa Office, Kaivalyadhama, Bombay, India, *Letter to Mr. Harry Dickman,* February 22, 1958.

83   Swami Kuvalayananda, *Pranayama,* 6th ed. (Science Press for The Sky Foundation, 1978), 54.

84   B. K. S. Iyengar, *Light on Yoga,* Mandala edition (George Allen & Unwin, 1976), 441.

85   Swami Sivananda, Divine Life Society, Rishikesh, India. *Letter to Sri Harry Dikman,* January 14, 1948.

86   Swami Sevananda, Yogoda Sat-Sanga, Self-Realization Fellowship, Shyamacharin Mission, Karar Ashram, Puri India, *Letter to Brother Dikman,* June 11, 1937.

87   Francis Yeats-Brown, *Lives of a Bengal Lancer* (Viking, 1930), possibly referring to chap. 18, "The Temple of the Undistracted Mind."

88   Swami Vishnu Tirth, Narain Kuti, Sanyas Ashram, Dewas, India. *Letter to Shri Dr. Hari Dickman,* May 24, 1967.

89   Author of this letter unknown; loose page.

90   Vasant G. Rele, *The Mysterious Kundalini,* (Bombay, India: D. B. Taraporevala Sons, 1983), 5–6, 9.

91   Vipin Raheja, on behalf of Yoga Niketan, email to author September 25, 2015.

92   Swami Yogeshwaranand Saraswati, Yogniketan Swaryogashram, Dehradun, U.P. India, *Letter to Dr. Harry Dickman,* undated but clearly prior to February 1963.

93   Swami Yogeshwaranand Saraswati, Gangotri, India, *Letter to Dear Harry,* September 19, 1967.

94   Yogeshwaranand Paramahansa, *First Steps to Higher Yoga,* 4th ed. (New Delhi: Yoga Niketan Trust, 2001).

95   Swami Yogeshwaranand Saraswati, Yogniketan Swaryogashram, Dehradun, U.P. India, *Letter to Dr. Harry Dickman,* undated, p 1.

96   Swami Yogeshwaranand Saraswati, Yogniketan Swaryogashram, Dehradun, U.P. India, *Letter to Dr. Harry Dickman,* undated, p 1.

97   Swami Yogeshwaranand Saraswati, *Letter to Dr. Harry Dickman,* undated, Yogniketan Swaryo-gashram, Dehradun, U.P. India, Yogniketan Swaryogashram, Dehradun, U.P. India, *Letter to Dr. Harry Dickman,* undated, p. 3.

98   Swami Yogeshwaranand Saraswati, Yogniketan Swaryogashram, Dehradun, U.P. India, *Letter to Dr. Harry Dickman,* undated, pp. 1–3.

99   Swami Yogeshwaranand Saraswati, *Letter to Priya Atman,* Oct 15, 1965, Yogniketan, Uttar-Kashi, Himalaya, India.

100   Swami Yogeshwaranand Saraswati, Yogniketan Swaryogashram, Dehradun, U.P. India, *Letter to Dr. Harry Dickman,* undated, p. 4.

101   Swami Yogeshwaranand Saraswati, Yogniketan Swaryogashram, Dehradun, U.P. India, *Letter to Dr. Harry Dickman,* undated, p. 4.

102   Swami Yogeshwaranand Saraswati, Yogniketan Swaryogashram, Dehradun, U.P. India, *Letter to Dr. Harry Dickman*, undated, p. 24.

103   Swami Shivananda Saraswati of Assam, Shivananda Yogasrarm, 471 Netaji Colony, Calcutta, 50, India, *Letter to My dear Dickman*, April 4, 1966, p. 6.

104   See Swami Vishnudevananda, *Commentary on The Hatha Yoga Pradipika*, 51.

105   Swami Yogeshwaranand Saraswati, Yogniketan Swaryogashram, Dehradun, U.P., India, *Letter to Dr. Harry Dickman*, undated, p. 5–6.

106   Swami Kuvalayananda, *Pranayama*, 28–29.

107   Swami Vishnu Tirth Maharaj, Narain Kuti, Sanyas Ashram, Dewas, India. *Letter to Dear Shri Hari Dickman*, Jan 29, 1958.

108   Swami Vishnudevananda, *Letter to Sri Harry Dikman, (Yogi Ruj)*, August 16, 1955.

109   Swami Vishnudevananda, Rishikesh, India, *Letter to Sri Yogi Raj Haridickman, NY*, undated, 1950s.

110   Swami Sivananda, Rishikesh, India, *Letter to Yogiraj Sri Harry Dikman*, September 21, 1949.

111   Vishnu Tirth, Narayan Kuti, Sanyas Ashram, Dewas, India, *Letter to Shri Hari Dickman*, May 16, 1966.

112   Swami Sivananda, Rishikesh, India, *Letter to Sri Harry Dikman, Location unknown*, October 3, 1947.

113   Hari Dickman, San Rafael, *Letter to Marion Kneẓacek*, July 23, 1977.

114   Swami Vishnudevananda, Yoga Vedanta Forest Academy, Rishikesh, India, *Letter to Sri Harry Dikman*, August 16, 1955.

115   Notes taken by author during studies with Hari Dickman, 1979, Pranayama, p. 1.

116   Swami Yogeshwaranand Saraswati, Yogniketan Swaryogashram, Dehradun, U.P., India, *Letter to Dr. Harry Dickman*, undated, p. 22.

117   Sri Swami Sivananda, *The Science of Pranayama*, 67.

118   Swami Suryadevananda, Florida, USA, email to Marion McConnell, dated April 29, 2015.

119   Swami Yogeshwaranand Saraswati, Yogniketan Swaryogashram, Dehradun, U.P., India, *Letter to Dr. Harry Dickman*, undated, p. 14.

120   Swami Vishnudevananda, *Commentary on The Hatha Yoga Pradipika*, 51.

121   Swami Vishnudevananda, *Commentary on The Hatha Yoga Pradipika*, 5.

122   Dr. Hari Dickman, San Rafael, CA, *Letter to Priya Bhanumati*, September 16, 1978.

123   B. K. S. Iyengar, *Light on Yoga*, 443.

124   Swami Vishnudevananda, *Commentary on The Hatha Yoga Pradipika*, 77.

125   Swami Kuvalayananda, *Pranayama*, 52.

126   Swami Kuvalayananda, *Pranayama*, 52.

127   Swami Yogeshwaranand Saraswati, *Letter to Dr. Harry Dickman*, undated, Yogniketan Swaryogashram, Dehradun, U.P., India, undated, pp. 7–8.

128   Swami Yogeshwaranand Saraswati, *Letter to Dr. Harry Dickman*, November 19, 1965, Yog Niketan, Swarg Ashrama, Rishikesh, India.

129   Notes taken by author during studies with Hari Dickman, 1979, Pranayama, p. 1.

130   Notes taken by author during studies with Hari Dickman, 1979, Pranayama, p. 1b.

131   Swami Sivananda, Rishikesh, India, *Letter to Sri Harry Dickman*, March 21, 1955.

132   Swami Yogeshwaranand Saraswati, Yogniketan Swaryogashram, Dehradun, U.P., India, *Letter to Dr. Harry Dickman*, undated, p. 7.

133   *The Hatha Yoga Pradipika, Commentary Jyotsna of Brahmananda* (Adyar, Madras, India: Adyar Library and Research Centre, The Theosophical Society, 1975), 34–35 (2:67).

134 Notes taken by author during studies with Hari Dickman, 1979, *Pranayama*, p. 1.

135 Swami Vishnudevananda, Yoga Vedanta Forest Academy, Rishikesh, India, *Letter to Sri Harry Dikman*, August 16, 1955.

136 *The Hatha Yoga Pradipika, Commentary Jyotsna of Brahmananda*, 34 (2:65).

137 Yogeshwaranand Paramahansa, *First Steps to Higher Yoga*, 324.

138 Swami Yogeshwaranand Saraswati, Yogniketan Swaryogashram, Dehradun, U.P. India, *Letter to Dr. Harry Dickman*, undated, pp. 1011.

139 *The Hatha Yoga Pradipika, Commentary Jyotsna of Brahmananda*, 25 (2:14–17).

140 Swami Shivapremananda, Centro Sivananda de Yoga Vedanta, Casilla 16062, Santiago, Chile-9, *Letter to Hari Maharaj*, January 11, 1978.

141 Swami Vishnudevananda, Rishikesh, India, *Letter to Sri Yogiraj Harry Dikman*, Germany, August 13, 1951.

142 *The Hatha Yoga Pradipika, Commentary Jyotsna of Brahmananda*, 33 (2:58).

143 *The Hatha Yoga Pradipika, Commentary Jyotsna of Brahmananda*, 32 (2:54–56).

144 Swami Kuvalayananda, *Pranayama*, 92–93.

145 Swami Yogeshwaranand Saraswati, Yogniketan Swaryogashram, Dehradun, U.P., India, *Letter to Dr. Harry Dickman*, undated, p. 12.

146 Swami Vishnudevananda, *Commentary on Hatha Yoga Pradipika*, 83.

147 Notes taken by author during studies with Hari Dickman, 1979, *Pranayama*, p. 1.

148 Swami Kuvalayananda, *Pranayama*, 98.

149 Swami Sivananda, Ananda Kutir, Rishikesh, India, *Letter to Sm. Hari Dickman*, February 2, 1946.

150 Yogamaharishi Dr. Swami Gitananda Giri Guru Maharaj, *Pranayama: The Science of Vital Control and Description of 99 Yoga Pranayama Techniques*, #42 and #43, date unknown.

151 Swami Satchidananda, Sivananda Thapovanam, Trincomalee, Ceylon, *Letter to Sri Harry Dickman*, Nov 23, 1953.

152 Swami Satchidananda, Sivananda Thapovanam, Trincomalee, Ceylon, *Letter to Sri Harry Dickman*, Nov 23, 1953.

153 Swami Yogeshwaranand Saraswati, Yogniketan Swaryogashram, Dehradun, U.P., India, *Letter to Dr. Harry Dickman*, undated, p. 8.

154 Swami Sivananda of Rishikesh, The Divine Life Society, Rishikesh, India, *Letter to Sri Harry Dikman*, August 3, 1947.

155 Rai Bahadur Srisa Chandra Vasu, *Commentary on the Gheranda Samhita*, 2nd ed. (New Delhi: Munshiram Manoharlal 1975), 49.

156 Dr. Minott W. Lewis, SRF, Encinitas, CA, *Letter to Mr. Harry Dikman*, September 25, 1953.

157 Thomas Ashley-Farrand, *Chakra Mantras* (San Francisco: Red Wheel/Weiser, 2006) 11.

158 Swami Sivananda, *Letter to Sm. Hari Dickman*, February 2, 1946, Ananda Kutir, Rishikesh.

159 William Harold Phillips, personal communication, "Comparison of Pranayama Techniques between Yogamaharishi Dr. Swami Gitananda Giri and Shyam Sundar Goswami," July 2013.

160 Swami Kuvalayananda, *Pranayama*, 102.

161 Swami Kuvalayananda, *Pranayama*, 28.

162 Rai Bahadur Srisa Chandra Vasu, *Commentary on The Siva Samhita*, 59.

163 Swami Sivananda, Ananda Kutir, Rishikesh, *Letter to Sm. Hari Dickman*, February 2, 1946.

164 Yogeshwaranand Paramahansa, *First Steps to Higher Yoga*, 322–23.

165 Swami Yogeshwaranand Saraswati, Yogniketan Swaryogashram, Dehradun, U.P., India, *Letter to Dr. Harry Dickman*, undated p. 9.

166 S. S. Goswami, Goswami Institute, Stockholm K, *Letter to Dr. Harry Dickman*, June 26, 1962.

167 Swami Vishnudevananda, *Commentary on The Hatha Yoga Pradipika*, 210.

168 Yogamaharishi Dr. Swami Gitananda Giri Guru Maharaj, *Pranayama: The Science of Vital Control and Description of 99 Yoga Pranayama Techniques*, *#75 and #76*, date unknown.

169 Swami Kuvalayananda, *Pranayama*, 104–5.

170 Swami Vishnudevananda, Rishikesh, India, *Letter to Sri Yogiraj Harry Dikman*, August 13, 1951.

171 Swami Kuvalayananda, *Pranayama*, 104.

172 Yogamaharishi Dr. Swami Gitananda Giri Guru Maharaj, *Pranayama: The Science of Vital Control and Description of 99 Yoga Pranayama Techniques*, *#75*, date unknown.

173 Notes taken by author during studies with Hari Dickman, 1979, Pranayama, p. 1b.

174 Swami Yogeshwaranand Saraswati, Yogniketan Swaryogashram, Dehradun, U.P., India, *Letter to Dr. Harry Dickman*, undated, p 13.

175 Swami Yogeshwaranand Saraswati, Yogniketan Swaryogashram, Dehradun, U.P., India, *Letter to Dr. Harry Dickman*, undated, unnumbered page.

176 Yogeshwaranand Paramahansa, *First Steps to Higher Yoga*, 340.

177 Swami Yogeshwaranand Saraswati, Yogniketan Swaryogashram, Dehradun, U.P., India, *Letter to Dr. Harry Dickman*, undated, pp. 13–14.

178 Yogeshwaranand Paramahansa, *First Steps to Higher Yoga*, 330.

179 Swami Yogeshwaranand Saraswati, Yog Niketan Swarg Ashrama, Rishikesh, Dehradun, India. *Letter to Dear Harry Dickman*, November 19, 1965.

180 Swami Yogeshwaranand Saraswati, Yogniketan Swargashram, Rishikesh, Dehradun, India, *Letter to Dear Dr. Harry Dickman*, January 1966.

181 Swami Yogeshwaranand Saraswati, Yogniketan Swaryogashram, Dehradun, U.P. India, *Letter to Dr. Harry Dickman*, undated, p. 16.

182 Korns, developer of website on History of Latvian Yoga Society, tradition.lf.lv/ljb.htm, February 24, 2007.

183 Rele, *The Mysterious Kundalini*, xxii–xxvi.

184 Rele, *The Mysterious Kundalini*, 5–6.

185 Faye Wright, Self-Realization Fellowship, Los Angeles, CA, *Letter to Mr. Harry Dikman*, July 11, 1947, p. 1.

186 William Harold Phillips, *Comparison of Pranayama Techniques between Yogamaharishi Dr. Swami Gitananda Giri and Swami Yogeshwaranand*, July 2013, pers. comm.

187 Brother Bhaktananda, Self-Realization Fellowship, Los Angeles, CA, *Letter to Dr. Harry Dickman*, June 28, 1967, p. 1.

188 Paramhansa Yogananda, Self-Realization Fellowship, Mount Washington Estates, Los Angeles, CA, *Letter to Mr Harry Dikman in Latvia*, February 10, 1939.

189 Swami Sivananda of Rishikesh, Divine Life Society, Rishikesh, India, *Letter to Sri Harry Dikman in Germany*, August 27, 1946.

190 Yogeshwaranand Paramahansa, *First Steps to Higher Yoga*, 338.

191 Swami Yogeshwaranand Saraswati, Yogniketan Swaryogashram, Dehradun, U.P., India, *Letter to Dr. Harry Dickman*, undated, unnumbered page.

192 Vasant G. Rele, *The Mysterious Kundalini*, xxii–xxvi.

193 Swami Yogeshwaranand Saraswati, Yogniketan Swaryogashram, Dehradun, U.P., India, *Letter to Dr. Harry Dickman*, undated, p. 25.

194 *The Upanishads*, trans. Juan Mascaró (London: Penguin Books, 1965), 83.

195 Paramhansa Yogananda, Self-Realization Fellowship, Los Angeles 31, California, USA, *Letter to Mr. Harry Dikman in Germany*, December 6, 1946.

196   Swami Sivananda Saraswati, Ananda Kutir, Rishikesh, Himalayas, India, *Letter to Sri Harry Dikman,* November 24, 1950.

197   *The Upanishads,* 83.

198   Swami Yogeshwaranand Saraswati, *Letter to Dr. Harry Dickman,* April 16, 1965, Yogniketan Swargashram, Rishikesh, Dehradun, U.P., India.

199   Swami Sivananda, Ananda Kutir, Rishikesh, Himalayas, India, *Letter to Sri Harry Dikman,* November 24, 1950.

200   Dr. Swami Gitananda, *Mudras* (Lawspet, Pondicherry, India: Satya Press, Ananda Ashram, undated), 18–20. Additional information for this section is from communications with Yogacharya Dr. Ananda Balayogi Bhavanani, son of Dr. Swami Gitananda and Chairman of the International Centre for Yoga Education and Research at Ananda Ashram, Pondicherry, India (www.icyer.com) and also Chairman of Yoganjali Natyalayam (www.rishiculture.org).

201   Dr. Swami Gitananda, *Mudras,* 18–20. Additional information for this section is from communications with Yogacharya Dr. Ananda Balayogi Bhavanani, son of Dr. Swami Gitananda and Chairman of the International Centre for Yoga Education and Research at Ananda Ashram, Pondicherry, India (www.icyer.com) and also Chairman of Yoganjali Natyalayam (www.rishiculture.org).

202   Swami Yogeshwaranand Saraswati, Yogniketan Swaryogashram, Dehradun, U.P., India, *Letter to Dr. Harry Dickman,* undated, p. 21.

203   Swami Yogeshwaranand Saraswati, Yogniketan Swaryogashram, Dehradun, U.P., India, *Letter to Dr. Harry Dickman,* undated, p. 26.

204   Swami Vishnudevananda, *Commentary on Hatha Yoga Pradipika,* 85 and 209.

205   Swami Sivananda of Rishikesh, The Divine Life Society, Rishikesh, India, *Letter to Sri Harry Dickman,* March 21, 1955.

206   *The Hatha Yoga Pradipika, Commentary Jyotsna of Brahmananda,* 36 (2:75).

207   Swami Yogeshwaranand Saraswati, Yogniketan Swaryogashram, Dehradun, U.P. India, *Letter to Dr. Harry Dickman,* undated, p 11.

208   Ganga White, *Yoga Beyond Belief, Insights to Awaken and Deepen Your Practice* (Berkeley, CA: North Atlantic Books), 63.

209   Swami Vishnudevananda, *Commentary on Hatha Yoga Pradipika,* 105 (3:6–7).

210   Swami Vishnudevananda, *Commentary on Hatha Yoga Pradipika,* 101.

211   Notes taken by author during studies with Hari, 1979. General, page 3b.

212   Swami Vishnudevananda, *Commentary on Hatha Yoga Pradipika,* 111.

213   Notes taken by author during studies with Hari Dickman, 1979, General, p. 18b.

214   Swami Vishnudevananda, *Commentary on Hatha Yoga Pradipika,* 110 (3:12).

215   Swami Narayanananda, Sri Narayana Niwas, Dehradun Road, Rishikesh, India, *Letter to Blessed Immortal Self,* January 5, 1960.

216   Swami Narayanananda, Jagrati-Niketan, RLY: Road, Rishikesh, India, *Letter to Blessed Immortal Self,* March 11, 1955.

217   Notes taken by author during studies with Hari Dickman, 1979, General, p. 18b.

218   Madhavananda, Bombay, India, *Letter to Blessed Self, Dr. Harry Dickman,* May 9, 1969.

219   Notes taken by author during studies with Hari Dickman, 1979, General, p. 19.

220   Swami Sivananda, Divine Life Society, Rishikesh, India, *Letter to Sri Harry Dikman,* January 14, 1948.

221   Notes taken by author during studies with Hari Dickman, 1979, General, p. 19.

222   Swami Narayanananda, Jagrati-Niketan, RLY: Road, Rishikesh, India, *Letter to Blessed Immortal Self,* June 30, 1955.

223 Swami Narayanananda, Jagrati-Niketan, RLY: Road, Rishikesh, India, *Letter to Blessed Immortal Self*, March 11, 1955.

224 Swami Vishnudevananda, *Commentary on Hatha Yoga Pradipika*, 113–14 (3:22–24).

225 Notes taken by author during studies with Hari Dickman, 1979, General p. 19.

226 Swami Vishnudevananda, *Commentary on Hatha Yoga Pradipika*, 115–16 (3:27–29).

227 Swami Vishnu Tirth, Rishikesh, District Dheradun, Uttar Pradesh, India, *Letter to Shri Dr. Hari Dickman*, March 6, 1967.

228 Swami Vishnudevananda, *Commentary on Hatha Yoga Pradipika*, 114 (3:25).

229 Notes taken by author during studies with Hari Dickman, 1979, General, p. 19.

230 Thomas Ashley-Farrand, *Chakra Mantras*, 165.

231 Swami Vishnudevananda, *Commentary on Hatha Yoga Pradipika*, 123 (3:49).

232 Swami Vishnudevananda, *Commentary on Hatha Yoga Pradipika*, 119 (3:37).

233 Swami Vishnudevananda, *Commentary on Hatha Yoga Pradipika*, 105 (3:6).

234 Madhavananda, Bombay, India, *Letter to Blessed Self, Dr. Harry Dickman*, May 9, 1969.

235 Madhavananda, Bombay, India, *Letter to Blessed Self, Dr. Harry Dickman*, February 16, 1969.

236 Notes taken by author during studies with Hari Dickman, 1979: Mudras, p. 3, General, p. 4.

237 Swami Vishnudevananda, Divine Life Society, Rishikesh, India, *Letter to Sri Yogi Raj Haridickman*, undated, 1950s.

238 Madhavananda, Bombay, India, *Letter to Blessed Self, Dr. Harry Dickman*, May 9, 1969.

239 Swami Sivananda of Rishikesh, *Letter to Yogiraj Sri Harry Dikman*, November 24, 1950.

240 Swami Vishnudevananda, *Commentary on Hatha Yoga Pradipika*, 141 (3:112).

241 Personal notes of author from teacher training course with Swami Vishnudevananda, 1978, and notes taken by author during studies with Hari Dickman, 1979, Mudras, p. 5.

242 Sir John Woodroffe, KT (a.k.a. Arthur Avalon), *The Serpent Power* (New York: Dover, 1974), 207.

243 Sir John Woodroffe, *The Serpent Power*, 207.

244 Swami Venkatesananda, c/o PMG, Mauritius, Indian Ocean, *Letter to Bhagavan, Dr. H. Dickman*, July 7, 1976.

245 Madhavananda, Bombay, India, *Letter to Blessed Self, Dr. Harry Dickman*, February 16, 1969.

246 Madhavananda, Bombay, India, *Letter to Blessed Self, Dr. Harry Dickman*, May 9, 1969.

247 Swami Vishnudevananda, Yoga Vedanta Forest University, Rishikesh, India, *Letter to Sri Harry Dikman*, August 16, 1955.

248 Swami Shivananda Saraswati of Assam, Shivananda Math, Umachal Hill, Kamakhya, Gauhati, Assam, India, *Letter to dear Dickman*, June 25, 1959.

249 Swami Sivananda of Rishikesh, Divine Life Society, Rishikesh, *Letter to Hari Om*, January 16, 1947.

250 Madhavananda, Bombay, India, *Letter to Blessed Self, Dr. Harry Dickman*, May 9, 1969.

251 Swami Venkatesananda, c/o PMG, Mauritius, Indian Ocean, *Letter to Bhagavan, Dr. H. Dickman*, Dec 6, 1971.

252 Swami Venkatesananda, c/o PMG, Mauritius, Indian Ocean, *Letter to Bhagavan, Dr. H. D ickman*, July 7, 1976.

253 Swami Yogeshwaranand Saraswati, *Letter to My dear Harry Dickman*, Yogniketan Swaryogashram, Dehradun, U.P., India, March 3, 1963.

254 Swami Yogeshwaranand Saraswati, *Letter to My dear Harry Dickman*, Yogniketan Swaryogashram, Dehradun, U.P., India, March 3, 1963.

255 Swami Yogeshwaranand Saraswati, *Letter to Mr. Harry Dickman*, Yogniketan Swaryogashram, Dehradun, U.P., India, December 12, 1963.

256   Swami Kriyananda, 220-16th Ave, San Francisco, Calif, *Letter to Mr. Dickman*, undated.

257   Swami Vishnudevananda, *Commentary on Hatha Yoga Pradipika*, 147 (3:125).

258   Swami Vishnudevananda, *Commentary on Hatha Yoga Pradipika*, 147 (4:35).

259   Swami Sivananda of Rishikesh, The Divine Life Society, Rishikesh, India, *Letter to Sri Harry Dickman*, April 7, 1948.

260   Swami Yogeshwaranand Saraswati, *Letter to My dear Harry Dickman*, Yogniketan Swaryogash-ram, Dehradun, U.P., India, March 31, 1963.

261   Swami Narayanananda, no return address, *Letter to Blessed Immortal Self*, undated, possibly in the 1960s.

262   Madhavananda, Bombay, India, *Letter to Blessed Self, Dr. Harry Dickman*, February 16, 1969.

263   Mudra information provided by Dr. Francisco Luid (Swami Tirthananda Saraswati), Centro de Yoga Satyananda Zaragoza, Madrid, and Yogacharya Dr. Ananda Balayogi Bhavanani, ICYER, Pondicherry, India.

264   Mudra information provided by Dr. Francisco Luid (Swami Tirthananda Saraswati), Centro de Yoga Satyananda Zaragoza, Madrid, and Yogacharya Dr. Ananda Balayogi Bhavanani, ICYER, Pondicherry, India.

265   Mudra information provided by Dr. Francisco Luid (Swami Tirthananda Saraswati), Centro de Yoga Satyananda Zaragoza, Madrid, and Yogacharya Dr. Ananda Balayogi Bhavanani, ICYER, Pondicherry, India.

266   Notes taken by author during time studying with Hari Dickman, 1979, Questions, p. 1.

267   Swami Shivananda Saraswati of Assam, L268 Netaji Colony, Calcutta 36, Bharat. *Letter to My Dear Harri Dickman*, April 16, 1959.

268   Swami Sivananda of Rishikesh, The Divine Life Society, Rishikesh, India, *Letter to Sri Harry Dickman*, March 21, 1955.

269   *The Upanishads*, 114

270   John 1:1 (Revised Standard Version).

271   *The Upanishads*, 83, Mandukya Upanishad.

272   Swami Thapovanam, Uttarkashi, India. *Letter to Dear and Devoted Sri H. Dickman!*, Jan 18, 1950. Reproduced courtesy of Central Chinmaya Mission Trust.

273   Swami Thapovanam, Uttarkashi, Tehri-Garhwal, (U.P.) Himalayas, *Letter to Dear Devoted Sree Dickman!* November 1, 1949. Reproduced courtesy of Central Chinmaya Mission Trust.

274   Swami Thapovanam, Uttarkashi, India, *Letter to Dear and Devoted Sri H. Dickman!*, January 18, 1950. Reproduced courtesy of Central Chinmaya Mission Trust.

275   Notes taken by author during time studying with Hari Dickman, 1979, General, p. 6.

276   Notes taken by author during time studying with Hari Dickman, 1979, Pratyahara, p. 1.

277   Swami Sivananda of Rishikesh, The Divine Life Society, Rishikesh, India, *Letter to Sri Harry Dickman*, March 21, 1955.

278   Swami Vishnudevananda, Divine Life Society, Rishikesh, India, *Letter to Sri YogiRaj Hari Dickman*, undated.

279   Swami Sivananda, The Divine Life Society, Rishikesh, India, *Letter to Sri Harry Dickman*, March 21, 1955.

280   Swami Sivananda, Ananda Kutir, Sivananda-nagar post, Dehra Dun, India, *Letter to Yogiraj Sri Harry Dickman in New York*. January 28, 1954.

281   Notes taken by author during time studying with Hari Dickman, 1979, Concentration, pp. 1–4.

282   Notes taken by author during time studying with Hari Dickman, 1979, General, p. 9b.

283   Swami Yogeshwaranand, Yog Nikitan, Uttarkashi, Himalaya, India, *Letter to Priya Atman*, October 15, 1965.

284 Notes taken by author during time studying with Hari Dickman, 1979, Meditation, p. 1.

285 Notes taken by author during time studying with Hari Dickman, 1979, Meditation, p. 1.

286 Swami Vishnu Tirth Maharaj, Narain Kuti, Sanyas Ashram, Dewas, India, *Letter to Dear Shri Hari Dickman*, May 16, 1966, quoting *Bhawartha Dipika*, 18:52, 1030–35.

287 Swami Vishnu Tirth Maharaj, Narain Kuti, Sanyas Ashram, Dewas, India, *Letter to Dear Shri Hari Dickman*, May 16, 1966.

288 Swami Vishnu Tirth Maharaj, Narain Kuti, Sanyas Ashram, Dewas, India, *Letter to Dear Shri Dr. Hari Dickman*, July 26, 1966.

289 Swami Vishnu Tirth Maharaj, Narayankuti, Sanyas Ashram, Dewas, India, *Letter to Dear Dr. Harry Dickman*, Oct. 24, 1966,

290 Notes taken by author during time studying with Hari Dickman, 1979, General, p. 3b.

291 Swami Vishnu Tirth Maharaj, Narain Kuti, Sanyas Ashram, Dewas, India, *Letter to Dear Shri Hari Dickman*, June 21, 1966.

292 Notes taken by author during time studying with Hari Dickman, 1979, Meditation, p. 1.

293 Swami Shivapremananda, *Letter to Hari Maharaj*, May 19, 1975, London England.

294 Swami Sivananda, Rishikesh, India, *Letter to Yogiraj Sri Harry Dikman, in Germany*, September 21, 1949.

295 Swami Sivananda, Rishikesh, India, *Letter to Yogiraj Sri Harry Dikman, in Germany*, September 21, 1949.

296 Swami Vishnudevananda, Rishikesh, India, *Letters to Sri Harry Dikman Yogi Raj*, August 16, 1955, March 20, 1956, and undated, stationary implies 1950s.

297 Swami Sivananda Radha, *Kundalini Yoga for the West* (Boulder, CO: Shambhala, 1978).

298 Sir John Woodroffe, *The Serpent Power*, 156–57.

299 Swami Vishnudevananda, Rishikesh, India, *Letter to Sri Yogiraj Haridickman*, undated, stationary implies 1950s.

300 Swami Vishnudevananda, Rishikesh, India, *Letter to Sri Yogiraj Hari Dickman*, March 20, 1956.

301 Swami Vishnudevananda, Divine Life Society, Rishikesh, India, *Letter to Sri YogiRaj Hari Dickman*, undated, stationary implies 1950s.

302 Author unknown, undated.

303 Author unknown, undated.

304 Swami Vishnu Tirth Maharaj, Narain Kuti, Sanyas Ashram, Dewas, India, *Letter to Shri Hari Dickman*, May 16, 1966.

305 Swami Vishnu Tirth Maharaj, Narain Kuti, Sanyas Ashram, Dewas, India, *Letter to Shri Hari Dickman*, undated, but mentions Hari's last letter was March 30, 1966.

306 Swami Shivananda Saraswati of Assam, Shivananda Math, Umachal Hill, Kamakhya, Gauhati, Assam, India, *Letter to Dear Harry Dickman*, May 10, 1972.

307 Swami Shivananda Saraswati of Assam, Shivananda Math, Umachal Hill, Kamakhya, Gauhati, Assam, India, *Letter to Dear Harry Dickman*, June 22, 1972.

308 Swami Vishnudevananda, *Commentary on The Hatha Yoga Pradipika*, 169 (4:39).

309 Tarachand Garg, Department of Anatomy, MGM Medical College Indore, India, *Letter to Shree Hari Dickman*, February 2, 1958.

310 Dr. Chandra Singh Yadav, MB, BS, NB Mills Maternity Home, Snehlataganj, Indore, India, answering on behalf of Swami Vishnu Tirth, *Letter to Mr. Hari Dickman*, October 27, 1957.

311 Tarachand Garg, Department of Anatomy, MGM Medical College Indore, India, *Letter to Shree Hari Dickman*, December 25, 1957.

312 Tarachand Garg, University of Minnesota, The Medical School, Minneapolis, *Letter to Dear and most Respected Brother*, May 21, 1959.

313   Swami Vishnu Tirth Maharaj, Narayan Kuti, Sanyas Ashram, Dewas, India, *Letter to Hari*, November 8, 1960.

314   Swami Vishnu Tirth Maharaj, Narayan Kuti, Sanyas Ashram, Dewas, India, *Letter to Hari*, December 7, 1960.

315   Swami Vishnu Tirth Maharaj, Narayan Kuti, Sanyas Ashram, Dewas, India, *Letter to Shri Dr. Hari Dickman*, July 26, 1966.

316   Swami Vishnu Tirth Maharaj, Narayan Kuti, Sanyas Ashram, Dewas, India, *Letter to Dear most Hari*, January 28, 1961.

317   *The Hatha Yoga Pradipika*, Commentary by Brahmananda, 74–75, (4:69–80).

318   Swami Vishnu Tirth Maharaj, Narayan Kuti, Sanyas Ashram, Dewas, India, *Letter to Dear Most Hari*, January 28, 1961

319   Swami Vishnu Tirth Maharaj, Narayan Kuti, Sanyas Ashram, Dewas, India, *Letter to Dear Most Hari*, January 28, 1961.

320   See *The Hatha Yoga Pradipika*, Commentary by Brahmananda, 74–76, (4:69–77).

321   See *The Hatha Yoga Pradipika*, Commentary by Brahmananda, 74, (4:68).

322   *The Hatha Yoga Pradipika*, Commentary by Brahmananda, 74, (4:67).

323   Shri Brahmananda Sarasvati, *Nada Yoga* (New York: George Leone Publication Center, Ananda Ashram Press, 1989) 18.

324   Source unknown. Possibly Swami Kriyananda.

325   Swami Shivananda Saraswati of Assam, Shivananda Math, Umachal Hill, Assam, *Letter to my dear Dickman*, June 25, 1959, p. 3.

326   Sri Satyakam, Amritayan Yogapeeth, Jadapur, Calcutta, India, *Letter to Priya Brahma [Hari Dickman]*, undated.

327   Sri Swami Sivananda, *Japa Yoga*, 7th ed. (Shivanandanagar, Distt. Tehri-Garhwal, U.P. Himalayas, India: Swami Krishnananda for the Divine Life Trust Society, Yoga-Vedanta Forest Academy Press, Shivanandanagar, 1972) 19.

328   Sri Swami Sivananda, *Japa Yoga*, xxxvii.

329   Sri Swami Sivananda, *Japa Yoga*, 18.

330   Sri Swami Sivananda, *Japa Yoga*, 80.

331   Sri Swami Sivananda, *Japa Yoga*, 77 and 82.

332   Rai Bahadur Srisa Chandra Vasu, *Commentary on The Gheranda Samhita*, 50 (5:84–85).

333   Swami Shivananda Saraswati of Assam, Shivananda Yogasram, 471 Netaji Colony, Calcutta, India, *Letter to My dear Dickman*, April 14, 1966.

334   Notes taken by author during time studying with Hari Dickman, 1979, Meditation, p. 2 and Questions, p. 5.

335   Swami Muktananda, *So'Ham Japa* (Ganeshpuri, Maharashtra, India: Shree Gurudev Ashram, 1972). Quote from notes taken by author during time studying with Hari Dickman, 1979, Meditation, p. 3.

336   Swami Sivananda of Rishikesh, The Divine Life Society, Rishikesh, India, *Letter to Sri Harry Dikman*, January 14, 1948.

337   Paramhansa Yogananda, Self-Realization Fellowship, Los Angeles, CA, *Letter to Mr. Harry Dikman*, December 6, 1946.

338   Sister Radharani for Rajasi Janakananda, Self Realization Fellowship, Los Angeles, CA, *Letter to Mr. Harry Dikman*, October 8, 1953.

339   Swami Sivananda of Rishikesh, The Divine Life Society, Rishikesh, India, *Letter to Yogiraj Harry Dikman*, August 19, 1948.

340   Swami Sivananda, Ananda Kutir, Rishikesh, India, *Letter to Sri Harry Dikman*, April 7, 1948.

341 Erich Schiffmann, *Yoga: The Spirit and Practice of Moving into Stillness* (New York: Pocket Books, 1996), 19.

342 Swami Sivananda, The Divine Life Society, Rishikesh, India, *Letter to Sri Harry Dikman*, April 7, 1948.

343 Swami Sivananda, Ananda Kutir, Rishikesh, *Letter to Yogiraj Sri Harry Dikman*, November 2, 1950.

344 Dr. Hari Dickman, San Rafael, CA. *Letter to Marion Kneẓacek*, September 16, 1978.

345 Sadhu Arunachala, "Sri Dakshinamurti and Sri Ramana" *The Maharshi* 15, no. 2 (March–April 2005). The article identifies Major A. W. Chadwick as Sadhu Arunachala. http://www.arunachala.org/newsletters/2005/mar-apr.

346 A. W. Chadwick, *Letter to Mr. Dikman*, Tiruvannamalai, March 6, 1951.

347 Swami Sevananda, Karar Ashram, Swargadwar, Puri, India, *Letter to Brother Mr. Dickman*, October 24, 1946.

348 T. K. Sundaresa Iyer, Tiruvannamalai, *Letter to Harry Dikman*, September 18, 1931.

349 Paramhansa Yogananda, Self-Realization Fellowship, Los Angeles 31, California, USA, *Letter to Mr. Harry Dikman*, September 13, 1949.

350 Vishnu Tirth, Narayan Kuti, Sanyas Ashram, Dewas, MP, *Letter to Dear Dr. Shri Hari Dickman*, June 29, 1967.

351 Paramhansa Yogananda, Self-Realization Fellowship, Los Angeles, CA, *Letter to Dear One*, September 22, 1947.

352 Paramhansa Yogananda, Self-Realization Fellowship, Los Angeles, CA, *Letter to Mr. Harry Dikman*, December 2, 1949.

353 Brother Chidananda of the Self-Realization Fellowship, personal communication, email December 28, 2015, on the excellent explanation of why the souls of suicides are not able to return "for long" until they have made many attempts at rebirth.

354 Boris Sacharow, c/o Schroeder, 31 Bismark Str. (13a) Bayreuth, Bavaria, Germany US Zone, *Letter to Shri Paramahansa Swami Yoganandaji*, November 4, 1947.

355 Paramhansa Yogananda, Self-Realization Fellowship, Los Angeles, CA, *Letter to Mr. Boris Sacharow*, January 22, 1948.

356 Paramhansa Yogananda, Self-Realization Fellowship, Los Angeles, CA, *Letter to Dear One*, September 22, 1947.

357 Swami Narayanananda, Rishikesh, India, *Letter to Mr. Harry Dickman*, March 11, 1955.

358 Swami Vishnu Tirth, District Dheradun, Rishikesh, UP, India, *Letter to Dear Shri Dr. Hari Dickman*, March 6, 1967.

359 Swami Vishnu Tirth, Dewas (M.P.) Bharat, India, *Letter to Shri Hari Dickman*, April 15, 1967.

360 Swami Vishnu Tirth, Dewas (M.P.) Bharat, India, *Letter to Shri Hari Dickman*, April 15, 1967.

361 Swami Vishnu Tirth, District Dheradun, Rishikesh, UP, India, *Letter to Dear Shri Dr. Hari Dickman*, April 15, 1967.

362 Swami Shivananda Saraswati of Assam, Shivananda Math, Umachal Hill, Kamakhya, Gauhati, Assam, India, *Letter to Dear Harry Dickman*, May 10, 1972.

363 Swami Shivananda Saraswati of Assam, Shivananda Math, Umachal Hill, Kamakhya, Gauhati, Assam, India, *Letter to Dear Harry Dickman*, May 10, 1972.

364 Yogindra Amar Nandy, District Hooghly, West Bengal, India, *Letter to Priya Gurubhai*, September 29, 1972.

365 Swami Vishnu Tirth, District Dheradun, Rishikesh, UP, India, *Letter to Dear Dr. Hari Dickman*, October 24, 1966.

366 Swami Vishnu Tirth, District Dheradun, Rishikesh, UP, India, *Letter to Dear Shri Dr. Hari Dickman*, March 6, 1967.

367 Swami Shivananda Saraswati of Assam, L268, Netaji Colony, Calcutta 36, Bharat, India, *Letter to My Dear Harri Dickman*, April 16, 1959.

368 Paramhansa Yogananda, Self-Realization Fellowship, Los Angeles, CA, *Letter to Mr.Harry Dikman*, December 6, 1948.

369 Paramhansa Yogananda, Self-Realization Fellowship, Los Angeles, CA, *Letter to Mr.Harry Dikman*, March 13, 1951.

370 Brahmachari Animananda Dharmacharya, Yogoda Sat-Sanga Society of India, Self-Realization Fellowship & Shyamacharan Mission under Paramhansa Yogananda, Ranchi, India, *Letter to Mr. Harry Dikman*, December 9, 1952.

371 Boris Sacharow, c/o Schroeder, 31 Bismark Str. (13a) Bayreuth, Bavaria, Germany US Zone, *Letter to Shri Paramahansa Swami Yoganandaji*, November 4, 1947.

372 Paramhansa Yogananda, Self-Realization Fellowship, Los Angeles, CA, *Letter to Mr. Boris Sacharow*, January 22, 1948.

373 Notes taken by author during time studying with Hari Dickman, 1979, General Notes, pp. 2 and 23b.

374 Notes taken by author during time studying with Hari Dickman, 1979, General Notes, pp. 2 and 23b.

375 Swami Sivananda of Rishikesh, The Divine Life Society, Rishikesh, India, *Letter to Sri Harry Dickman*, August 27, 1946.

376 Notes taken by author during time studying with Hari Dickman, 1979, General notes, pp. 2 and 23b.

377 Swami Sivananda of Rishikesh, The Divine Life Society, Rishikesh, India, *Letter to Sri Harry Dickman*, Oct 25, 1946.

378 Notes taken by author during time studying with Hari Dickman, 1979, General notes, p. 2.

379 Surath Kumar Sarkar, *Indo-Christian Legend* (no publication information, undated).

380 *The Upanishads*, 83, and John 1:1 (Revised Standard Version.

381 John 14:6–11 and 17–20 (Revised Standard Version).

382 *The Bhagavad Gita*, trans. Juan Mascaró (London: Penguin 1962), 43–46 (9:1–3, 11, 13, 17, 18, and 29).

383 Thais Thomas, Madurai S. India, *Letter to Dear Sri Hari*, January 3, 1977.

384 Swami Shivananda Saraswati of Assam, Shivananda Math, Umachal Yogashram, Kamakhya, Gauhati, India, *Letter to Dear Dickman*, undated, but likely early 1961—precludes following letter of October 1961.

385 Swami Shivananda Saraswati of Assam, Shivananda Math, Umachal Hill, Kamakhya, Assam, India, *Letter to Dickman*, October 14, 1961.

386 Brahmachari Punyabrata, Shivananda Math, Umachal Hill, Kamakhya, Assam, India. *Letter to Harry Dickman*, undated, but likely late 1959; Shivananda Math, Umachal Hill, Kamakhya, Assam, India.

387 Swami Shivananda Saraswati of Assam, Shivananda Math, Umachal Hill, Kamakhya, Assam, India, *Letter to Dickman*, May 10, 1972.

388 Swami Shivananda Saraswati of Assam, Shivananda Math, Umachal Hill, Kamakhya, Assam, India, *Letter to Dickman*, June 22, 1972.

389 Swami Shivananda Saraswati of Assam, Shivananda Math, Umachal Hill, Kamakhya, Gauhati, Assam, India, *Letter to dear Dickman*, June 25, 1959.

390 Swami Shivananda Saraswati of Assam, Swami Shivananda Saraswati of Assam, Shivananda Math, Umachal Hill, Kamakhya, Gauhati, Assam, India, *Lecture written and sent to Hari*, 1967.

391   Swami Shivananda Saraswati of Assam, Shivananda Math, Umachal Hill, Kamakhya, Gauhati, Assam, India, *Letter to My dear Harry Dickman*, January 25, 1967.

392   Swami Shivananda Saraswati of Assam, Shivananda Math, Umachal Hill, Kamakhya, Gauhati, Assam, India, *Letter to My dear Harry Dickman*, January 25, 1967, and March 13, 1967.

393   Swami Shivananda Saraswati of Assam, Shivananda Math, Umachal Hill, Kamakhya, Gauhati, Assam, India, *Letter to My dear Dickman*, March 13, 1967, and April 30, 1967.

394   Swami Shivananda Saraswati of Assam, Shivananda Math, Umachal Hill, Kamakhya, Gauhati, Assam, India, *Letter to My dear Dickman*, April 30, 1967.

395   Swami Shivananda Saraswati of Assam, Shivananda Math, Umachal Hill, Kamakhya, Gauhati, Assam, India, *Letter to My dear Dr. Hari*, February 19, 1968.

396   Swami Sivananda of Rishikesh, *Letter to Yogiraj Sri Harry Dikman*, November 24, 1950.

397   Swami Shivananda Saraswati of Assam, Umachal Yogashram, Kamakhya, Gauhati, Assam, India, *Letter to Priya Dr. Harrydickman*, February 21, 1975.

398   Swami Shivananda Saraswati of Assam, Shivananda Math, Umachal Yogashram, Kamakhya, Gauhati, India, *Letter to Priya Dickman*, April 9, 1975.

399   Swami Shivananda Saraswati of Assam, Shivananda Math, Umachal Yogashram, Kamakhya, Gauhati, India, *Letter to Dr. Harry Dickman*, April 16, 1976.

400   Margaret Knezacek, *Letter to Marion Knezacek*, February 21, 1979.

401   Mantra translation and source from *Sadguru Dattatreya* by Sadguru Sant Keshavadas (Vishwa Dharma Publications, 1988), www.templeofcosmicreligion.org.

PERMISSIONS

For those permissions not listed here, every effort was made to obtain permission, but requests sent by the author did not receive a response. If you have any information, please contact North Atlantic Books.

Acharya Dr. Ananda Balayogi Bhavanani, ICYER Ananda Ashram, Pondicherry, India (hand mudras for vibhaga pranayama and references to his father Dr. Swami Gitananda Giri Maharaj)

William Harold Phillips, Okanangan Falls, BC Canada, (personal communications)

Arunachala Ashram, Tiruvannamalai Temple, Tamil Nadu, India (permission to use letters from disciples of Ramana Maharshi)

Self-Realization Fellowship, Los Angeles, CA (permission to use letters from Paramhansa Yogananda and his disciples)

Sigmund Feurabendt, Germany (permission to use letters to Boris Sacharow)

Brieanne Mikuska, Calgary, Alberta (graphic of three bandhas in meditation)

Ann Gordon on behalf of the College of Divine Metaphysics, Indianapolis, (letters of certification for Hari)

Divine Life Society, Rishikesh, India (quotes drawn from Divine Life Society books)

Dr. Francisco Luid (aka Swami Tirthananda Saraswati), Zaragoza, Spain, (permission to use mudras for emotional balance, psychic balance and humility)

Dr. Vijayendra Pratap, SKY Foundation, Philadelphia, (quotes from *Skylight Journal of Yoga*)

Dzintars Vilinis Korns, Latvia, (various items used from his Latvian website on the history of the Latvian Yoga Society, and personal communication)

Dr. Phil. Solveiga Krumina-Konkova, leading researcher, Institute of Philosophy and Sociology, University of Latvia, (personal communication).

Health Research Books, Pomeroy, Washington (permission to reprint quotes from The Mysterious Kundalini)

Erich Schiffmann, Santa Monica, CA, (permission to quote from personal discussions)

Ganga White, Santa Barbara, CA (permission for quote from his book *Yoga Beyond Belief*)

Jo. C. Willems, Revelstoke, BC (permission to use all line drawings she created for book)

Katherine DaSilva Jain, San Rafael, CA (permission to copy all letters to Hari)

Ananda Sangha, Nayaswami Lakshman for Nayaswamis Jyotish and Devi) (permission to use letters from Swami Kriyananda)

Kaivalyadhama Yoga Institute, Kaivalyadhama, India for use of letters from Swami Kuvalayananda and quotes from *Yoga Mimamsa* magazine and the book, *Pranayama*.

Narayan Press, Rishikesh, India (permission to use letters from Swami Narayanananda)

Integral Yoga Institute, New York, New York (permission to use letters from Swami Satchidananda)

Satyabhama Ashley-Farrand, Albuquerque, NM (permission to use quotes from the book Chakra Mantras by Namadeva Acharya, aka Thomas Ashley-Farrand)

Swami Suryadevananda, Florida, (permission to quote from personal communication)

Central Chinmaya Mission, Powai, Mumbai, India (permission to quote letters from Swami Thapovanam)

Chiltern Yoga Trust, Fremantle, Western Australia, (permission to use letters from Swami Venkatesananda)

Vyankatesh Sapar, Maharashtra, India (painting created for story of Jesus as a yogi)

Swami Shivom Tirth, India (permission to use letters from Swami Vishnu Tirth)

Shivananda Yogsadhan Ashram, Belda, West Bengal (permission to use letters from Swami Shivananda Saraswati of Assam)

S. S. Goswami Institute, Sweden, (permission to use letters from Shyam Sundar Goswami)

Yoga Niketan Trust, Rishikesh, India (permission to use letters from Swami Yogeshwaranand Saraswati and quotes from his book *First Steps of Higher Yoga*

Swami Shivapremananda, Buenos Aires, Argentina, (permission to use letters from himself)

Sivananda Ashram Yoga Headquarters, Val Morin, PQ, Canada, (permission to use quotes from letters from Swami Vishnudevananda and quotes from his book *Hatha Yoga Pradipika*. Copyright.)

INDEX

ABOUT
THE AUTHOR

Marion (Mugs) McConnell, E-RYT500

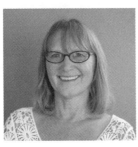 MARION (MUGS) McCONNELL was first introduced to yoga as a teenager in 1973. She has been practicing yoga ever since, and teaching since 1978. Her passion for this ancient practice and its many boundless layers of wisdom beyond the physical led her to study under Swami Vishnudevananda. She graduated from the Sivananda Yoga Vedanta Centre as a Yoga Acharya in 1978. In 1977 Mugs became a student of Yogiraj Dr. Hari Dickman, a disciple of Swami Sivananda and Paramhansa Yogananda.

Mugs has been the Canadian Representative for the International Yoga Teachers Association (IYTA) since 1982. She is a founding member (1995) of the South Okanagan Yoga Academy and cocreator of its teacher-training program, a Yoga Alliance Registered Yoga School (RYS200/300 advanced), unique in its adherence to IYTA standards. She is an Experienced Registered Teacher with Yoga Alliance (E-RYT500) and has served on the Yoga

Alliance Standards Committee since 2012. In 2012 Mugs received a Queen Elizabeth II Diamond Jubilee Medal for offering yoga in Canada and abroad for nearly forty years. In 2013 she was the recipient of a Certificate of Appreciation from IYTA in recognition of her contributions to yoga around the world.

Although Mugs is a disciple of the Sivananda tradition, her more recent teachers have included Namadeva Acharya in mantra therapy and Erich Schiffmann in Freedom Yoga, as well as Rod Stryker, Dharma Mittra, Mark Stephens, Ganga White, and Tracey Rich. These teachers have created a platform for Mugs to take her great love and respect of classical yoga and weave it together with modern-day wisdom, ensuring her students are always exposed to yoga right back to its roots.

Mugs has been leading yoga teacher trainings for twenty years. She currently holds trainings four times a year and manages SOYA teacher trainings, which are held annually in four additional SOYA satellite locations in British Columbia, Alberta, and Mexico. She presents workshops in Canada, the United States, Spain, Mexico, and Australia. Mugs is a regular contributor to the IYTA *International Light* magazine and manager of the SOYA monthly e-newsletter for the past eight years.

Mugs lives with her husband, Robert, in British Columbia and Mexico. *Letters from the Yoga Masters* is her first book.